Gastrointestinal Drug Absorption

Gastrointestinal Drug Absorption

Editor: Jeremy Artley

AMERICAN
MEDICAL PUBLISHERS
www.americanmedicalpublishers.com

AMERICAN
MEDICAL PUBLISHERS
www.americanmedicalpublishers.com

Cataloging-in-Publication Data

Gastrointestinal drug absorption / edited by Jeremy Artley.
p. cm.
Includes bibliographical references and index.
ISBN 978-1-63927-674-5
1. Gastrointestinal system--Diseases. 2. Gastrointestinal agents. 3. Clinical pharmacology.
4. Pharmacokinetics. 5. Drugs--Metabolism. 6. Drugs--Physiological effect. I. Artley, Jeremy.
RC817 .G37 2023
616.33--dc23

American Medical Publishers,
41 Flatbush Avenue,
1st Floor, New York,
NY 11217, USA

ISBN 978-1-63927-674-5 (Hardback)

Contents

Preface

Gastrointestinal absorption of a drug is a complex process which involves a series of sub-processes. It is also subject to different variables such as physiological factors and disease states. Passive non-ionic diffusion is the most prominent mechanism that plays a prominent role in the process of drug absorption. The difference in the concentration or the chemical potential across the membrane helps in the process of absorption. The cell membrane incorporates the non-ionized hydrophobic molecules between the long hydrocarbon chains through a dissolution-like process. As a result, the hydrophobic molecules are transferred into the absorptive cell. There are some other mechanisms that play a minor role in drug absorption. These mechanisms include pinocytosis, facilitated transport and passage through membrane pores. This book is compiled in such a manner, that it will provide in-depth knowledge about the mechanism of gastrointestinal drug absorption. A number of latest researches have been included to keep the readers updated with the latest concepts in this area of study. The book is a vital tool for all researching this biological process.

The information contained in this book is the result of intensive hard work done by researchers in this field. All due efforts have been made to make this book serve as a complete guiding source for students and researchers. The topics in this book have been comprehensively explained to help readers understand the growing trends in the field.

I would like to thank the entire group of writers who made sincere efforts in this book and my family who supported me in my efforts of working on this book. I take this opportunity to thank all those who have been a guiding force throughout my life.

Editor

1

BCS Class IV Oral Drugs and Absorption Windows: Regional-Dependent Intestinal Permeability of Furosemide

Milica Markovic [1], Moran Zur [1], Inna Ragatsky [1], Sandra Cvijić [2] and Arik Dahan [1,*]

[1] Department of Clinical Pharmacology, School of Pharmacy, Faculty of Health Sciences, Ben-Gurion University of the Negev, Beer-Sheva 8410501, Israel; milica@post.bgu.ac.il (M.M.); moranfa@post.bgu.ac.il (M.Z.); inna.ragatsky@gmail.com (I.R.)

[2] Department of Pharmaceutical Technology and Cosmetology, Faculty of Pharmacy, University of Belgrade, Vojvode Stepe 450, 11221 Belgrade, Serbia; sandra.cvijic@pharmacy.bg.ac.rs

* Correspondence: arikd@bgu.ac.il

Abstract: Biopharmaceutical classification system (BCS) class IV drugs (low-solubility low-permeability) are generally poor drug candidates, yet, ~5% of oral drugs on the market belong to this class. While solubility is often predictable, intestinal permeability is rather complicated and highly dependent on many biochemical/physiological parameters. In this work, we investigated the solubility/permeability of BCS class IV drug, furosemide, considering the complexity of the entire small intestine (SI). Furosemide solubility, physicochemical properties, and intestinal permeability were thoroughly investigated in-vitro and in-vivo throughout the SI. In addition, advanced in-silico simulations (GastroPlus®) were used to elucidate furosemide regional-dependent absorption pattern. Metoprolol was used as the low/high permeability class boundary. Furosemide was found to be a low-solubility compound. Log D of furosemide at the three pH values 6.5, 7.0, and 7.5 (representing the conditions throughout the SI) showed a downward trend. Similarly, segmental-dependent in-vivo intestinal permeability was revealed; as the intestinal region becomes progressively distal, and the pH gradually increases, the permeability of furosemide significantly decreased. The opposite trend was evident for metoprolol. Theoretical physicochemical analysis based on ionization, pK_a, and partitioning predicted the same trend and confirmed the experimental results. Computational simulations clearly showed the effect of furosemide's regional-dependent permeability on its absorption, as well as the critical role of the drug's absorption window on the overall bioavailability. The data reveals the absorption window of furosemide in the proximal SI, allowing adequate absorption and consequent effect, despite its class IV characteristics. Nevertheless, this absorption window so early on in the SI rules out the suitability of controlled-release furosemide formulations, as confirmed by the in-silico results. The potential link between segmental-dependent intestinal permeability and adequate oral absorption of BCS Class IV drugs may aid to develop challenging drugs as successful oral products.

Keywords: BCS class IV drugs; segmental-dependent intestinal permeability; intestinal absorption; oral drug delivery; biopharmaceutics; physiologically-based pharmacokinetic (PBPK) modeling; furosemide

1. Introduction

The biopharmaceutical classification system (BCS) developed by Amidon et al. revealed that the solubility/dissolution of the drug and its intestinal permeability are the two key factors that dictate drug absorption following oral administration [1,2]. Drug solubility in the gastrointestinal milieu may change in different intestinal segments, e.g., due to pH changes, in a fairly predictable manner; depending on the pKa, the solubility of acidic drugs may increase as the luminal pH rises in more distal regions of the small intestine, and vice versa for basic drugs [3–5]. On the other hand, time- and segmental-dependent intestinal permeability is more complicated and harder to predict [1]. Mechanisms contributing to segmental-dependent permeability throughout the gastrointestinal tract (GIT) include different morphology along the GIT, variable intestinal mucosal cell differentiation, changes in the drug concentration (in case of carrier-mediated transport), modulation of tight junction permeability, and luminal contents and properties, e.g., pH, transporter expression, variability in the structure/composition of the intestinal membrane itself, and more [6–11].

The four BCS classes highlight the limiting factors of the absorption process: (1) Class I, high-solubility high-permeability drugs, indicate the easier and straightforward development process, and complete absorption is expected; (2) Class II, low-solubility high-permeability drugs, indicate that a solubility/dissolution limitation is expected; (3) Class III, high-solubility low-permeability drugs, indicate that the intestinal absorption of this class of drugs will be limited by the permeability rate; and (4) Class IV, low-solubility low-permeability drugs [12]. Since Class IV drugs suffer from inadequate solubility and permeability, they have very poor oral bioavailability and are inclined to exhibit very large inter- and intrasubject variability. Therefore, unless the drug dose is very low, they are generally poor oral drug candidates. Yet, according to some estimates, ~5% of the world's top oral drugs belong to this class [13–15]. In some cases, this is due to the absorption window, which is often critical for the success or failure of a certain drug. In order to gather information about the drug absorption window, extensive work and thorough analysis of luminal conditions and drug absorption is needed, within different locations throughout the GIT. Here, we present such analysis for BCS class IV drug, furosemide [16].

Furosemide is a powerful loop diuretic and is indicated for treating edematous conditions associated with heart, renal, and hepatic failure, as well as for the treatment of hypertension [17,18]. Drug therapy with furosemide is often complex, due to apparent erratic oral systemic availability and unpredictable responses to an administered dose [19]. Even though furosemide is a class IV drug, it is a very common and widely prescribed drug on the market.

In this work, we aimed to investigate the reason for apparent success of furosemide as a marketed product, despite its poor biopharmaceutical properties, and classification as BCS class IV drug, in order to allow development of future class IV compounds. We posit that segmental-dependent permeability of furosemide may contribute to its absorption complexity and provide a certain absorption window in which the drug has suitable permeability and, hence, gets absorbed. For this reason, we investigated the in-vivo intestinal permeability of furosemide throughout different segments of the small intestine. Solubility studies, as well as theoretical physicochemical analysis of furosemide and advanced modern in-silico GastroPlus® simulations, were performed, in order to elucidate the mechanistic reasons behind the experimental results. Furosemide data were compared to the β-blocker metoprolol, the Food and Drug Administration (FDA) reference drug for the low/high permeability class boundary. Overall, this experimental setup allowed us to reveal important insights on the performance of furosemide, despite its unfavorable drug-like properties, and discuss extrapolation of these insights to other BCS class IV drug candidates.

2. Methods

2.1. Materials

Furosemide, metoprolol, phenol red, potassium chloride, potassium phosphate monobasic, potassium phosphate dibasic, sodium chloride, acetic acid, maleic acid, *n*-octanol, and trifluoroacetic acid (TFA) were all purchased from Sigma Chemical Co. (St. Louis, MO, USA). Acetonitrile and water, ultra-performance liquid chromatography (UPLC) grade were purchased from Merck KGaA, Darmstadt, Germany. Remaining chemicals were of analytical reagent grade.

2.2. Solubility Studies

The pH-dependent solubility studies were performed using the shake flask method, as previously reported [20–23]. The equilibrium solubility of furosemide was determined at both 37 °C and at room temperature (25 °C), in phosphate buffer pH 7.5, acetate buffer pH 4.0, and maleate buffer pH 1.0. Surplus quantity of furosemide was introduced to glass vials holding buffer solutions with different pH; the pH of those solutions was measured following drug addition to the buffers and, consequently, placed in the shaking incubator (100 rpm) at 37 °C. The vials were centrifuged (10,000 rpm, 10 min), and the supernatant was instantly analyzed by UPLC. The dose number for furosemide was calculated using the established equation: $D_0 = M/V_0/C_s$; M being the highest single-unit dose strength of furosemide (taken as 80 mg [24]), V_0 is the initial volume of water (250 mL), and C_s is the solubility at each pH; the drug is considered highly soluble if the $D_0 < 1$.

2.3. Evaluation of Octanol-Buffer Partition Coefficients (Log D)

Furosemide and metoprolol experimental octanol-buffer partition coefficients (Log D) were studied at pH 6.5, 7.0, and 7.5 using the shake-flask method [8,11]. Drug solutions in octanol-saturated phosphate buffer (pH 6.5, 7.0, 7.5) were equilibrated at 37 °C for 48 h. The octanol and water phase were divided via centrifugation, and the drug content in the water phase was quantified using UPLC; the furosemide/metoprolol concentration in the octanol phase was determined by mass balance.

2.4. Physicochemical Analysis

The theoretical fraction extracted into octanol (f_e) was calculated using the following equation [25,26].

$$f_e = \frac{f_u P}{1 + f_u P},$$

in which P represents the octanol-water partition coefficient of the unionized drug form, and f_u is the fraction unionized of the drug at a certain pH. Experimental Log P values were taken from the literature for both furosemide (2.29) [27] and metoprolol (2.19) [28]. The f_u versus pH was plotted according to the Henderson-Hasselbalch equation, using the pK_a literature values: 9.68 for metoprolol [29] and 3.8 for furosemide [24].

2.5. Rat Single-Pass Intestinal Perfusion

Effective permeability coefficient (P_{eff}) of furosemide versus metoprolol in various intestinal segments was assessed using the single-pass rat intestinal perfusion (SPIP) in-vivo model. The murine studies were completed according to the approved protocol by Ben-Gurion University of the Negev Animal Use and Care Committee (Protocol IL-08-01-2015). The animals (male Wistar rats weighing 230–260 g, Harlan, Israel) were housed and handled according to Ben-Gurion University of the Negev Unit for Laboratory Animal Medicine Guidelines. All animals were fasted overnight (12–18 h) with free access to water; rats were randomly allocated to different experimental groups. The intestinal perfusion study was performed according to the previous reports [7,9,30–32]. Animals were anesthetized via intramuscular injection of 1 mL/kg ketamine-xylazine solution (9%:1%) and placed on a heated (37 °C) surface (Harvard Apparatus Inc., Holliston, MA, USA); the rat abdomen was uncovered via a midline incision (~3 cm). Permeability (P_{eff}) was measured in proximal jejunum (starting 2 cm lower from the ligament of Treitz), mid-small intestine (SI) segment (isolated between the end of the upper and the beginning of the lower segments), and distal segment of the ileum (ending 2 cm above the cecum) accounting for the complexity of the entire SI [7]. Intestinal segments were cannulated on both ends and perfused with drug-free buffer. Working solutions containing furosemide (320 μg/mL), metoprolol (400 μg/mL), and phenol red (a non-absorbable marker for water flux measurements) were prepared with potassium phosphate monobasic and sodium phosphate dibasic, to achieve pH of 6.5, 7.0 and 7.5; osmolarity (290 mOsm/L) and ionic strength in all buffers was maintained throughout the study.

Drug solutions were incubated in a 37 °C water bath. Steady-state environment was ensured by perfusing the drug-containing buffer for 1 h, followed by additional 1 h of perfusion, during which sampling was done every 10 min. The pH of the collected samples was measured in the outlet sample to verify that there was no pH change throughout the perfusion. All samples were assayed by UPLC. The length of each perfused intestinal segment was measured in the end of the experiment. The effective permeability (P_{eff}; cm/s) through the rat SI wall was calculated according to the following equation:

$$P_{eff} = \frac{-Q\ln\left(C'_{out}/C'_{in}\right)}{2\pi RL},$$

in which Q is the perfusion buffer flow rate (0.2 mL/min); C'_{out}/C'_{in} is the ratio of the outlet/inlet drug concentration adjusted for water transport; R is the radius of the intestinal segment (conventionally used as 0.2 cm); and L is the exact length of the perfused SI segment as was measured at the experiment endpoint [7,33,34].

2.6. Analytical Methods

Concentration of furosemide and metoprolol was evaluated using an UPLC instrument Waters Acquity UPLC H-Class (Milford, MA, USA), with a photodiode array detector and Empower software. Furosemide and metoprolol were separated on Acquity UPLC XTerra C18 3.5 μm 4.6 mm × 250 mm column (Waters Co., Milford, MA, USA). Gradient mobile phase, going from 70:30% to 90:10% *v/v* 0.1% trifluoroacetic acid in water/acetonitrile, respectively, on a flow rate of 1 mL/min (25 °C). The inter- and intraday coefficients of variation were < 1.0% and 0.5%, respectively.

2.7. Statistics

Solubility studies were performed in four replicates; Log D studies were performed in six replicates, whereas animal perfusion studies were $n = 4$. Values are expressed as means ± standard deviation (SD). To determine statistically significant differences among the experimental groups, a 2-tailed nonparametric Mann–Whitney U test for 2-group comparison was used; $p < 0.05$ was termed significant.

2.8. In-Silico Simulations

Computer simulations of furosemide absorption and concomitant plasma concentrations following oral administration in humans were conducted using GastroPlus™ software package (v. 9.7.0009, 2019, Simulations Plus Inc., Lancaster, CA, USA). The required input data regarding drug physicochemical and pharmacokinetic properties were experimentally determined, taken from literature or in-silico predicted. Human permeability values throughout the SI were calculated from the experimental rat single-pass intestinal perfusion data, using the software integrated "permeability converter". Drug disposition was best described by three-compartmental pharmacokinetic model, whereas the relevant parameters (clearance (*CL*), volume of distribution (*V*d) and distribution constants between central and peripheral compartments) were estimated using PKPlus software module, based on the in-vivo plasma concentration data for an intravenous (i.v.) bolus dose [35]. The application of three-compartmental model to describe furosemide pharmacokinetics has already been reported in literature [36,37]. Graphical data from literature were digitized using DigIt™ program (version 1.0.4, 2001–2008, Simulations Plus, Inc., Lancaster, CA, USA). Physiological parameters were the software default values representing fasted state physiology of a healthy human representative.

The software simulates drug absorption from the GIT using the integrated Advanced Compartment Absorption and Transit (ACAT) GIT model that consists of nine compartments (stomach, duodenum, two segments of jejunum, three segments of ileum, caecum, and ascendant colon). These compartments are linked in series, and the amount of drug dissolved and absorbed from each compartment is calculated by the system of differential equations. More details on the ACAT model can be found in the literature [38,39]. Regarding the fact that furosemide is a poorly-soluble drug, the model accounted for the effect of bile salt on drug solubility and diffusion coefficient. Drug dissolution rate under physiological conditions was predicted using the software default Johnson dissolution equation (based on modified Nernst-Bruner equation) [40].

The validity of the model (i.e., the selection of input values) was validated by comparison of the prediction results (bioavailability (F), maximum plasma concentration (C_{max}), time to reach C_{max} (t_{max}), and area under the plasma concentration-time curve ($AUC_{0-\infty}$)) with published data from the in-vivo studies for peroral (p.o.) drug administration. Percent prediction error (%PE) between the predicted and mean in-vivo observed data from a clinical study was calculated using the following equation:

$$\%PE = \frac{(\text{Observed value} - \text{Predicted value}) \times 100}{\text{Observed value}}.$$

In the next step, the generated model was used to mechanistically interpret furosemide regional absorption pattern, and to estimate the outcomes for various hypothetical drug dissolution scenarios (illustrating drug dissolution from immediate-release (IR) and controlled-release (CR) oral formulations). In the last case, hypothetical dissolution profiles were used as additional inputs to describe drug release rate in-vivo, and the selected dosage form was "CR dispersed" to allow input of the tabulated dissolution data.

3. Results

The solubility values obtained for furosemide at 37 °C and at room temperature (25 °C) are summarized in Table 1, as well as the corresponding dose number (D_0). Furosemide showed pH-dependent solubility, in accordance with its acidic nature. It can be seen that, while, at pH 7.5, furosemide has suitable solubility (as evident by D_0 lower than 1), at the lower pH values, 1.0 and 4.0, it is poorly soluble. When taking 80 mg as the highest dose strength, although $D_0 < 1$ was obtained at pH 7.5, at pH 1.0 and 4.0, the D_0 is higher than 1; hence, furosemide was found to be a low-solubility compound according to the BCS.

Table 1. Furosemide solubility values (µg/mL) at the tree pH values 1.0, 4.0, and 7.5, at 37 °C (upper panel), and at room temperature (25 °C; lower panel), as well as the corresponding dose number (D_0) calculated for an 80-mg dose. Data presented as mean ± SD; $n = 6$.

	At 37 °C	
pH	**Solubility (µg/mL)**	**Corresponding D_0**
1	19.4 ± 3.7	16.5
4	65.5 ± 9.0	4.8
7.5	8340.1 ± 81.6	0.04
	At 25 °C	
pH	**Solubility (µg/mL)**	**Corresponding D_0**
1	40.3 ± 16.2	7.9
4	56.7 ± 12.2	5.6
7.5	8550.6 ± 149.4	0.04

Octanol-buffer partition coefficient values of furosemide and metoprolol at the three pH values 6.5, 7.0, and 7.5 (representing the conditions throughout the small intestine) are presented in Figure 1. Both drugs presented a clear pH-dependent Log D values across the studied pH range, with opposite trends; while furosemide's partitioning decreases as the pH rises, metoprolol shows higher partitioning into octanol at higher pH (metoprolol is the acceptable reference drug for the low/high permeability class boundary). In addition, furosemide's Log D at pH 6.5 was higher than that of metoprolol at the same pH; this is a surprising finding since Log D may sometimes be used as a surrogate for passive permeability. Indeed, at higher pH values (7.0 and 7.5), metoprolol Log D increases, while furosemide decreases, and metoprolol Log D becomes higher than furosemide.

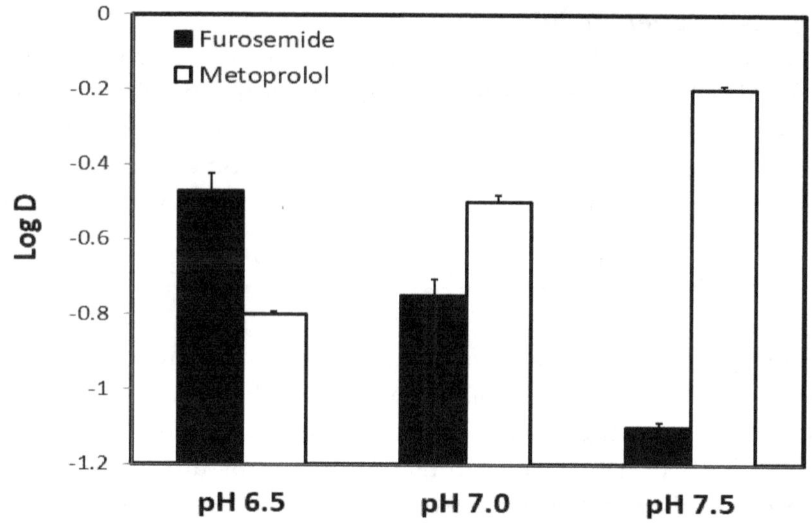

Figure 1. The octanol-buffer partition coefficients, Log D, for furosemide and metoprolol at the three pH values 6.5, 7.0, and 7.5. Data are presented as the mean ± S.D.; $n = 6$ in each experimental group.

Furosemide and metoprolol physicochemical properties are presented in Table 2. Figure 2 presents furosemide versus metoprolol theoretical fraction unionized (f_u) and fraction extracted into octanol (f_e) as a function of pH. The plots have a standard sigmoidal shape, with opposite trends for furosemide vs. metoprolol. The f_e vs. pH plot follows the same pattern to the f_u plot, only with a shift to the right (higher pH values) for acidic drug (furosemide), and to the left (lower pH values) for basic (metoprolol) drugs. The shift magnitude in both cases equals Log(P − 1) at the midpoint of the f_e and f_u curves [25,26]. The experimental drug octanol-buffer partitioning at the three pH values (6.5, 7.0, and 7.5) are illustrated in Figure 2, as well, and it can be seen that they were in excellent agreement with the theoretical plots.

Table 2. Physicochemical parameters and chemical structure of furosemide and metoprolol.

Drug	Chemical Structure	pK_a	Log P	PSA
Furosemide	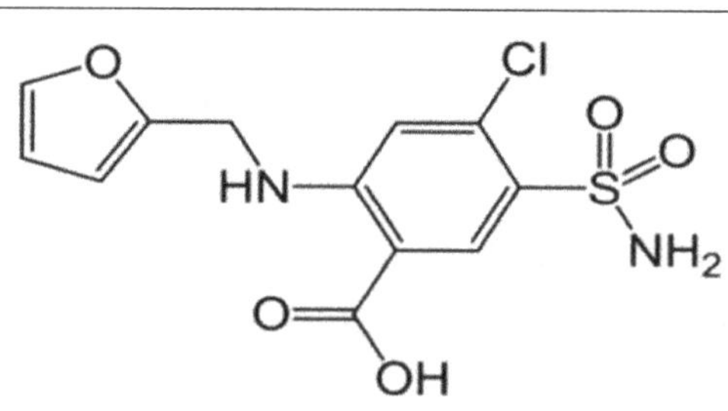	3.8	2.3	127.7
Metoprolol	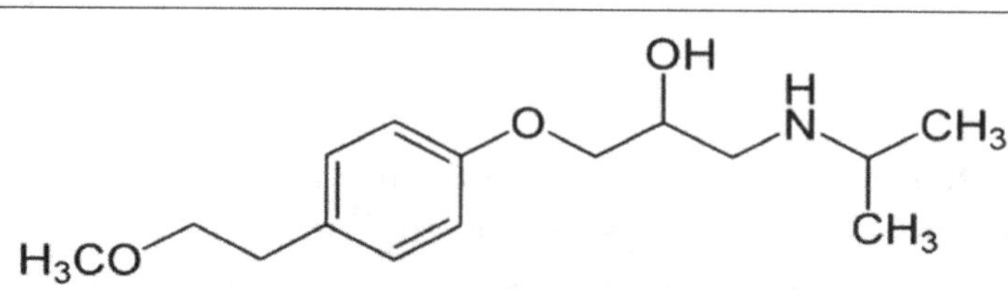	9.7	2.2	53.2

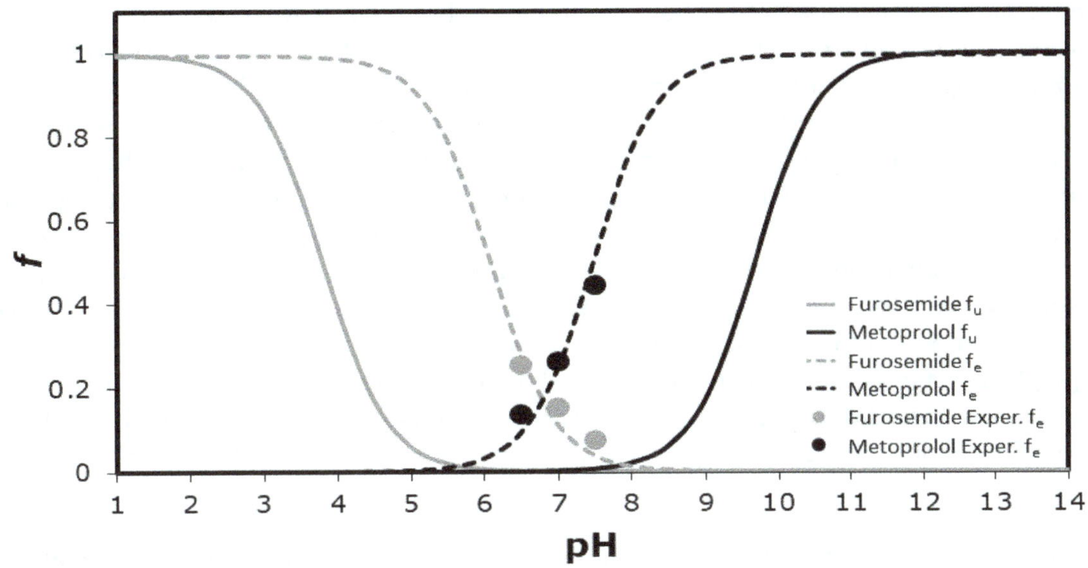

Figure 2. The theoretical fraction unionized (f_u) and fraction extracted into octanol (f_e) plots as a function of pH for furosemide and metoprolol, as well as experimental buffer-octanol partitioning of the drugs in the three pH values 6.5, 7.0, and 7.5 ($n = 5$).

The effective permeability coefficient (P_{eff}, cm/sec) values of furosemide and metoprolol determined using the single-pass intestinal perfusion (SPIP) rat model, in three intestinal segments, namely proximal jejunum (pH 6.5), mid small intestine (pH 7.0), and distal ileum (pH 7.5), are presented in Figure 3. It can be seen that significant regional-dependent permeability of furosemide throughout the small intestine was evident: the permeability of furosemide gradually decreases, while the permeability of metoprolol gradually increases, as the SI segments become more distal.

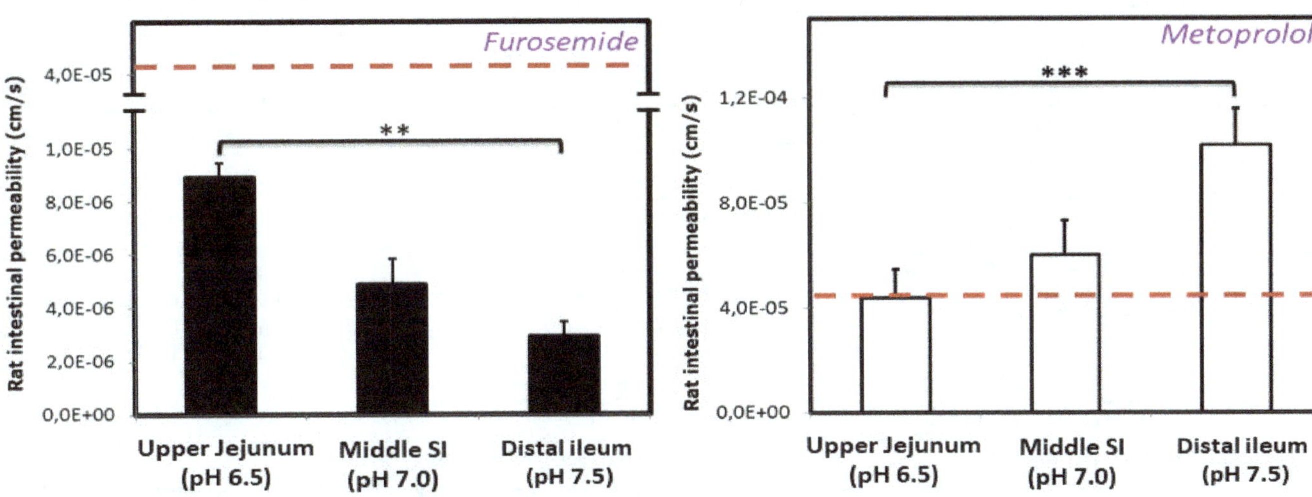

Figure 3. Effective permeability values (P_{eff}; cm/s) obtained for furosemide and metoprolol after in-situ single pass perfusion to the rat proximal jejunum at pH 6.5, mid-small intestine at pH 7.0, and to the distal ileum at pH 7.5. Mean ± S.D.; $n = 4$ in each experimental group; ** $p < 0.01$, *** $p < 0.001$.

The input data regarding drug physicochemical and pharmacokinetic properties, used for in-silico simulations, are presented in Table 3. The simulated furosemide plasma concentration profile following p.o. administration is depicted in Figure 4, along with the mean profiles observed in the in-vivo studies. In addition, the observed and model predicted pharmacokinetic parameters are compared in Table 4. The presented data demonstrate that the generated model adequately describes furosemide absorption and disposition. The course of the predicted plasma profile fairly resembles the observed data. However, certain variations are observed between the mean in-vivo data from different studies referring to the same drug dose (Figure 4, Table 4). Indeed, it has been reported that furosemide oral absorption is highly variable between individuals, e.g., C_{max} varied three-fold, and t_{max} varied five-fold [36,37,41]; moreover, individual AUC values for 40 mg furosemide oral dose varied between 1.57 and 3.76 μg·h/mL (more than two-fold) [36,37,41], and even larger AUC values were observed in another study with the same drug dose (2.23–6.10 μg·h/mL) [42], indicating that, regardless of the high PE(%) values in Table 4, the model predicted value of 3.66 μg·h/mL is not an overestimate of the extent of drug absorption. In addition, extensive intrasubject variability was observed for orally dosed furosemide, and these variations were attributed to the absorption process (i.e., day to day variations in physiological factors) since the repeated i.v. doses showed only marginal intrasubject variability [36,37,41]. Considering pronounced inter- and intraindividual variability in furosemide oral absorption, the simulated profile can be seen as a reasonable estimate (Figure 4). Moreover, the predicted fraction of oral drug absorption (cc. 52%) is in accordance with the values reported in the literature [36,37].

Table 3. The selected input parameters for furosemide absorption GastroPlus® simulation.

Parameter	Value	Source
Molecular weight (g/mol)	330.75	/
Log D (pH 7.5)	−1.0818	experimental values
Solubility at 37 °C (μg/mL)	19.4 (pH 1.0) 65.5 (pH 4.0) 8340.1 (pH 7.5)	
pK_a (acid)	3.8	[24]
Human effective permeability, P_{eff} (cm/s)	0.4043×10^{-4} (duodenum, jejunum) 0.2246×10^{-4} (ileum 1 and 2) 0.1392×10^{-4} (ileum 3, caecum, colon)	values converted using GastroPlus™ integrated "permeability converter" based on experimental rat perfusion data
Diffusion coefficient (cm^2/s)	0.7289×10^{-5}	GastroPlus™ calculated value (based on molecular weight)
Mean precipitation time (s)	900	GastroPlus™ default values
Particle density (g/mL)	1.2	
Particle radius (μm)	25	
Blood/plasma concentration ratio	1	
Plasma fraction unbound (%)	1	[24]
Clearance, CL (L/h/kg)	0.121	calculated using GastroPlus™ PKPlus module, based on the i.v. data [35]
Volume of distribution, Vd (L/kg)	0.043	
Distribution constant k_{12} (1/h)	0.964	
Distribution constant k_{21} (1/h)	1.614	
Distribution constant k_{13} (1/h)	0.925	
Distribution constant k_{32} (1/h)	0.708	
Regional pH in the GIT	1.3; 6.0; 6.2; 6.4; 6.6; 6.9; 7.4; 6.4; 6.8	GastroPlus™ default values for stomach, duodenum, jejunum 1, jejunum 2, ileum 1, ileum 2, ileum 3, caecum, and ascendant colon
Regional volume of fluid in the GIT (mL)	46.56; 40.54; 150.00; 119.30; 91.71; 68.88; 48.57; 46.44; 49.21	
Regional transit time in the GIT (h)	0.25; 0.26; 0.93; 0.74; 0.58; 0.42; 0.29; 4.13; 12.38	

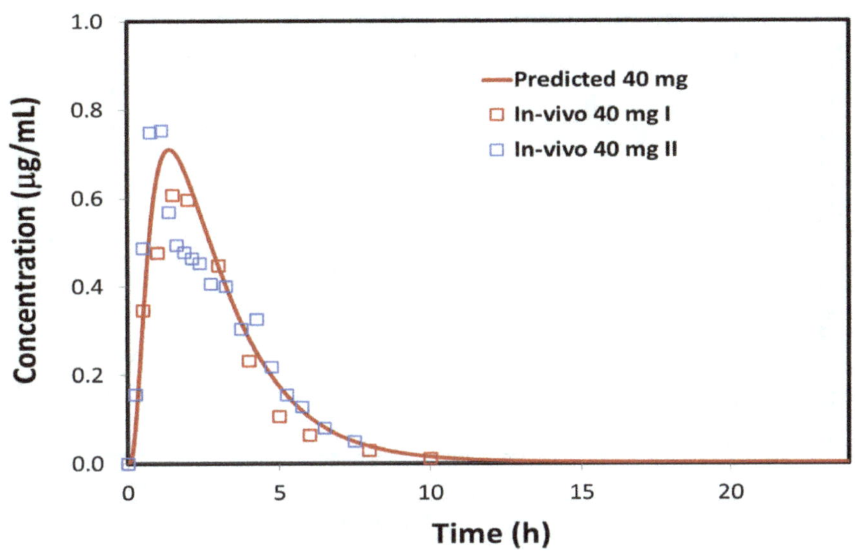

Figure 4. GastroPlus® simulated (line) versus mean observed (markers) plasma concentration profiles following p.o. administration of furosemide. Mean observed values represent 40 mg immediate-release (IR) tablet profile I [43] and 40 mg IR tablet profile II [37].

Table 4. Comparison between GastroPlus® simulated and in-vivo observed furosemide pharmacokinetic parameters following p.o. drug administration.

40 mg p.o. Dose					
Parameter	**In-Vivo I [a]**	**In-Vivo II [b]**	**Predicted**	**PE(%) I**	**PE(%) II**
C_{max} (μg/mL)	0.61	0.75	0.71	−17.14	5.54
t_{max} (h)	1.5	1.12	1.36	9.33	−22.22
$AUC_{0\to\infty}$ (μg·h/mL)	2.13	2.44	3.66	−71.25	−50.06
$AUC_{0\to 24\ h}$ (μg·h/mL)	2.11	2.33	2.52	−19.25	−8.15
F (%)	NA	NA	52.2	NA	NA

[a] Refers to the mean plasma profile from [43] (40 mg IR tablet); [b] refers to the mean plasma profile from [37] (40 mg IR tablet); NA, not available/not applicable.

The predicted furosemide dissolution and absorption profiles following an IR oral formulation (IR tablet) are illustrated in Figure 5. The generated profiles clearly indicate that drug permeability is the limiting factor for absorption under fasted state GIT conditions. Namely, although furosemide is a low-solubility drug, due to ionization at the elevated pH conditions in the proximal SI, drug dissolution from an IR formulation is expected to be fast (>85% in 30 min). Therefore, furosemide absorption from an IR formulation is mainly governed by poor permeability. The predicted regional-dependent absorption distribution (Figure 6) further highlights the role of furosemide segmental absorption on the overall drug bioavailability. As implied by the regional-dependent permeability data, but also considering the surface area available for absorption, furosemide absorption predominantly happens in the proximal parts of the SI (76.6% of the total amount absorbed into the enterocytes), and only a minor fraction of drug (23.2% of the total amount absorbed into the enterocytes) passes into systemic circulation through mid and distal GIT regions.

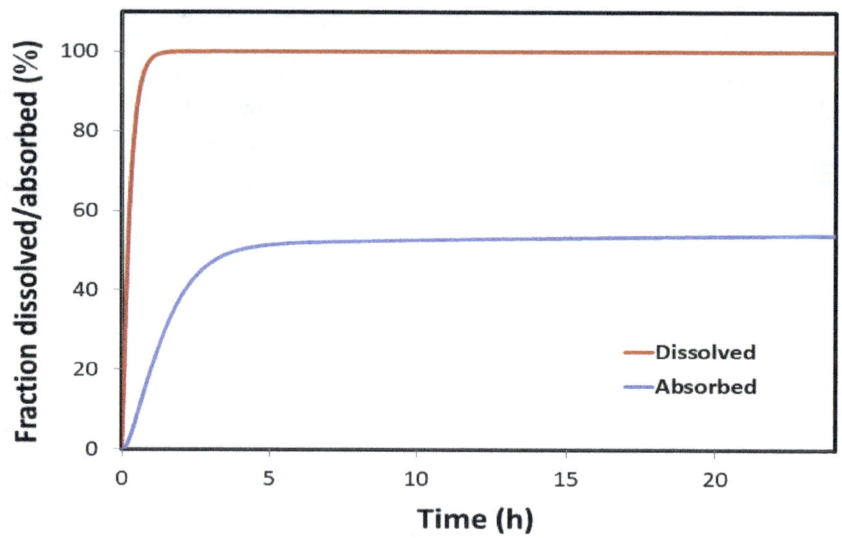

Figure 5. GastroPlus® simulated dissolution and absorption profiles following p.o. administration of 40 mg furosemide dose (dissolution profile was simulated using the software default Johnson equation).

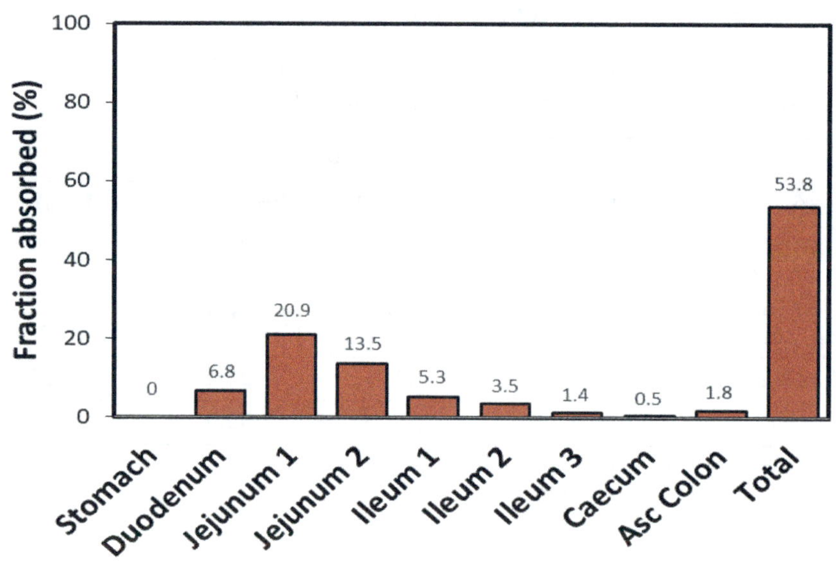

Figure 6. GastroPlus® simulated regional absorption of furosemide following p.o. administration of 40 mg drug dose (the simulated values refer to the fraction of drug dose that entered into the enterocytes).

The prediction results corresponding to various dissolution scenarios are presented in Figure 7b–d and Table 5. According to the simulated data, furosemide release rate from an oral formulation highly impacts the concomitant absorption process, whereas prolonged drug release rate leads to marked delay in the rate and extent of drug absorption. The estimated pharmacokinetic parameters (Table 5) indicate that furosemide bioavailability would show more than a 10-fold decrease in case the complete drug dissolution is achieved within 24 h in comparison to 15 min. A similar trend is observed for C_{max} and AUC values (17.75- and 17.38-fold decrease, respectively), while t_{max} would be prolonged (about two-fold). It is interesting to note that t_{max} increases with decrease in drug dissolution up to some point, but further decrease in drug dissolution (e.g., 85% in more than 6 h) would not cause additional delay in peak plasma concentration. This is because, after cc. 2 h, the drug leaves proximal parts of the intestine, where majority of furosemide absorption takes place, and, later on, in mid and especially distal intestine, only a small fraction of drug can be absorbed, as illustrated in Figure 7d.

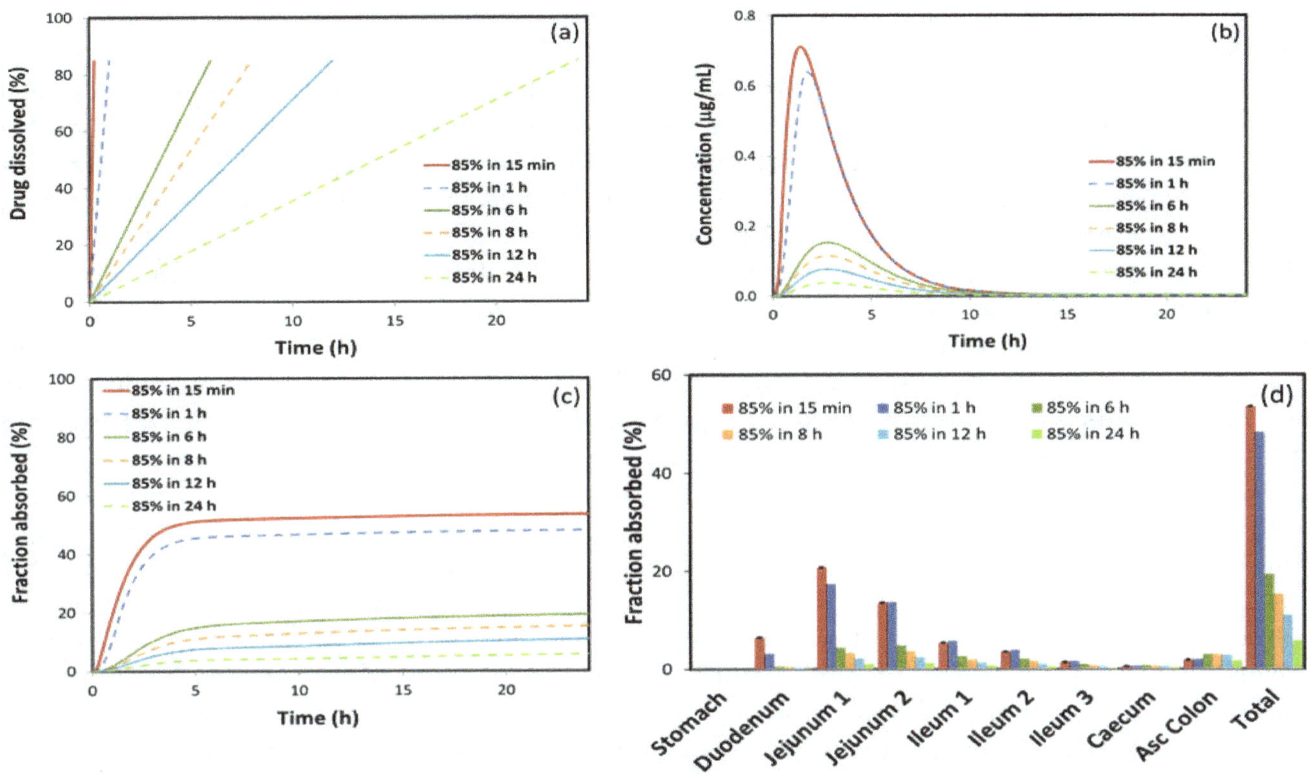

Figure 7. GastroPlus® simulated furosemide dissolution profiles (**a**); and (**b**) the corresponding simulated plasma profiles; (**c**) absorption profiles; and (**d**) regional absorption distribution.

Table 5. GastroPlus® predicted pharmacokinetic parameters for different furosemide virtual dissolution profiles from 40 mg p.o. dosage forms.

Dissolution	C_{max} (μg/mL)	t_{max} (h)	$AUC_{0\to\infty}$ (μg·h/mL)	F (%)
85% in 15 min	0.71	1.36	3.65	51.91
85% in 1 h	0.64	1.76	3.71	46.35
85% in 6 h	0.15	2.80	0.80	16.64
85% in 8 h	0.11	2.80	0.61	12.73
85% in 12 h	0.08	2.80	0.41	8.65
85% in 24 h	0.04	2.80	0.21	4.36

4. Discussion

BCS class IV drugs (e.g., sulfamethoxazole, ritonavir, paclitaxel, and furosemide) exhibit numerous unfavorable characteristics (low solubility and permeability, high presystemic metabolism, efflux transport), which make their oral drug delivery challenging. In addition to this, class IV drugs often demonstrate inter/intra-subject variability. Indeed, following oral administration, the absorption and bioavailability of furosemide are highly variable (37–51%) [35,41]. It has been suggested that this variability is highly depend on the absorption process [41], which in turn is dependent on drug aqueous solubility and intestinal permeability following oral administration [1,44]. It has also been hypothesized that variable gastric/intestinal first-pass metabolism can be a factor in causing incomplete and irregular furosemide absorption in humans [45]. Despite the unfavorable class IV drug characteristics, furosemide was shown to be exceptionally useful and successful marketed drug product for the treatment of edema [17]. For this reason, we decided to investigate furosemide's solubility and in-vivo regional-dependent permeability throughout the GIT, as main parameters that guide absorption of oral drugs.

It was shown that a correlation between human P_{eff} in the jejunum and physicochemical parameters advocates that there is a high pH-dependent influence on the passive intestinal permeability in-vivo [46]. Indeed, furosemide in-vivo permeability data demonstrate a downward trend towards the distal intestinal segments as the pH gradually increases, a trend that can be expected for acidic drugs, since the pH in the intestinal lumen gradually increases towards distal SI regions (Figure 3). Many BCS class IV drugs are substrates for efflux transporters [47]. There is some evidence that furosemide might be a substrate for efflux transporters [48,49]; thus, such permeability trend could also be influenced by the P-glycoprotein (P-gp) transporter in which expression levels are increased from proximal to distal SI segments [6,50–52]. Since metoprolol's intestinal permeability is passive and does not involve carrier-mediated absorption, it exhibited pH-dependent intestinal permeability, with reverse tendency compared to furosemide; as a basic drug, metoprolol showed upward increase in permeability towards distal SI segments with rising pH values (Figure 3). At any point throughout the SI, furosemide exhibited significantly lower permeability than the benchmark (metoprolol's jejunum permeability), which confirms its BCS low-permeability classification and incomplete absorption. Despite the fact that furosemide is a low-permeability drug, the higher permeability in the proximal intestinal regions provides a window for furosemide absorption, and we posit that this is one of the main reasons for furosemide's sufficient bioavailability and success as a marketed drug. Theoretical f_u and f_e as a function of pH were found to be in excellent correlation to these in-vivo data. In addition, in-silico modeling indicated that furosemide dissolution from an IR formulation would be fairly complete before the drug leaves proximal SI (Figure 5), although the drug is generally classified as low-soluble, enabling timely delivery of the dissolved drug to the distinct absorption site. Complete furosemide dissolution under physiological conditions is also confirmed by the experimental solubility results (Table 1).

Furosemide Log D studies showed higher partition coefficient in comparison to metoprolol at pH 6.5, whereas, in the in-vivo intestinal perfusion experiment, furosemide showed significantly lower jejunum permeability than metoprolol (Figure 1). A possible reason for this difference in the partitioning and in-vivo permeability can be the polar surface area (PSA) of both drugs [53]. A sigmoidal relationship between the fraction absorbed following oral administration and the dynamic polar surface area was reported in the past [54–56]. It was shown that orally administered drugs with large PSA (>120) are hardly absorbed by the passive transcellular route, while drugs with a small PSA (<60) are almost completely absorbed [55,56]. This is in agreement with our results, as furosemide has much higher PSA (127.7) than metoprolol (53.2) [54,55]. Another reason for the difference in the partitioning and in-vivo permeability may be the presence of active efflux transport involved in the intestinal permeability. The influence of efflux transport at pH 6.5 (proximal intestinal segments) could decrease furosemide's permeability in-vivo, which was not accounted for in the octanol partitioning studies.

The Log P value of furosemide (2.3) is in the close proximity to that of metoprolol (2.2), pointing to high permeability (Table 2). However, the Log P calculation is based on the unionized drug fraction, and, since furosemide has acidic nature it is likely that, once it passes the acidic stomach environment, it will mostly be in ionized form (the pH throughout the GIT varies from 5.9–6.3 in the proximal SI to 7.4–7.8 in distal SI segments; pH in the colon is fluctuating between pH 5–8 [57]); therefore the high furosemide Log P is not in correspondence with permeability in-vivo. Thus, we posit that no single parameter can be used for measuring the drug absorption process, but rather, a combination of physicochemical parameters and in-vitro and in-vivo findings, as well as careful consideration of inclusion criteria prior to making decisions. Despite the high Log P value for furosemide, it was indeed confirmed that furosemide is a BCS class IV drug, based on both the solubility data (Table 1) and the intestinal permeability (Figure 3).

Suitable formulation is the main approach to create an efficacious drug product for the administration of BCS class IV drugs [47]. Absorption windows in the proximal intestinal segments can restrict the oral drug bioavailability and can be a significant limitation for the development of CR drug formulation. The underlying reasons are mechanistically explained by our in-silico results (Figure 7). As mentioned, furosemide permeability results revealed acceptable permeability in the proximal segments of the SI, which is presumably the reason why furosemide has appropriate drug bioavailability, despite being a BCS class IV drug. However, since CR products release the drug over 12–24 h, mostly in the colon, (transit time throughout the small intestine is 3–4 h [58]), the fact that furosemide is mainly absorbed from proximal SI segments, (with decreased permeability at distant GIT segments) prevents the formulation of furosemide as a CR product, as shown previously [21,59,60]. However, we believe that formulations based on gastro-retentive dosage forms (GRDF) can be shown as prosperous for furosemide [61]. There are several similar examples in the literature where absorption window occurs in the upper GI, and this has been used to create GDRF formulations to improve the drug absorption, such as riboflavin [62] and levodopa [59,63].

Several types of bariatric surgeries (specifically Roux-en-Y gastric bypass and mini bypass) result in bypassing the upper SI. In cases where the absorption window is indeed in this upper SI region, the absorption following the bariatric surgery can be hampered vastly, since the actual segment responsible for the majority of absorption is bypassed [64–66].

5. Conclusions

Regional-dependent permeability throughout the small intestine was evident for furosemide. The permeability of furosemide gradually decreases throughout the small intestine as a function of the pH change in the intestinal lumen. However, at any point throughout the small intestine, furosemide exhibited significantly lower permeability than the benchmark of metoprolol's permeability in the jejunum, which may explain the incomplete absorption of the drug. We propose that, for a drug to be classified as BCS low-permeability, its intestinal permeability should not match/exceed the low/high class benchmark anywhere throughout the intestinal tract, as well as is not restricted necessarily to the jejunum. Nevertheless, low-permeable drugs should not be treated as 'unfavorable' by default; instead, therapeutic potential and suitable formulation strategies should be considered on a case-by-case basis, taking into account the overall results of in-vitro, in-vivo, and in-silico testing, throughout the entire gastrointestinal tract.

Author Contributions: M.M., M.Z., I.R., S.C. and A.D. worked on conceptualization, methodology, investigation, analyzed the data, and outlined the manuscript. S.C. worked on software investigation. Writing: S.C., A.D. and M.M. prepared the original draft of the article, and M.Z. and I.R. contributed to the writing-review and editing of the full version. All authors have read and agreed to the published version of the manuscript.

References

1. Amidon, G.L.; Lennernäs, H.; Shah, V.P.; Crison, J.R. A theoretical basis for a biopharmaceutic drug classification: The correlation of in vitro drug product dissolution and in vivo bioavailability. *Pharm. Res.* **1995**, *12*, 413–420. [CrossRef]
2. Dahan, A.; Miller, J.M.; Amidon, G.L. Prediction of solubility and permeability class membership: Provisional BCS classification of the world's top oral drugs. *AAPS J.* **2009**, *11*, 740–746. [CrossRef]
3. Dahan, A.; Beig, A.; Lindley, D.; Miller, J.M. The solubility-permeability interplay and oral drug formulation design: Two heads are better than one. *Adv. Drug Deliv. Rev.* **2016**, *101*, 99–107. [CrossRef]
4. Dahan, A.; Miller, J.M. The solubility-permeability interplay and its implications in formulation design and development for poorly soluble drugs. *AAPS J.* **2012**, *14*, 244–251. [CrossRef]
5. Miller, J.M.; Beig, A.; Carr, R.A.; Webster, G.K.; Dahan, A. The solubility-permeability interplay when using cosolvents for solubilization: Revising the way we use solubility-enabling formulations. *Mol. Pharm.* **2012**, *9*, 581–590. [CrossRef]
6. Dahan, A.; Amidon, G.L. Segmental dependent transport of low permeability compounds along the small intestine due to P-Glycoprotein: The role of efflux transport in the oral absorption of BCS class III drugs. *Mol. Pharm.* **2009**, *6*, 19–28. [CrossRef]
7. Dahan, A.; West, B.T.; Amidon, G.L. Segmental-dependent membrane permeability along the intestine following oral drug administration: Evaluation of a triple single-pass intestinal perfusion (TSPIP) approach in the rat. *Eur. J. Pharm. Sci.* **2009**, *36*, 320–329. [CrossRef]

8. Fairstein, M.; Swissa, R.; Dahan, A. Regional-dependent intestinal permeability and BCS classification: Elucidation of pH-related complexity in rats using pseudoephedrine. *AAPS J.* **2013**, *15*, 589–597. [CrossRef]
9. Lozoya-Agullo, I.; Zur, M.; Beig, A.; Fine, N.; Cohen, Y.; Gonzalez-Alvarez, M.; Merino-Sanjuan, M.; Gonzalez-Alvarez, I.; Bermejo, M.; Dahan, A. Segmental-dependent permeability throughout the small intestine following oral drug administration: Single-pass vs. Doluisio approach to in-situ rat perfusion. *Int. J. Pharm.* **2016**, *515*, 201–208. [CrossRef]
10. Markovic, M.; Zur, M.; Dahan, A.; Cvijić, S. Biopharmaceutical characterization of rebamipide: The role of mucus binding in regional-dependent intestinal permeability. *Eur. J. Pharm. Sci.* **2020**, *152*, 105440. [CrossRef]
11. Zur, M.; Hanson, A.S.; Dahan, A. The complexity of intestinal permeability: Assigning the correct BCS classification through careful data interpretation. *Eur. J. Pharm. Sci.* **2014**, *61*, 11–17. [CrossRef]
12. U.S. Department of Health and Human Services, Food and Drug Administration; Center for Drug Evaluation and Research (CDER). *Waiver of In-Vivo Bioavailability and Bioequivalence Studies for Immediate-Release Solid Oral Dosage Forms Based on a Biopharmaceutics Classification System; Guidance for Industry*; Center for Drug Evaluation and Research (CDER): Silver Spring, MD, USA, 2017.
13. Dahan, A.; Wolk, O.; Kim, Y.H.; Ramachandran, C.; Crippen, G.M.; Takagi, T.; Bermejo, M.; Amidon, G.L. Purely in silico BCS classification: Science based quality standards for the world's drugs. *Mol. Pharm.* **2013**, *10*, 4378–4390. [CrossRef]
14. Takagi, T.; Ramachandran, C.; Bermejo, M.; Yamashita, S.; Yu, L.X.; Amidon, G.L. A provisional biopharmaceutical classification of the top 200 oral drug products in the United States, Great Britain, Spain, and Japan. *Mol. Pharm.* **2006**, *3*, 631–643. [CrossRef]
15. Wolk, O.; Agbaria, R.; Dahan, A. Provisional in-silico biopharmaceutics classification (BCS) to guide oral drug product development. *Drug Des. Dev. Ther.* **2014**, *8*, 1563–1575. [CrossRef]
16. Lindenberg, M.; Kopp, S.; Dressman, J.B. Classification of orally administered drugs on the World Health Organization model list of essential medicines according to the biopharmaceutics classification system. *Eur. J. Pharm. Biopharm.* **2004**, *58*, 265–278. [CrossRef]
17. Furosemide Tablets, United States Pharmacopeia Label. Available online: https://www.accessdata.fda.gov/drugsatfda_docs/label/2016/018487s043lbl.pdf (accessed on 11 July 2020).
18. Ellison, D.H.; Felker, G.M. Diuretic Treatment in Heart Failure. *N. Engl. J. Med.* **2017**, *377*, 1964–1975. [CrossRef]
19. Hammarlund-Udenaes, M.; Benet, L.Z. Furosemide pharmacokinetics and pharmacodynamics in health and disease—An update. *J. Pharmacokinet. Biopharm.* **1989**, *17*, 1–46. [CrossRef]
20. Dahan, A.; Wolk, O.; Zur, M.; Amidon, G.L.; Abrahamsson, B.; Cristofoletti, R.; Groot, D.W.; Kopp, S.; Langguth, P.; Polli, J.E.; et al. Biowaiver monographs for immediate-release solid oral dosage forms: Codeine phosphate. *J. Pharm. Sci.* **2014**, *103*, 1592–1600. [CrossRef]
21. Markovic, M.; Zur, M.; Fine-Shamir, N.; Haimov, E.; González-Álvarez, I.; Dahan, A. Segmental-dependent solubility and permeability as key factors guiding controlled release drug product development. *Pharmaceutics* **2020**, *12*, 295. [CrossRef]
22. Zur, M.; Cohen, N.; Agbaria, R.; Dahan, A. The biopharmaceutics of successful controlled release drug product: Segmental-dependent permeability of glipizide vs. metoprolol throughout the intestinal tract. *Int. J. Pharm.* **2015**, *489*, 304–310. [CrossRef]
23. Zur, M.; Gasparini, M.; Wolk, O.; Amidon, G.L.; Dahan, A. The low/high BCS permeability class boundary: Physicochemical comparison of metoprolol and labetalol. *Mol. Pharm.* **2014**, *11*, 1707–1714. [CrossRef]
24. Granero, G.E.; Longhi, M.R.; Mora, M.J.; Junginger, H.E.; Midha, K.K.; Shah, V.P.; Stavchansky, S.; Dressman, J.B.; Barends, D.M. Biowaiver monographs for immediate release solid oral dosage forms: Furosemide. *J. Pharm. Sci.* **2010**, *99*, 2544–2556. [CrossRef] [PubMed]
25. Wagner, J.G.; Sedman, A.J. Quantitaton of rate of gastrointestinal and buccal absorption of acidic and basic drugs based on extraction theory. *J. Pharmacokinet. Biopharm.* **1973**, *1*, 23–50. [CrossRef]
26. Winne, D. Shift of pH-absorption curves. *J. Pharmacokinet. Biopharm.* **1977**, *5*, 53–94. [CrossRef]
27. Berthod, A.; Carda-Broch, S.; Garcia-Alvarez-Coque, M.C. Hydrophobicity of ionizable compounds. A theoretical study and measurements of diuretic octanol−water partition coefficients by countercurrent chromatography. *Anal. Chem.* **1999**, *71*, 879–888. [CrossRef]

28. Henchoz, Y.; Guillarme, D.; Martel, S.; Rudaz, S.; Veuthey, J.L.; Carrupt, P.A. Fast log P determination by ultra-high-pressure liquid chromatography coupled with UV and mass spectrometry detections. *Anal. Bioanal. Chem.* **2009**, *394*, 1919–1930. [CrossRef]
29. Teksin, Z.S.; Hom, K.; Balakrishnan, A.; Polli, J.E. Ion pair-mediated transport of metoprolol across a three lipid-component PAMPA system. *J. Control. Release Off. J. Control. Release Soc.* **2006**, *116*, 50–57. [CrossRef]
30. Lozoya-Agullo, I.; Gonzalez-Alvarez, I.; Zur, M.; Fine-Shamir, N.; Cohen, Y.; Markovic, M.; Garrigues, T.M.; Dahan, A.; Gonzalez-Alvarez, M.; Merino-Sanjuán, M.; et al. Closed-loop doluisio (colon, small intestine) and single-pass intestinal perfusion (colon, jejunum) in rat—Biophysical model and predictions based on Caco-2. *Pharm. Res.* **2017**, *35*, 2. [CrossRef]
31. Lozoya-Agullo, I.; Zur, M.; Fine-Shamir, N.; Markovic, M.; Cohen, Y.; Porat, D.; Gonzalez-Alvarez, I.; Gonzalez-Alvarez, M.; Merino-Sanjuan, M.; Bermejo, M.; et al. Investigating drug absorption from the colon: Single-pass vs. Doluisio approaches to in-situ rat large-intestinal perfusion. *Int. J. Pharm.* **2017**, *527*, 135–141. [CrossRef]
32. Lozoya-Agullo, I.; Zur, M.; Wolk, O.; Beig, A.; Gonzalez-Alvarez, I.; Gonzalez-Alvarez, M.; Merino-Sanjuan, M.; Bermejo, M.; Dahan, A. In-situ intestinal rat perfusions for human Fabs prediction and BCS permeability class determination: Investigation of the single-pass vs. the Doluisio experimental approaches. *Int. J. Pharm.* **2015**, *480*, 1–7. [CrossRef]
33. Dahan, A.; Miller, J.M.; Hilfinger, J.M.; Yamashita, S.; Yu, L.X.; Lennernas, H.; Amidon, G.L. High-permeability criterion for BCS classification: Segmental/pH dependent permeability considerations. *Mol. Pharm.* **2010**, *7*, 1827–1834. [CrossRef]
34. Wolk, O.; Markovic, M.; Porat, D.; Fine-Shamir, N.; Zur, M.; Beig, A.; Dahan, A. Segmental-dependent intestinal drug permeability: Development and model validation of in silico predictions guided by in vivo permeability values. *J. Pharm. Sci.* **2019**, *108*, 316–325. [CrossRef]
35. Kelly, M.R.; Cutler, R.E.; Forrey, A.W.; Kimpel, B.M. Pharmacokinetics of orally administered furosemide. *Clin. Pharmacol. Ther.* **1974**, *15*, 178–186. [CrossRef]
36. Benet, L.Z. Pharmacokinetics/pharmacodynamics of furosemide in man: A review. *J. Pharmacokinet. Biopharm.* **1979**, *7*, 1–27. [CrossRef]
37. Hammarlund, M.M.; Paalzow, L.K.; Odlind, B. Pharmacokinetics of furosemide in man after intravenous and oral administration. Application of moment analysis. *Eur. J. Clin. Pharmacol.* **1984**, *26*, 197–207. [CrossRef]
38. Agoram, B.; Woltosz, W.S.; Bolger, M.B. Predicting the impact of physiological and biochemical processes on oral drug bioavailability. *Adv. Drug Deliv. Rev.* **2001**, *50*, S41–S67. [CrossRef]
39. Lin, L.; Wong, H. Predicting oral drug absorption: Mini review on physiologically-based pharmacokinetic models. *Pharmaceutics* **2017**, *9*, 41. [CrossRef]
40. Lu, A.T.K.; Frisella, M.E.; Johnson, K.C. Dissolution modeling: Factors affecting the dissolution rates of polydisperse powders. *Pharm. Res.* **1993**, *10*, 1308–1314. [CrossRef]
41. Grahnén, A.; Hammarlund, M.; Lundqvist, T. Implications of intraindividual variability in bioavailability studies of furosemide. *Eur. J. Clin. Pharmacol.* **1984**, *27*, 595–602. [CrossRef]
42. Waller, E.S.; Hamilton, S.F.; Massarella, J.W.; Sharanevych, M.A.; Smith, R.V.; Yakatan, G.J.; Doluisio, J.T. Disposition and absolute bioavailability of furosemide in healthy males. *J. Pharm. Sci.* **1982**, *71*, 1105–1108. [CrossRef]
43. Beermann, B.; Midskov, C. Reduced bioavailability and effect of furosemide given with food. *Eur. J. Clin. Pharmacol.* **1986**, *29*, 725–727. [CrossRef]
44. Dahan, A.; Lennernäs, H.; Amidon, G.L. The fraction dose absorbed, in humans, and high jejunal human permeability relationship. *Mol. Pharm.* **2012**, *9*, 1847–1851. [CrossRef]
45. Lee, M.G.; Chiou, W.L. Evaluation of potential causes for the incomplete bioavailability of furosemide: Gastric first-pass metabolism. *J. Pharm. Biopharm.* **1983**, *11*, 623–640. [CrossRef]
46. Dahlgren, D.; Lennernas, H. Intestinal permeability and drug absorption: Predictive experimental, computational and in vivo approaches. *Pharmaceutics* **2019**, *11*, 411. [CrossRef]
47. Ghadi, R.; Dand, N. BCS class IV drugs: Highly notorious candidates for formulation development. *J. Control. Release Off. J. Control. Release Soc.* **2017**, *248*, 71–95. [CrossRef]
48. Flanagan, S.D.; Cummins, C.L.; Susanto, M.; Liu, X.; Takahashi, L.H.; Benet, L.Z. Comparison of furosemide and vinblastine secretion from cell lines overexpressing multidrug resistance protein (P-glycoprotein) and multidrug resistance-associated proteins (MRP1 and MRP2). *Pharmacology* **2002**, *64*, 126–134. [CrossRef]

49. Takahashi, M.; Washio, T.; Suzuki, N.; Igeta, K.; Fujii, Y.; Hayashi, M.; Shirasaka, Y.; Yamashita, S. Characterization of gastrointestinal drug absorption in cynomolgus monkeys. *Mol. Pharm.* **2008**, *5*, 340–348. [CrossRef]
50. Cao, X.; Yu, L.X.; Barbaciru, C.; Landowski, C.P.; Shin, H.C.; Gibbs, S.; Miller, H.A.; Amidon, G.L.; Sun, D. Permeability dominates in vivo intestinal absorption of P-gp substrate with high solubility and high permeability. *Mol. Pharm.* **2005**, *2*, 329–340. [CrossRef]
51. Englund, G.; Rorsman, F.; Rönnblom, A.; Karlbom, U.; Lazorova, L.; Gråsjö, J.; Kindmark, A.; Artursson, P. Regional levels of drug transporters along the human intestinal tract: Co-expression of ABC and SLC transporters and comparison with Caco-2 cells. *Eur. J. Pharm. Sci.* **2006**, *29*, 269–277. [CrossRef]
52. Zimmermann, C.; Gutmann, H.; Hruz, P.; Gutzwiller, J.-P.; Beglinger, C.; Drewe, J. Mapping of multidrug resistance gene 1 and multidrug resistance-associated protein isoform 1 to 5 mRNA expression along the human intestinal tract. *Drug Metab. Dispos.* **2005**, *33*, 219. [CrossRef]
53. Winiwarter, S.; Bonham, N.M.; Ax, F.; Hallberg, A.; Lennernäs, H.; Karlén, A. Correlation of human jejunal permeability (in vivo) of drugs with experimentally and theoretically derived parameters. A multivariate data analysis approach. *J. Med. Chem.* **1998**, *41*, 4939–4949. [CrossRef]
54. Clark, D.E. Rapid calculation of polar molecular surface area and its application to the prediction of transport phenomena. 1. Prediction of intestinal absorption. *J. Pharm. Sci.* **1999**, *88*, 807–814. [CrossRef]
55. Palm, K.; Luthman, K.; Ungell, A.-L.; Strandlund, G.; Beigi, F.; Lundahl, P.; Artursson, P. Evaluation of dynamic polar molecular surface area as predictor of drug absorption: Comparison with other computational and experimental predictors. *J. Med. Chem.* **1998**, *41*, 5382–5392. [CrossRef]
56. Ertl, P.; Rohde, B.; Selzer, P. Fast calculation of molecular polar surface area as a sum of fragment-based contributions and its application to the prediction of drug transport properties. *J. Med. Chem.* **2000**, *43*, 3714–3717. [CrossRef]
57. Koziolek, M.; Grimm, M.; Becker, D.; Iordanov, V.; Zou, H.; Shimizu, J.; Wanke, C.; Garbacz, G.; Weitschies, W. Investigation of pH and temperature profiles in the GI tract of fasted human subjects using the intellicap(®) system. *J. Pharm. Sci.* **2015**, *104*, 2855–2863. [CrossRef]
58. Davis, S.S.; Hardy, J.G.; Fara, J.W. Transit of pharmaceutical dosage forms through the small intestine. *Gut* **1986**, *27*, 886–892. [CrossRef]
59. Streubel, A.; Siepmann, J.; Bodmeier, R. Drug delivery to the upper small intestine window using gastroretentive technologies. *Curr. Opin. Pharmacol.* **2006**, *6*, 501–508. [CrossRef]
60. Clear, N.J.; Milton, A.; Humphrey, M.; Henry, B.T.; Wulff, M.; Nichols, D.J.; Anziano, R.J.; Wilding, I. Evaluation of the Intelisite capsule to deliver theophylline and frusemide tablets to the small intestine and colon. *Eur. J. Pharm. Sci. Off. J. Eur. Fed. Pharm. Sci.* **2001**, *13*, 375–384. [CrossRef]
61. Darandale, S.S.; Vavia, P.R. Design of a gastroretentive mucoadhesive dosage form of furosemide for controlled release. *Acta Pharm. Sin. B* **2012**, *2*, 509–517. [CrossRef]
62. Kagan, L.; Lapidot, N.; Afargan, M.; Kirmayer, D.; Moor, E.; Mardor, Y.; Friedman, M.; Hoffman, A. Gastroretentive accordion pill: Enhancement of riboflavin bioavailability in humans. *J. Control. Release Off. J. Control. Release Soc.* **2006**, *113*, 208–215. [CrossRef]
63. Klausner, E.A.; Eyal, S.; Lavy, E.; Friedman, M.; Hoffman, A. Novel levodopa gastroretentive dosage form: In-vivo evaluation in dogs. *J. Control. Release* **2003**, *88*, 117–126. [CrossRef]
64. Israel, S.; Elinav, H.; Elazary, R.; Porat, D.; Gibori, R.; Dahan, A.; Azran, C.; Horwitz, E. Case report of increased exposure to antiretrovirals following sleeve gastrectomy. *Antimicrob. Agents Chemother.* **2020**, *64*. [CrossRef]
65. Porat, D.; Dahan, A. Medication management after bariatric surgery: Providing optimal patient care. *J. Clin. Med.* **2020**, *9*, 1511. [CrossRef]
66. Porat, D.; Markovic, M.; Zur, M.; Fine-Shamir, N.; Azran, C.; Shaked, G.; Czeiger, D.; Vaynshtein, J.; Replyanski, I.; Sebbag, G.; et al. Increased paracetamol bioavailability after sleeve gastrectomy: A crossover pre- vs. post-operative clinical trial. *J. Clin. Med.* **2019**, *8*, 1949. [CrossRef]

2

Liquid and Solid Self-Emulsifying Drug Delivery Systems (SEDDs) as Carriers for the Oral Delivery of Azithromycin: Optimization, In Vitro Characterization and Stability Assessment

Reem Abou Assi [1,2,†], Ibrahim M. Abdulbaqi [1,2,†], Toh Seok Ming [1], Chan Siok Yee [1,*], Habibah A. Wahab [1,*], Shaik Mohammed Asif [1,3] and Yusrida Darwis [1,*]

1 The Discipline of Pharmaceutical Technology, School of Pharmaceutical Sciences, Universiti Sains Malaysia, Penang 11800, Malaysia; drmeer1@gmail.com (R.A.A.); ibrahimm.abdulbaqi@gmail.com (I.M.A.); smtoh@usm.my (T.S.M.); asif81ind@gmail.com (S.M.A.)

2 The Discipline of Pharmaceutical Technology, College of Pharmacy, Al-Kitab University, Altun kupri, Kirkuk 36001, Iraq

3 Pharma Research, Wockhardt Research Center, Aurangabad 431002, India

* Correspondence: sychan@usm.my (C.S.Y.); habibahw@usm.my (H.A.W.); yusrida@usm.my (Y.D.)

† Authors have equally contributed to this work.

Abstract: Azithromycin (AZM) is a macrolide antibiotic used for the treatment of various bacterial infections. The drug is known to have low oral bioavailability (37%) which may be attributed to its relatively high molecular weight, low solubility, dissolution rate, and incomplete intestinal absorption. To overcome these drawbacks, liquid (L) and solid (S) self-emulsifying drug delivery systems (SEDDs) of AZM were developed and optimized. Eight different pseudo-ternary diagrams were constructed based on the drug solubility and the emulsification studies in various SEDDs excipients at different surfactant to co-surfactant (Smix) ratios. Droplet size (DS) < 150 nm, dispersity ($Đ$) ≤ 0.7, and transmittance (T)% > 85 in three diluents of distilled water (DW), 0.1 mM HCl, and simulated intestinal fluids (SIF) were considered as the selection criteria. The final formulations of L-SEDDs (L-F1$_{(H)}$), and S-SEDDs (S-F1$_{(H)}$) were able to meet the selection requirements. Both formulations were proven to be cytocompatible and able to open up the cellular epithelial tight junctions (TJ). The drug dissolution studies showed that after 5 min > 90% and 52.22% of the AZM was released from liquid and solid SEDDs formulations in DW, respectively, compared to 11.27% of the pure AZM, suggesting the developed SEDDs may enhance the oral delivery of the drug. The formulations were stable at refrigerator storage conditions.

Keywords: liquid SEDDs; solid SEDDs; drug delivery; self-emulsifying; cytotoxicity; MTT assay; tight junctions; Caco-2 cell; stability

---

1. Introduction

Oral drug delivery is the most widely used and the common route of drug administration because it is convenient, economical, comfortable, and requires no special training for use [1,2]. However, despite these advantages, problems such as poor solubility, low dissolution rates, and limited drug diffusion through the paracellular pathways before eventually entering the systemic circulation making it challenging for many drugs to reach the therapeutic levels via this route [3,4].

Azithromycin (AZM) is a semisynthetic 15-membered macrolide antibiotic [5], with a lipophilic nature (log P = 4), (pKa = 8.74), and a molecular weight of 749 g/mol [6,7]. The drug, which is included in the model list of essential medicines on the World Health Organization website [7], is classified as the first azalide subclass among its family members [8,9] with a superior antibacterial activity in the market for the last three decades. This makes AZM the drug of choice for the treatment of various gastrointestinal, respiratory, and genitourinary infections. Recently it has gained increased popularity owing to its suggested important role in improving the ability of hydroxychloroquine to eradicate the global outbreak of COVID-19 virus at clinical levels [10]. However, the oral intake of AZM is associated with a relatively low bioavailability of 37%. The exact reasons for this low oral bioavailability are not specified. However, many reports are suggesting that it might be attributed to different factors such as the low aqueous solubility (AZM is practically insoluble in water) which may lead to erratic dissolution rates [11–15], the drug relatively high molecular weight, the low stability at the acidic gastric pH (AZM have a high potential of decomposition in acidic medium) [16], and the incomplete gastrointestinal tract (GIT) absorption [17]. Pharmacokinetically, most poorly water-soluble drugs have low bioavailability. Furthermore, AZM is recognized to be a substrate for the P-glycoprotein (P-gp) efflux transporters, which can potentially restrict its transcellular diffusion and permeability [18–20]. To the best of our knowledge, cellular studies on the paracellular permeability of AZM and its nanoformulation(s) on colon adenocarcinoma human cells (Caco-2) line are scanty. Nevertheless, some reports are suggesting that AZM may increase the transepithelial electrical resistance (TEER) values when studied in certain cell lines such as human airway epithelial cell lines [21,22], which could be linked to changing the processing of tight junction proteins [22,23]. This may lead to a negative impact on AZM paracellular transport and permeability. All these drawbacks led to higher oral AZM dosing regimens and longer times of treatment that, in turn, intensified the associated GIT side effects, including diarrhea, nausea, and abdominal pain. The only other available dosage form of AZM is the intravenous infusion, which is also associated with severe adverse effects, including pain at the injection site and local inflammation [24].

Increasing the solubility and dissolution rates of poorly water-soluble drugs are of the most challenging tasks in drug development nowadays for enhancing their oral bioavailability. Different strategies and techniques were employed for this purpose such as complexation, chemical modification, solid dispersions, and the use of nanocarriers and drug delivery systems. Solid dispersions [11,15,25], nanosuspensions [26], and niosomes [27] of AZM were employed to enhance its solubility and dissolution rates.

Lipid-based carriers have been used successfully to enhance the oral delivery of various drugs. These formulations are generally classified into four types (I, II, III, and IV) [28,29]. In particular, type III carriers, which are also known as self-emulsifying drug delivery systems (SEDDs), have been driving a profound interest by the pharmaceutical researchers and industries for their efficacy in enhancing oral delivery of various therapeutic agents of different physiochemical properties [30–34]. SEDDs are used as effective tools to enhance the GIT absorption and oral bioavailability of poorly water-soluble drugs by significantly increasing their solubility and improving their dissolution behavior [35]. Furthermore, SEDDs are also existing as liquid (L-SEDDs) and solid (S-SEDDs) formulations. The S-SEDDs are suggested to provide better stability, reproducibility, and patient compliance, in addition to ease of process control [36].

The present study aimed to develop L-SEDDs and S-SEDDs formulations for potentially enhancing the oral delivery of AZM by increasing its solubility and dissolution rates using excipients that are able to solubilize the highest amounts of the drug and at the same time have a previously reported capacity to loosen the intestinal TJ. In this work, AZM-loaded L-SEDDs were prepared and characterized. The optimized liquid SEEDs were converted to solid SEDDs using various solidifying agents. All the prepared AZM-loaded liquid and solid SEEDs formulations were characterized in terms of droplet size (DS), dispersity (*Đ*), zeta potential (ZP), maximum drug content (DC) which is also called solubilization capacity, and in vitro release behaviors. The cytotoxicity and the potential abilities of the optimized liquid and solid formulations to open the epithelial TJ by reducing the trans-epithelial electrical resistance (TEER) for better drug permeability were investigated. Furthermore, the stability of the optimized formulations was evaluated at different storage conditions.

2. Materials and Methods

2.1. Materials

Azithromycin (purity > 97.2%) was a kind gift from Wockhardt research center (Aurangabad, India). Labrasol®, Labrafac PG®, Labrafil® M 1944 CS, Capryol 90® and Transcutol HP® were purchased from Gattefossé (Lyon, France). Span 20®, Span 80®, Tween 20®, Tween 80®, octanoic acid ≥ 99%, castor oil, potassium phosphate monobasic ≥ 99%, Trypsin-EDTA solution 1× (0.25% trypsin, 0.02% EDTA), dimethyl sulfoxide ≥ 99.5% (DMSO), thiazolyl blue tetrazolium bromide 98% (MTT) and Corning® transwell polycarbonate membrane cell culture inserts 24 well plates were obtained from Sigma-Aldrich (St. Louis, MO, USA). Cremophor 40®, Cremophor EL® were bought from BASF (Ludwigshafen, Germany). Pureco® 76 was purchased from Abitec corporation (Janesville, WIS, USA). Aerosil 200® ≥ 99.8% was obtained from Evonik Inc. (Essen, Germany). Calcium carbonate, mannitol, and sodium hydroxide pellets were brought from R & M chemicals Ltd. (Essex, UK). HMS lactose was ordered from B.V. Hollandsche Melksuikerfabriek (Uitgeest, Holland). The medium used for the cell culture was Gibco® Dulbecco's modified eagle's medium (DMEM (1×) + GlutaMAXTM-1), penicillin-streptomycin solution (Pen-Strep) (which contains 10,000 units of penicillin, and 10 mg of streptomycin), and Gibco® fetal bovine serum (FBS) (New Zealand origin), along with Gibco® Dulbecco's phosphate-buffered saline (1×) (DPBS), and hydrochloric acid (HCl) were bought from ThermoFisher scientific (Waltham, MA, USA). Caco-2 cells line was obtained from the American Type Culture Collection (ATCC) (Manassas, VA, USA). Palm oil was purchased from a local Malaysian market. All other used organic solvents or chemicals were either of analytical or HPLC grades.

2.2. Methods

2.2.1. HPLC Analysis

AZM solubility, drug content, and the in vitro release studies were determined using a previously validated HPLC method which was specially developed for these purposes [37]. In brief, the separation was done using Hypersil GOLD C-18 analytical column packed with deactivated silica (250 mm × 4.6 mm ID × 5 μm) kept at 60 °C. A mixture of ammonium acetate solution (30 mmol/L, pH = 6.8) and acetonitrile at the ratio of (18:82, *v/v*) was used as the mobile phase. The UV detection was done at 210 nm. Samples were eluted isocratically at a flow rate of 0.7 mL/min. The theoretical plate (N > 1500), tailing factor (T ≤ 1.5), and resolution (Rs > 3) were as per the United States Pharmacopeia (USP) [5]. The linearity was observed over the concentration range of 5–200 μg/mL ($R^2 > 0.9999$). The limit of detection (LOD) and limit of quantification (LOQ) were 0.476 μg/mL and 1.443 μg/mL, respectively. The developed method was statistically confirmed to be accurate, precise, and reproducible.

2.2.2. Preparation and Characterization of Blank Liquid SEDDs

- Excipients selection and screening

Excipients selection was mainly based on their ability to solubilize the highest amounts of the AZM. The impact of lipids classes as long carbon chain triglycerides (LCT) and medium carbon chain triglycerides (MCT) was observed, as such differences in carbon chain lengths were reported to have an influence on drug solubilization potential and the ability to facilitate the emulsification process [38,39]. Extra attention was given to include excipients with previously reported abilities to loosen the cellular TJ for the possibility of enhancing the drug paracellular route diffusion. Besides, certain compounds were reported to have other cellular activities (such as P-gp inhibition) along with the TJ loosening were also investigated. Other excipients which have not been reported for owning any such cellular activity were also included for their potentials in enhancing AZM solubility, as illustrated in Table 1.

Table 1. Screened excipients' role, characteristics, and previously reported cellular activities.

Name	Role	HLB	Chain Length	Reported Cellular Activity (s)	References
Capryol 90®		5	Medium-chain (C8)	TJ opening	[33,40,41]
Castor Oil		-	Long-chain (C18)	-	-
Octanoic acid (caprylic acid or caprylate)	Oil	-	Medium-chain (C8)	TJ opening	[42,43]
Palm Oil		-	Long-chain. Mixture of C16 and C18	-	-
Pureco 76®		-	Medium-chain (C8–C10)	-	-
Cremophor EL®		12–14	Medium-chain C8	TJ opening and P-gp inhibitor	[44]
Cremophor RH40®		14–16	Medium-chain C10	TJ opening and P-gp inhibitor	[45]
Labrafac PG®	Surfactant	1	Medium-chain. Mixture of C8 and C10	-	-
Labrafil® M 1944 CS		9	Long-chain C18	-	-
Labrasol®		12–14	Medium-chain (C8–C10)	TJ opening and P-gp inhibitor	[44,46]
Tween 20®		16.7	Medium-chain C12	P-gp inhibitor	[47–49]
Tween 80®		15	Long-chain C18	TJ opening and P-gp inhibitor	[50–52]
Span 20®		8.6	Medium-chain C12	P-gp inhibitor	[53]
Span 80®	Co-surfactant	4.3	Long-chain C18	-	-
Transcutol HP®		-	-	P-gp inhibitor	[54]

(HLB, Hydrophile-lipophile balance; TJ, Tight Junctions; P-gp, P-glycoprotein).

- Solubility study

The solubilization capacities of various excipients were investigated using the equilibrium method to ensure the selection of excipients that can solubilize the maximum amount of AZM. In brief, an excess amount of AZM (300 mg) was weighed in multiple 5 mL screw-capped bottles, then 3 mL of the different oils, surfactants, or co-surfactants were added separately into each bottle and vortexed for 2 min using ZX3 vortex mixer (VELP Scientifica, Italy). The filled bottles were then placed in a reciprocating shaker bath (Braun, Melsungen, Germany) at 500 oscillations/min for 72 h and maintained at 37 ± 2 °C. The bottles were centrifuged at 3000 rpm for 15 min to remove the undissolved AZM, and the resulted supernatant layer was filtered through a 0.45 μm syringe driven filter (Whatman, USA). Drug concentration in each vehicle was determined by HPLC.

- Emulsification studies

Based on the results of the AZM solubility study, the selected surfactants and co-surfactants were further screened for their emulsification abilities in the selected oils. Various surfactant to co-surfactant (Smix) ratios of (1:1), (2:1), (3:1), (4:1), (5:1), (6:1) and (1:2) (*v*/*v*) were mixed in separate vials and vortexed for few seconds until homogenous mixtures were obtained. A fixed oil ratio of 10% was added to each Smix ratio (90%); the mixtures were then gently vortexed and allowed to equilibrate at a reciprocating shaker bath for 2 h at room temperature. The produced mixtures had a range of hydrophilic–lipophilic balance (HLB) values within the range of 6.55 to 14.22. Although the characterization of SEDDs is mainly conducted using either distilled or deionized water as the dispersing medium [34,55–57], yet, in this work, the self-emulsification efficiency of various mixtures was evaluated on the bases of the produced droplet size (DS), dispersity (*Đ*) and transmittance percentage (T%), in three different diluents namely: distilled water (DW), 0.1 mM HCl (pH = 4), and simulated intestinal fluids (SIF) (pH = 6.8) for mimicking the oral route of administration and select the most physically stable formulation(s) [58,59]. All the used diluents were freshly prepared and filtered through a 0.45 μm nylon membrane filter before use. Each formulation underwent a standard dilution of 1:1000 ratio (10 μL sample to 10 mL diluent) then gently stirred with a magnetic stirrer and allowed to equilibrate before loading into a cuvette in a thermostatic chamber to measure DS and Đ through Photon Correlation Spectroscopy (PCS) using laser light scattering spectrometer Zetasizer 1000HSA (Malvern Instrument, UK). The measurement of T% was conducted at a dilution ratio of 10:1000 (100 μL sample to 10 mL diluent), then evaluated at 650 nm using a UV-Vis Spectrophotometer U-2000 (Hitachi, Japan) [60]. Only mixtures that produced DS < 150 nm, Đ ≤ 0.7, and T% > 85 in the three different diluents were selected for the construction of the pseudo-ternary diagram.

- Pseudo-ternary diagram construction

This step was done to identify the self-emulsifying regions of the L-SEDDs, where the total concentration of the three constituents (oil, surfactant, co-surfactant) was always 100%. A series of 19 blank L-SEDDs formulations were prepared by mixing the oil with the previously selected Smix ratios in different vials and volume ratios (1:9, 1:8.5, 1:8, 1:7.5, 1:7, 1:6.5, 1:6, 1:5.5, 1:5, 1:4.5, 1:4, 1:3.5, 1:3, 1:2.5, 1:2, 1:1.5, 1:1, 1.5:1 and 2:1). The vials were gently vortexed for 20 s and kept in the reciprocating shaker bath for two hours at room temperature. The blank L-SEDDs formulations were assessed for visual appearance and DS after preforming the employed standard dilution with filtered DW [61,62]. Only clear-transparent dispersions with DS < 150 nm were considered in the self-emulsified region of the phase diagrams for this study. The phase diagrams were plotted using CHEMIX® ternary plot software (CHEMIX School Ver. 3.60, Pub. Arne Standnes, Bergen, Norway).

2.2.3. Preparation and Characterization of AZM-Loaded L-SEDDs

Out of each identified self-emulsification area, three transparent formulations with DS < 150 nm were selected at three oil concentrations (low, medium, and high) for the maximum DC (or solubilization capacity) studies. There was a 5% difference between the three oil concentrations. A total of 24 L-SEDDs formulations were chosen for the DC studies. To perform the experiment, an excess amount of AZM (200 mg) was accurately weighed in multiple 5 mL screw-capped bottles, then 2 mL of each blank L-SEDDs formulation was added to each bottle. The samples were then treated as per the procedure of the AZM solubility studies, and the DC was measured. Both blank L-SEDDs and their corresponding AZM loaded L-SEDDs (AZM-L-SEDD) formulations were further characterized in terms of DS, Đ, T%, and zeta potential (ZP) in three diluents (DW, 0.1 mM HCl, and SIF). ZP was measured using Zetasizer nanoseries Nano-Z, (Malvern Instrument, UK). The AZM-L-SEDDs formulations with the highest AZM content, DS < 150 nm, Đ ≤ 0.7, T% > 85, and highest ZP value were selected for the solidification process.

2.2.4. Preparation and Characterization of AZM-Loaded S-SEDDs

Various solidification methods such as adsorption to solid carriers, spray drying, freeze-drying, rotary evaporation, melt extrusion-spheronization, and melt granulation are available for the preparation of S-SEDDs [63,64]. In this work, adsorption to solid carriers' method was adopted, as the technique is simple, which involves the addition of the L-SEDDs to the selected carriers with suitable mixing. Furthermore, the produced S-SEDDs by this method are stable and freely flowing [65,66]. Various water-soluble (mannitol and lactose) and water-insoluble (calcium carbonate and Aerosil 200®) solidifying agents were screened to select the suitable one for the conversion of the optimized blank L-SEDDs and AZM-L-SEDDs into blank solid SEDDs (S-SEDDs) and AZM loaded solid SEDDs (AZM-S-SEDDs), respectively.

At first, the adsorption capacity (expressed as a weight ratio of L-SEDDs: solidifying agent) of each solidifying agent was studied through a drop-wise addition and mixing of a fixed portion of blank L-SEDDs (0.5 mL~535.6 mg) with an equivalent portion(s) of the solidifying agent (~535.6 mg) in a porcelain mortar until a non-sticky solid powder was produced. The mixing was done using a glass rod after each addition to ensure uniform distribution of the formulation. The obtained S-SEDDs were left for 24 h at room temperature to dry before further characterization for their DS, Đ, and ZP [67–69]. For DS and Đ measurements, 10 mg of the prepared S-SEDDs were dispersed in 10 mL of filtered diluent (DW, 0.1 mM HCl, or SIF). The S-SEDDs formulations solidified with a water-soluble solidifying agent were gently stirred with a magnetic stirrer for 10 min, then allowed to equilibrate and loaded into a cuvette in a thermostatic chamber. While those S-SEDDs solidified with a water-insoluble solidifying agent, the dispersions were first centrifuged using MiniSpin® plus Eppendorf centrifuge (Eppendorf Ag, Hamburg, Germany) at 8000 rpm for 10 min to remove the water-insoluble solids then the samples were loaded into a cuvette in a thermostatic chamber [70].

The solidifying agent that produced S-SEDDs formulation with the lowest DS, Đ, and highest ZP was selected for solidifying AZM-L-SEDDs. Formulations were further examined for their DS, Đ, and ZP in the previously mentioned three diluents. AZM concentration in AZM-S-SEDDs formulation was quantified by dissolving the solid formulation (1.51 g) in 10 mL methanol and stirring it with a magnetic stirrer for 30 min. The solution was then sonicated in an ultrasonic bath (Branson 5510, Las Animas, CA, USA) for 2 min. Suitable aliquots were taken and diluted with the diluting solution and filtered with a 0.2 µm pore size nylon filter, then injected into HPLC.

2.2.5. Transmission Electron Microscope (TEM)

The morphology and shape of the final selected SEDD formulations in their liquid and solid forms were studied by TEM. A drop of the dispersed liquid or solid formulation in DW (as per the dispersing procedures for DS and Đ measurements) was placed onto 400 mesh carbon-coated copper grid, air dried, then negatively stained with 2% phosphotungstic acid for 5 min at room temperature. After that, the excess sample was removed using a filter paper and allowed to dry before observation. Images were taken under the transmission electron microscope TEM (LIBRA 120, Carl Zeiss, Oberkochen, Germany).

2.2.6. Cell Culture Studies

- Cell stock preparation

Caco-2 cells with passage numbers of 25 and 26 were grown and maintained on culture flask in DMEM supplemented with 10% *v/v* of FBS and 1% *v/v* of 1% Pen-Strep (named as the complete medium) and were maintained at 37 °C in an atmosphere of 5% CO_2 and 90% relative humidity in a Binder® constant climate chamber (Tuttlingen, Germany) [71]. Once 80% of the flask surface is covered by cell monolayer, cells were split and washed twice with DPBS, then the trypsin-EDTA solution was added and gently swirled, ensuring the complete covering of trypsin to all the cells. The flask was then incubated for 10 min in an atmosphere of 5% CO_2 and 90% relative humidity. Cells stock was prepared by aspirating out the trypsin-EDTA, and adding the complete medium, then centrifuging this cells stock in HERAEUS® LABOFUGE 400R centrifuge ThermoFisher Scientific (Waltham, MA, USA) at 900 rpm for 5 min to create a pellet at the bottom of the centrifuge tube. The cell pellet was re-suspended in 3 mL of fresh complete medium for further use as a cell stock. All cell culture buffers and solutions were pre-warmed to 37 °C prior to contact with the cells, and all protocols involved the handling of Caco-2 cells in cultures were performed aseptically.

- Cytotoxicity assay

The cytocompatibility of the optimized blank L-SEDDS and S-SEDDs formulas was investigated using the microtiter tetrazolium assay (MTT). The assay was done according to previously described methods [72,73], with slight modifications. Proper dilutions of the cell stock with the complete medium were made to get the required seeding density of 51,000 cells/cm^2 on Biofil® tissue culture 96 well plates (Guangzhou, China).

After 24 h of seeding on the 96 well plates at 37 °C in an incubator with 5% CO_2 and 90% relative humidity, the attached cells were washed twice with DPBS, then concentrations of blank L-SEDDS (0.25, 0.5, 1, and 2% *v/v*) and blank S-SEEDs (0.39, 0.77, 1.54, and 3.08% *w/v*) were selected for the study. The SEDDs were dispersed in DMEM solution, gently vortexed, filtered using a 0.2 µm sterile filter membrane, and added to the 96 wells plates then incubated for 4 h. DMEM alone was employed as blank. After incubation, the supernatant layer was discarded, and all cells were washed twice with DPBS. To observe cells' vibrant reductive activity, a final concentration of 1 mg/mL of thiazolyl blue tetrazolium bromide dye solution (MTT solution) was dissolved in DPBS within a tube wrapped in aluminum foil to protect it from light, and the cells in the well plates were loaded with 100 μL of sterile and filtered MTT solution and incubated for another 4 h. Then the supernatant layers were removed, the precipitated formazan crystals were dissolved in DMSO, and the plates were gently rotated on an orbital shaker for 5 min. The color of the resulted formazan solutions in DMSO was measured at 570 nm with background subtraction at 690 nm by a Multiskan™ FC microplate photometer (Thermo Scientific, Waltham, MA, USA) with Skanit software version 3.2. The percentage of cells viability was calculated with respect to the control [74], as follows:

$$Viability\ \% = \frac{Abs\ sample - Abs\ blank}{Abs\ control - Abs\ blank} * 100 \quad (1)$$

where, $Abs_{\ sample}$: Absorbance of cells treated with formulations. $Abs_{\ control}$: Absorbance of cells not treated with formulations. $Abs_{\ blank}$: Absorbance of blank.

- Transepithelial electrical resistance evaluation

Transepithelial electrical resistance (TEER) is a widely accepted quantitative technique to measure the integrity of tight junction dynamics in cell culture models of epithelial monolayers where the TJ proteins in the paracellular route contribute to an ohmic resistance (RTEER) in the equivalent circuit [75]. The TJ opening was investigated as per the previous protocol [76]. Cells suspension corresponding to 51,000 cells/cm^2 was prepared from the cells' stock and added to the apical transwell compartments of all plates. The plates were maintained at 37 °C in an incubator with 5% CO_2 and 90% relative humidity until they formed a polarized/differentiated monolayer, which took approximately a period of 21–23 days. During that period, a regular replacement of cells medium in both chambers (every 48 h), and monolayer's integrity monitoring were conducted by measuring the TEER using an EVOM2® epithelial volt ohmmeter with STX100 electrodes (World Precision Instruments Ltd., Stevenage, UK). Figure 1 shows a schematic diagram of the measuring procedure of the TEER. The Caco-2 cell monolayer with average TEER values ≥ 300 Ω.cm^2 indicated that cells are intact [69], and accordingly, they were used in this study. Raw data were measured in Ohm (Ω) and converted to Ω × cm^2 based on the area of transwell plate inserts, which is equal to 0.4 cm^2 for the used 24-well plate [77].

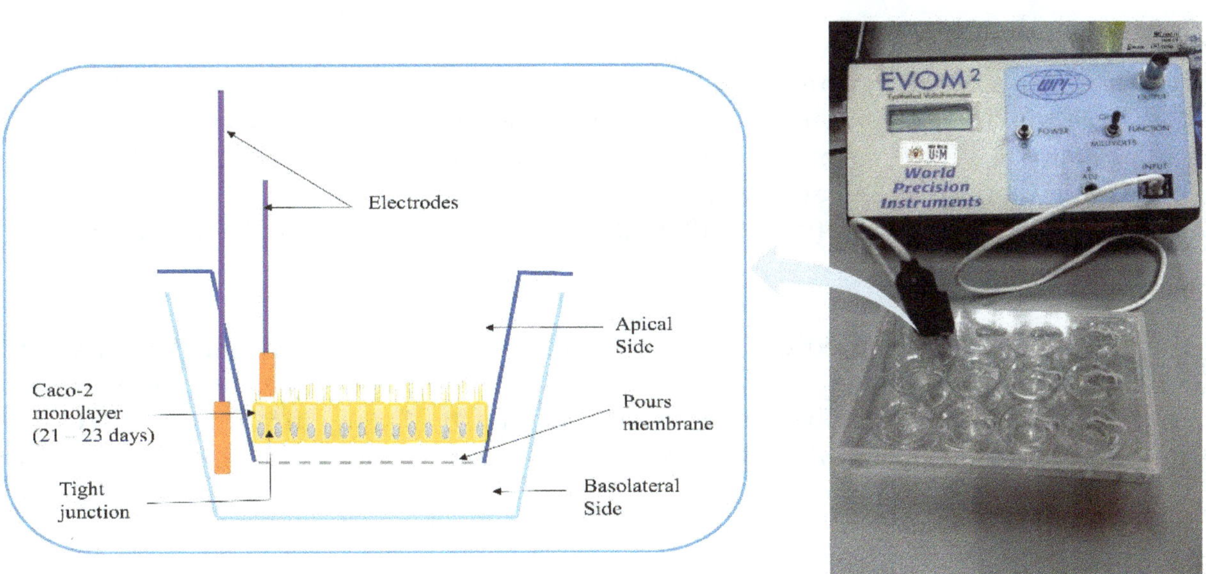

Figure 1. Schematic diagram for the measuring procedure of transepithelial electrical resistance (TEER).

On the day of the experiment, the cell cultures medium was removed, the monolayers were washed with DPBS, and fresh medium was placed in both chambers; cell cultures were left for 15 min. to equilibrate before starting the measurements. The monolayers TEER values were measured in all the studied plates for the first 10 min of the test before adding any samples, including DMSO as control, DMEM as blank, pure AZM, blank and AZM incorporated L-SEDDs, as well as blank and AZM incorporated S-SEDDs formulations.

The selected studied concentration was based on the MTT assay results. The blank and AZM incorporated L-SEDDs at the concentration of 0.5%, and an equivalent concentration of blank and AZM incorporated S-SEDDs formulations, as well as pure AZM, were dispersed in DMEM. All samples were filtered using a 0.2 μm sterile filter membrane immediately before use. At the apical side, 10 μL of the medium was replaced with 10 μL of each of the seven studied solutions, and once the addition is made, TEER values were measured at different time intervals including, every minute for 30 min, and then every hour for a period of 4 h. The resistance of the monolayer was calculated using the following equation:

$$\boldsymbol{R}\ \textit{cell layer} = \boldsymbol{R}\ \textit{sample} - \boldsymbol{R}\ \textit{blank} \tag{2}$$

where, ***R** cell layer*: Resistance of the Caco-2 monolayer. ***R** sample*: Resistance reading of the studied sample. ***R** blank*: Resistance reading of the blank.

2.2.7. The In Vitro AZM Release Studies

The in vitro release of the optimized L-SEDDs and S-SEDDs formulations was performed in comparison to the pure AZM powder using Varian® 7000 USP dissolution apparatus II (Santa Clara, CA, USA), paddle method, as recommended by USFDA [78]. Three different dissolution media were employed, namely: DW, 0.1 mM HCl (pH = 4), and SIF (pH = 6.8). The SIF was prepared by mixing 250 mL of 0.2 M potassium phosphate monobasic solution with 118 mL of 0.2 M sodium hydroxide solution then diluted with DW to 1000 mL [79]. A volume of 900 mL of the selected dissolution medium was placed in each vessel of the dissolution apparatus and was kept at 37 ± 2 °C with a paddle rotating speed of 100 rpm. An amount of 100 mg of pure AZM powder, and equivalent volume and weight of AZM-loaded L-SEDDs and S-SEDDs formulations that are containing 100 mg of the drug were placed in the vessels [15,80]. From each vessel, 5 mL aliquot was drawn at selected time intervals of 5, 15, 30, 60, 90, 120, 180, and 240 min, respectively, and were filtered through 0.45 μm polytetrafluoroethylene (PTEF) filters (Titan®, West Springfield, MA, USA). The drawn aliquots were directly replaced with an equal volume of the same fresh dissolution media, and AZM was quantified by HPLC.

2.2.8. Stability Studies

Stability studies of the optimized AZM incorporated L-SEDDS and S-SEDDS formulas were conducted for three months under three different temperatures and relative humidity conditions, namely refrigerator (4 ± 2 °C), room condition (25 ± 2 °C and 60 ± 5 relative humidity %), and humidity chamber (40 ± 2 °C and 75 ± 5 relative humidity %). The samples were analyzed for their DS, Đ, ZP, DC %, and the in vitro release profiles at different time intervals of 0, 0.5, 1, 2, and 3 months.

2.2.9. Statistical Analysis

All experiments were carried out for at least in triplicate. To test the statistical significance, a one-way analysis of variance (ANOVA) with Tukey's HSD (honest significant difference) tests were used. The difference in all the analyses was considered statistically significant when $p < 0.05$. All the statistical tests were done using (Minitab® statistical software, version 17.2.1.0, Minitab Inc., USA).

3. Results and Discussion

3.1. Excipients Selection and Solubility Studies

In this study, excipients of different carbon chain lengths were employed for better screening of SEDDs ingredients. Figure 2 illustrates the solubility of AZM in the screened excipients.

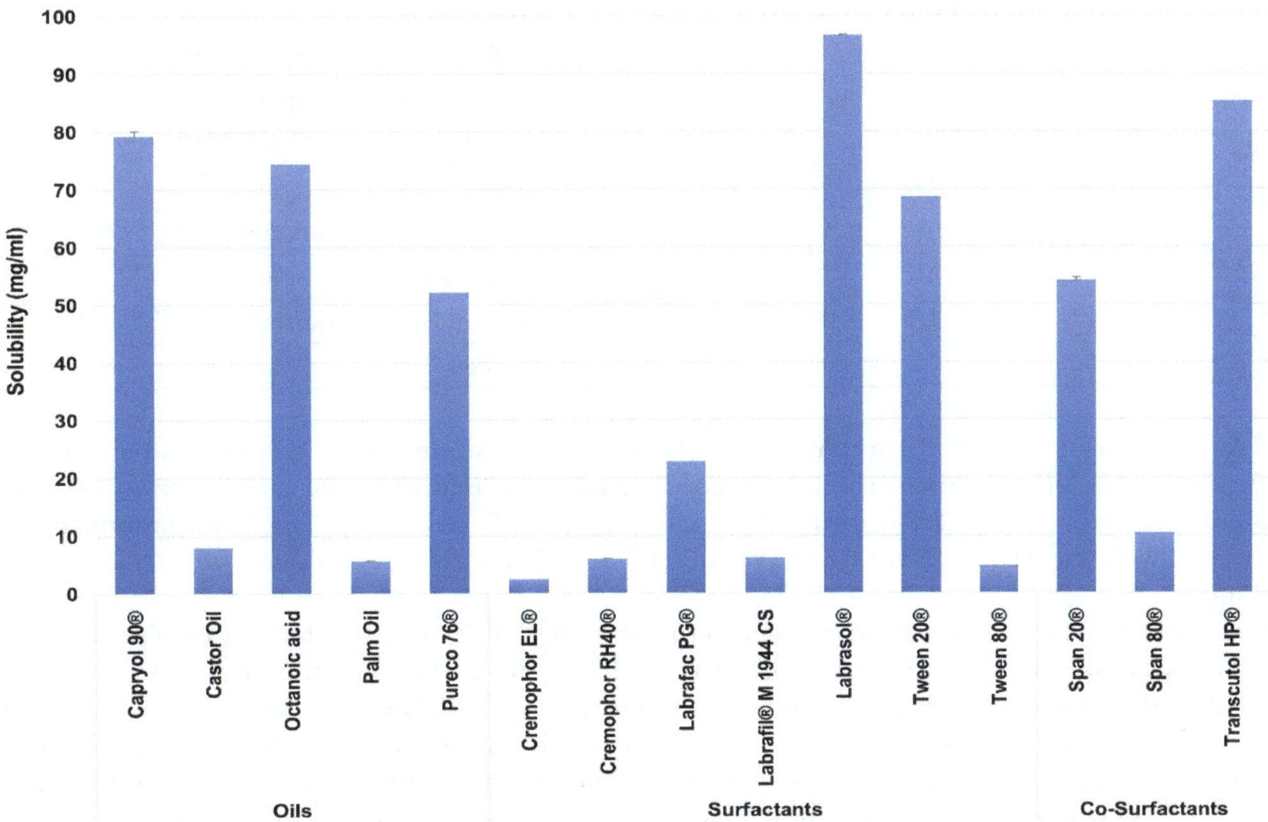

Figure 2. The solubility of Azithromycin (AZM) in the different screened excipients. Mean ± SD, n = 3.

Among the studied excipients, the highest solubility of AZM was observed in the oils of Capryol 90® (80.16 ± 0.83 mg/mL), and Octanoic acid (74.5 ± 0.035 mg/mL), in the surfactants of Labrasol® (97.44 ± 0.7 mg/mL), and Tween 20® (69.43 ± 0.81 mg/mL) and in the co-surfactants of Transcutol® HP (85.41 ± 0.27 mg/mL), and Span 20® (53.48 ± 0.75 mg/mL).

Based on the literature review, many reports showed that drugs' solubilities in various oils and surfactants might vary based on the carbon chain lengths of the oils and surfactants [81], including MCT [82–84], and LCT [85,86]. This attitude is probably linked to the employed drug physicochemical properties [82,87]. Among the studied excipients, AZM showed higher solubility in the MCT rather than the LCT. This may be linked to the high log p-value of AZM (4.02), where such drugs are shown to be more soluble in MCT than LCT [88]. Furthermore, MCT are reported to have a higher solvent capacity [89,90]. In contrast, AZM showed poor solubility in Cremophor RH40® and Cremophor EL® despite being medium-chain surfactants; this is likely because these surfactants are derived from edible oil (castor oil), where some lipophilic drugs reported to have very low solubility in such oils during SEDDs formulation studies [91–93].

3.2. Emulsification Efficiency Studies

Based on the solubility study results, all possible combinations of the various excipients were investigated for emulsification efficiency, as illustrated in Table 2. As more than two types of chemicals were incorporated in the SEDDs formulations, then one of the components was used at a fixed ratio (oil) [94], while others (Smix) were studied at the previously mentioned ratios in the method section. Precisely, a fixed ratio of 10% of the oil was employed as recommended to produce spontaneous L-SEDDs formulations with small DS upon dispersion [28].

Table 2. The combination of the selected components in liquid self-emulsifying drug delivery systems (L-SEDDs) formulations.

No.	Formulation Code	Oil	Surfactant	Co-Surfactant
1	A1	Capryol 90®	Labrasol®	Transcutol HP®
2	B1		Labrasol®	Span 20®
3	C1		Tween 20®	Transcutol HP®
4	D1		Tween 20®	Span 20®
5	A2	Octanoic acid	Labrasol®	Transcutol HP®
6	B2		Labrasol®	Span 20®
7	C2		Tween 20®	Transcutol HP®
8	D2		Tween 20®	Span 20®

As the present SEDDs formulations are designed for oral delivery, the potential effects of GIT conditions on SEDDs emulsification were considered by performing the emulsification studies in different diluents, namely DW, 0.1 mM HCl (pH = 4), and SIF (pH = 6.8). The formulations that were able to maintain their DS < 150 nm, $Đ \leq 0.7$, and T% > 85 in all the three diluents were selected for the next steps.

The selection criteria are based on the fact that the smaller DS is associated with greater absorption, and faster release, facilitated hydrophobic drug solubilization, and quick transport from the stomach and distribution along the GIT [38,95–97]. Furthermore, the L-SEDDS formulations with DS < 150 nm showed higher size robustness upon dilutions in the different media in the emulsification study. On the other hand, smaller $Đ$ values were required to get a better system homogeneity [98,99]. While T% > 85 was considered, as it indicates good emulsification in terms of rapid and reproducible equilibrium [100–102].

By performing the emulsification studies, Tween 20® was shown to be superior to Labrasol® in emulsifying Capryol 90® or Octanoic acid in A1, A2, and B1, B2 formulations. This ability might be attributed to the higher HLB value of Tween 20® (16.7) than the HLB value of Labrasol® (12–14) [103,104].

Based on the discussed selection criteria, C1 and C2 formulations at the Smix ratios of (2:1), (5:1), (6:1) and (2:1), (3:1), (4:1), (5:1), (6:1), respectively were selected for further studies through the construction of pseudo-ternary diagram.

3.3. Construction of Pseudo-Ternary Phase Diagram

Ternary phase diagrams are constructed to determine self-emulsification areas at which various concentrations of the excipients (oil, surfactant, and co-surfactant) would possess a transparent appearance and DS < 150 nm. These parameters were considered for selecting the optimum L-SEDDs formulations. Based on the emulsification study, eight diagrams were constructed (Figure 3).

Different blank L-SEDDs samples with three levels of oil: Smix ratios including (8:1), (5:1), and (3.5:1) that meet the set selection criteria were further investigated. These ratios represent high (H), medium (M), and low (L) concentrations on the pseudo-ternary diagram as described in Table 3. This approach was considered to avoid the use of a high concentration of surfactants (>60%), which is associated with GIT irritation when used in L-SEDDS formulations [105,106]. In the pseudo ternary phase diagram, each blue dot represents a formulation with various combination ratios of (oil: surfactant: co-surfactant) where all set criteria are met.

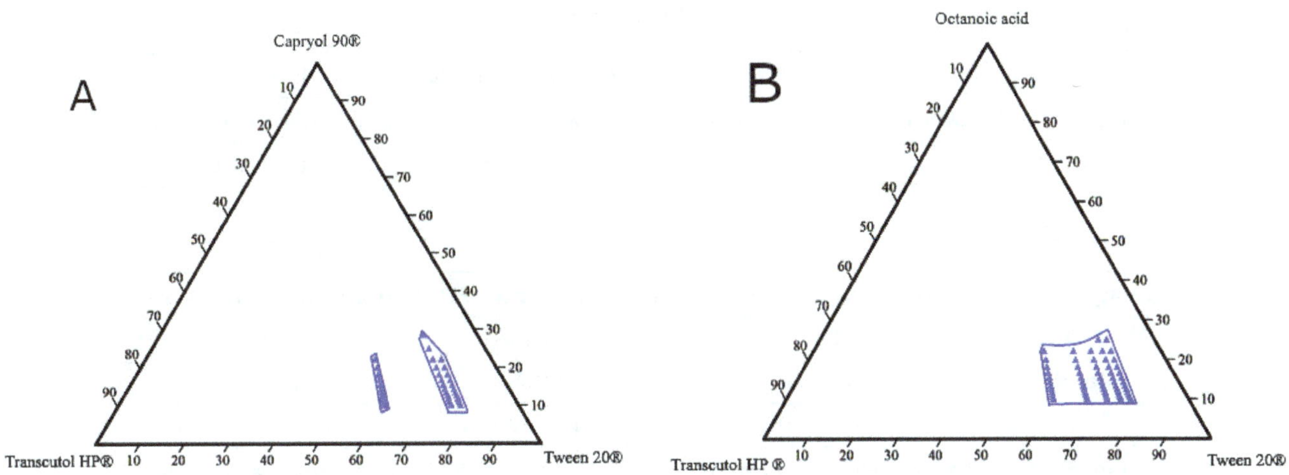

Figure 3. The pseudo-ternary diagram plots for the L-SEDDs formulations. (**A**) For the L-SEDDs formulation composed of Capryol 90® (oil), Tween 20® (surfactant), and Transcutol HP® (co-surfactant) at different Smix ratios. (**B**) For the L-SEDDs formulations composed of Octanoic acid (oil), Tween 20® (surfactant), and Transcutol HP® (co-surfactant) at different Smix ratios.

Table 3. The selected L-SEDDs components' concentrations and droplet size (DS) out of the constructed pseudo-ternary diagrams. Mean ± SD, n = 3.

Oil %	Surfactant %	Co-Surfactant %	DS (nm)
Diagram 1: Capryol 90®, Tween 20®, and Transcutol HP® at Smix ratio of 2:1			
11.11111	59.25926	29.62963	113.6 ± 1.3
16.66667	55.55556	27.77778	126.03 ± 1.3
22.22222	51.85185	25.92593	139.2 ± 0.69
Diagram 2: Capryol 90®, Tween 20®, and Transcutol HP® at a Smix ratio of 5:1			
11.11111	74.07407	14.81481	56.17 ± 0.76
16.66667	69.44444	13.88889	76 ± 1
22.22222	64.81481	12.96296	94 ± 1
Diagram 3: Capryol 90®, Tween 20®, and Transcutol HP® at a Smix ratio of 6:1			
11.11111	76.19048	12.69841	10.1 ± 0.3
16.66667	71.42857	11.90476	12.13 ± 0.31
22.22222	66.66667	11.11111	60.27 ± 1.1
Diagram 4: Octanoic acid, Tween 20®, and Transcutol HP® at a Smix ratio of 2:1			
11.11111	59.25926	29.62963	125.1 ± 1.1
16.66667	55.55556	27.77778	140.03 ± 0.95
22.22222	51.85185	25.92593	145 ± 1
Diagram 5: Octanoic acid, Tween 20®, and Transcutol HP® at a Smix ratio of 3:1			
11.11111	66.66667	22.22222	98.13 ± 0.91
16.66667	62.5	20.83333	112.73 ± 1.14
22.22222	58.33333	19.44444	144.23 ± 0.93

Table 3. *Cont.*

Oil %	Surfactant %	Co-Surfactant %	DS (nm)
Diagram 6: Octanoic acid, Tween 20®, and Transcutol HP® at a Smix ratio of 4:1			
11.11111	71.11111	17.77778	86.37 ± 1.1
16.66667	66.66667	16.66667	103.6 ± 0.36
22.22222	62.22222	15.55556	112.2 ± 0.72
Diagram 7: Octanoic acid, Tween 20®, and Transcutol HP® at a Smix ratio of 5:1.			
11.11111	74.07407	14.81481	63.67 ± 1.5
16.66667	69.44444	13.88889	87.1 ± 1.2
22.22222	64.81481	12.96296	109.07 ± 0.86
Diagram 8: Octanoic acid, Tween 20®, and Transcutol HP® at a Smix ratio of 6:1			
11.11111	76.19048	12.69841	10.13 ± 0.15
16.66667	71.42857	11.90476	13.43 ± 0.35
22.22222	66.66667	11.11111	97.43 ± 1.09

(DS, Droplet size; Smix, Surfactant to co-surfactant ratio).

3.4. Preparation of AZM Loaded L-SEDDs

AZM Incorporation and Its Impact on L-SEDDs Properties

The optimal drug incorporation into the L-SEDDs formulations depends on the compatibility between the added drug and the physicochemical properties of the formulation. The results of AZM incorporation and its related impacts on the L-SEDDs characteristics are shown in Tables 4 and 5.

The results of exploring DC or solubilization capacity of various formulations showed that it is directly proportional to the oil concentration increment where L-F1$_{(L)}$, L-F1$_{(M)}$, and L-F1$_{(H)}$ formulations were found to have a DC of 12.3 ± 0.05, 32.23 ± 0.07, and 60.42 ± 0.4 mg/mL, respectively. While the DC of L-F2$_{(L)}$, L-F2$_{(M)}$, and L-F2$_{(H)}$ formulations were 18.68 ± 0.16, 29.97 ± 0.14 and 46.9 ± 0.67 mg/mL, respectively. L-F1$_{(H)}$ and L-F2$_{(H)}$ formulations of both oils with Smix of Tween 20® and Transcutol HP® at 2:1 ratio showed the highest DC, and their characteristics were within the selection criteria. The higher was the oil concentration, the more was the amount of AZM incorporated in the formulations. This finding is probably related to the higher solubility of AZM in the oil phase than to its solubility in the used surfactant (Figure 2). However, L-F1$_{(H)}$ formulation (prepared with Capryol 90® oil) showed higher drug content (60.42 ± 0.4 mg/mL) than L-F2$_{(H)}$ formulation (prepared with Octanoic acid) (46.9 ± 0.674 mg/mL); this might be attributed to the higher solubility of AZM in Capryol 90® than in octanoic acid oil.

AZM addition to the blank L-SEDDs formulations also caused some changes in their DS, Đ, ZP, and T% characteristics (Tables 4 and 5). These changes might be linked to the entering of the drug molecule into the interfacial surface where surfactant molecules exist [98]. Unlike formulations constructed with octanoic acid, formulations with Capryol 90® oil showed characteristics robustness upon drug incorporation. Such observations were in line with previously reported data using high oil concentrations of 25% Capmul 808G EP/NF [107], as well as 30% of oil mixture (Maisine® 35-1 and Labrafac® CC (1:1)) [108,109].

Increasing oil concentration was associated with significant increases in DS and Đ, as well as a decrease in T% in all formulations. These effects could be attributed to the presence of an insufficient amount of surfactant and co-surfactant in the mixture to reduce the DS, and Đ values.

Table 4. Characterization of blank and AZM-L-F1 formulations at Capryol 90® oil concentrations of low, medium, and high analyzed in the three diluents. Mean ± SD, n = 3.

	Blank L-SEDDs				AZM-L-SEDDs			
	DW							
Code	DS (nm)	Đ	ZP (mV)	T%	DS (nm)	Đ	ZP (mV)	T%
L-F1$_{(L)}$	112.63 ± 1.02	0.56 ± 0.05	−18.5 ± 0.96	90.17 ± 0.56	112.17 ± 1.26	0.41 ± 0.01	−21.73 ± 0.96	91.51 ± 0.19
L-F1$_{(M)}$	125.4 ± 1.02	0.57 ± 0.002	−23.3 ± 1.4	90.01 ± 0.66	124.9 ± 1.65	0.47 ± 0.01	−23.1 ± 0.96	90.33 ± 0.31
L-F1$_{(H)}$	138.6 ± 0.85	0.59 ± 0.009	−23.03 ± 1.1	90.1 ± 0.11	141.57 ± 1.1	0.52 ± 0.004	−26.47 ± 0.65	90.1 ± 0.1
	0.1 mM HCl (pH = 4)							
L-F1$_{(L)}$	116.83 ± 1.3	0.56 ± 0.004	1.24 ± 1.5	94.75 ± 0.11	97.6 ± 1.6	0.52 ± 0.003	0.33 ± 1.7	98.2 ± 0.23
L-F1$_{(M)}$	112.63 ± 1.4	0.54 ± 0.01	−0.89 ± 0.28	94.45 ± 0.11	91.23 ± 0.76	0.54 ± 0.003	−0.896 ± 0.35	98.04 ± 0.06
L-F1$_{(H)}$	93.5 ± 1.3	0.62 ± 0.002	0.24 ± 0.47	94.75 ± 0.05	86.6 ± 1.44	0.52 ± 0.003	0.567 ± 2.2	97.99 ± 0.09
	SIF (pH = 6.8)							
L-F1$_{(L)}$	89.43 ± 0.53	0.628 ± 0.005	−3.23 ± 0.11	93.3 ± 0.1	166.27 ± 1.96	0.824 ± 0.01	−3.27 ± 0.55	97.47 ± 0.08
L-F1$_{(M)}$	86.63 ± 1.25	0.63 ± 0.01	−5.86 ± 0.68	93.48 ± 0.13	154.67 ± 2.1	0.83 ± 0.02	−6.05 ± 1.3	95.23 ± 0.12
L-F1$_{(H)}$	95.47 ± 1.7	0.657 ± 0.04	−5.28 ± 0.89	93.38 ± 0.13	148.1 ± 1.6	0.68 ± 0.006	−5.97 ± 1.8	94.55 ± 0.48

(Blank L-SEDDs, Blank liquid self-emulsifying drug delivery systems; AZM-L-SEDDs, Azithromycin-loaded self-emulsifying drug delivery systems; DW, Distilled water; DS, Droplet size; *Đ*, Dispersity; ZP, Zeta potential; T%, Transmittance percentage; HCl, Hydrochloric acid).

Table 5. Characterization of blank and AZM-L-F2 formulations at Octanoic acid oil concentrations of low, medium, and high analyzed in the three diluents. Mean ± SD, n = 3.

	Blank L-SEDDs				AZM-L-SEDDs			
	DW							
Code	DS (nm)	Đ	ZP (mV)	T%	DS (nm)	Đ	ZP (mV)	T%
L-F2$_{(L)}$	124.93 ± 1.5	0.64 ± 0.003	−17 ± 0.76	89.44 ± 0.26	143.1 ± 1.4	0.84 ± 0.02	−16.3 ± 0.87	90.47 ± 0.24
L-F2$_{(M)}$	139.73 ± 1.31	0.59 ± 0.005	−17.1 ± 0.53	88.69 ± 0.08	148.43 ± 1.3	0.71 ± 0.003	−17.77 ± 0.96	89.03 ± 0.15
L-F2$_{(H)}$	143.9 ± 1.64	0.68 ± 0.002	−18.23 ± 0.59	88.83 ± 0.32	267.8 ± 1.9	1 ± 0	−18.43 ± 0.97	77.96 ± 0.48
	0.1 mM HCl (pH = 4)							
L-F2$_{(L)}$	104.65 ± 0.5	0.45 ± 0.002	0.27 ± 1.8	94.75 ± 0.1	113.7 ± 1.8	0.61 ± 0.07	0.086 ± 1.1	97.17 ± 0.55
L-F2$_{(M)}$	113.53 ± 1.8	0.47 ± 0.003	−2.6 ± 0.4	93.77 ± 0.04	127.6 ± 1.5	0.54 ± 0.009	−0.58 ± 0.83	96.56 ± 0.57
L-F2$_{(H)}$	130.37 ± 0.6	0.55 ± 0.002	0.24 ± 0.5	90.75 ± 0.07	136.7 ± 1.9	0.54 ± 0.02	0.62 ± 0.8	91.76 ± 0.58
	SIF (pH = 6.8)							
L-F2$_{(L)}$	126.77 ± 1.2	1 ± 0	−3.61 ± 0.5	93.03 ± 0.11	149.77 ± 1.5	0.68 ± 0.01	−1.53 ± 0.17	89.1 ± 0.68
L-F2$_{(M)}$	115.6 ± 1.1	1 ± 0	−4.18 ± 0.7	93.47 ± 0.12	159.47 ± 0.93	1 ± 0	−4.16 ± 1.02	86.62 ± 0.29
L-F2$_{(H)}$	127.2 ± 1.4	1 ± 0	−4.44 ± 0.7	93.35 ± 0.13	226.3 ± 2.01	0.99 ± 0.006	−3.88 ± 0.69	75.02 ± 0.08

(Blank L-SEDDs, Blank liquid self-emulsifying drug delivery systems; AZM-L-SEDDs, Azithromycin-loaded self-emulsifying drug delivery systems DW, Distilled water; DS, Droplet size; Đ, Dispersity; ZP, Zeta potential; T%, Transmittance percentage; HCl, Hydrochloric acid).

The ZP measurement results showed that the charge of the prepared L-SEDDs formulations was negative when dispersed in DW and SIF. This may be linked to the presence of free fatty acids in the oil phase and/or surfactant [110]. However, upon the dilution of L-SEDDs formulations with 0.1 mM HCl, the ZP charge was shifted to be positive. This could be due to the neutralization of fatty acids and their negatively charged hydroxyl groups (OH^-) by the available positively charged hydrogens (H^+) in such acidic medium.

Furthermore, increasing oil(s) concentration was associated with a significant increase in the ZP values of the formulations, yet, relatively lower ZP values were obtained for formulations constructed with octanoic acid oil compared with those constructed with Capryol 90® oil. This might be related to the presence of a carboxyl group in the structure of octanoic acid [104]. The blank L-F1$_{(H)}$ formulation as well as its drug-loaded form AZM-L-F1$_{(H)}$ were shown to have the highest ZP values of (−23.03 ± 1.1 mV)) and (−26.47 ± 0.65 mV) respectively.

Based on all the previously described characterizations, L-F1$_{(H)}$ and its drug-loaded AZM-L-F1$_{(H)}$ formulations were found to meet the selection criteria and were selected for further study. The formulation was composed of 22.22%, 51.85%, and 25.93% (*v/v*) of Capryol 90®, Tween 20®, and Transcutol HP® respectively.

3.5. Preparation of Solid Self-Emulsifying Drug Delivery System (S-SEDDs)

The water-insoluble solidifying agents such as Aerosil 200® and calcium carbonate as well as the water-soluble solidifying agents such as mannitol and lactose are the most common solidifiers used for the production of S-SEDDs formulations [111–116]. In this study, the adsorption capacity (expressed as a weight ratio of L- SEDDs (L-F1$_{(H)}$): Solidifying agent) of these solidifying agents were investigated. It was observed that each solidifying agent had a different adsorption capacity to yield a non-sticky solid powder of S-SEDDs formulations, as illustrated in Table 6.

Table 6. Adsorption capacity and characterization of blank S-SEDDs (S-F1$_{(H)}$) formulation. Mean ± SD, n = 3.

Solidifying Agent	Adsorption Capacity (L-F1$_{(H)}$): Solidifying Agent	DS (nm)	Đ	ZP (mV)
Calcium carbonate	(1:4)	1863.67 ± 10.3	1 ± 0	−14.47 ± 1.001
Aerosil 200®	(2:1)	156.67 ± 1.5	0.62 ± 0.004	−21.7 ± 1.4
Lactose	(1:3)	384.7 ± 4.04	1 ± 0	−40.33 ± 1.07
Mannitol	(1:2)	845.63 ± 6.2	1 ± 0	−23.4 ± 1.3

(DS, Droplet size; Đ, Dispersity; ZP, Zeta potential).

Aerosil200® was found to have the highest adsorption capacity of 2:1. Furthermore, it produced blank S-SEDDs formulation with the lowest DS (156.67 ± 1.5 nm) and Đ (0.62 ± 0.004). Accordingly, Aerosil200® was selected as the optimized solidifier for production of the solid SEDDs (S-F1$_{(H)}$) formulation. The characterization results of the solidified blank and AZM-loaded S-F1$_{(H)}$ formulations are shown in Table 7.

The results of the solidification process showed that S-F1$_{(H)}$ formulation had bigger DS, higher Đ values, and significantly lower AZM DC (38.79 ± 0.52 mg/g) in comparison to the L-F1$_{(H)}$ formulation which had smaller DS, lower Đ values and higher AZM DC (60.42 ± 0.4 mg/mL). Such effects are linked to the need of using large amounts of Aerosil 200® (~535.6 mg) to produce solid S-SEDDs formulation. The same pattern of characteristic change was previously reported upon solidifying L-SEDDs formulation [117].

Table 7. Characterization of the optimized blank and AZM loaded S-F1(H) formulations in DW, 0.1 mM HCl, and SIF diluents. Mean ± SD, n = 3.

Blank S-SEDDs (S-F1$_{(H)}$)			AZM S-SEDDs (S-F1$_{(H)}$)		
DW					
DS (nm)	Đ	ZP (mV)	DS (nm)	Đ	ZP (mV)
157.1 ± 1.85	0.61 ± 0.01	−22.67 ± 2.3	155.3 ± 1.91	0.62 ± 0.03	−19.43 ± 0.15
0.1 mM HCl (pH = 4)					
139.03 ± 1.8	1 ± 0	2.1 ± 0.2	136.6 ± 1.9	0.73 ± 0.01	0.88 ± 0.02
SIF (pH = 6.8)					
195.32 ± 1.9	1 ± 0	−5.93 ± 1.1	191.5 ± 1.4	1 ± 0	−7.43 ± 0.81

(DW, Distilled water; DS, Droplet size; Đ, Dispersity; ZP, Zeta potential; HCl, Hydrochloric acid; SIF, Simulated intestinal fluid).

3.6. Transmission Electron Microscope (TEM)

The TEM images of the optimized AZM-loaded L-F1$_{(H)}$ and S-F1$_{(H)}$ formulations have revealed the formation of emulsion upon their dispersion (Figure 4A,B). The dispersed droplets of the prepared liquid and solid SEDDs formulations were spherical in shape with no signs of aggregation (Figure 4C,D). These findings are in line with previous TEM studies of liquid and solid SEDDS formulations [118–121].

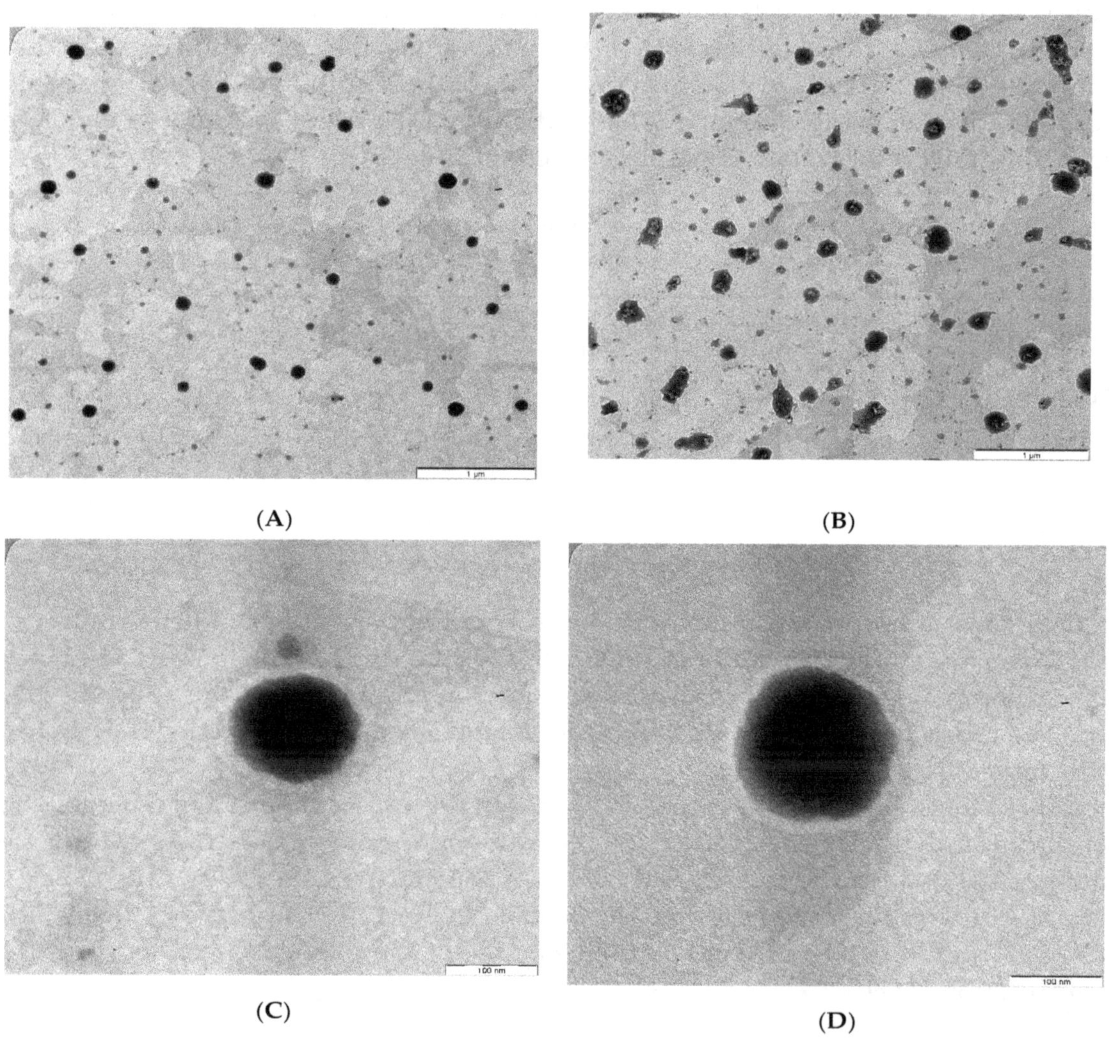

Figure 4. TEM images of the optimized AZM-loaded liquid and solid SEDDs formulations. (**A**) AZM-L-F1$_{(H)}$ Dispersion; (**B**) AZM-S-F1$_{(H)}$ Dispersion; (**C**) Individual droplet of AZM-L-F1$_{(H)}$; (**D**) Individual droplet of AZM-S-F1$_{(H)}$.

3.7. Cell Culture

3.7.1. Cytotoxicity Assay

Despite the fact that AZM is known to be cytocompatible [122,123] and the used excipients are considered relatively safe where they are used in the food, cosmetics or pharmaceutical industries (such as Transcutol® HP [124], Tween 20® [125], and Capryol 90® [126]), However, the cytotoxicity study in this work was conducted before proceeding to the TEER assay to make sure that the SEDDs effects on TEER must not be linked to the cytotoxicity of the excipients or their combination in the developed SEDDs formulations. Caco-2 cell monolayer model was used in this study because it is a reliable in vitro model, an approved standard by USFDA and pharmaceutical companies to investigate the cytotoxicity and behavior of developed formulations and/or drug in the intestinal tract [127,128]. The MTT assay is one of the most popular in vitro cytotoxicity assays. Its mechanism is based on the conversion of the water-soluble thiazolyl blue tetrazolium bromide dye to an insoluble purple-colored formazan, which is quantified by a microplate photometer [129]. The amount of formed crystals and the obtained readings represent the metabolic activities, and thus the number of the present viable cells [129,130]. The selected concentrations of the finally optimized blank formulations were chosen so that both formulations would have the same drug concentration when later preforming the TEER evaluation.

The results of the MTT assay indicated that the blank L-F1$_{(H)}$ and S-F1$_{(H)}$ formulations had low cytotoxicity with no induced toxic effects during the 4 h incubation period and at the different studied concentrations. As shown in Figure 5, the cells viabilities were above ~90% and ~86% for the tested blank L-F1$_{(H)}$ and S-F1$_{(H)}$ formulations, respectively.

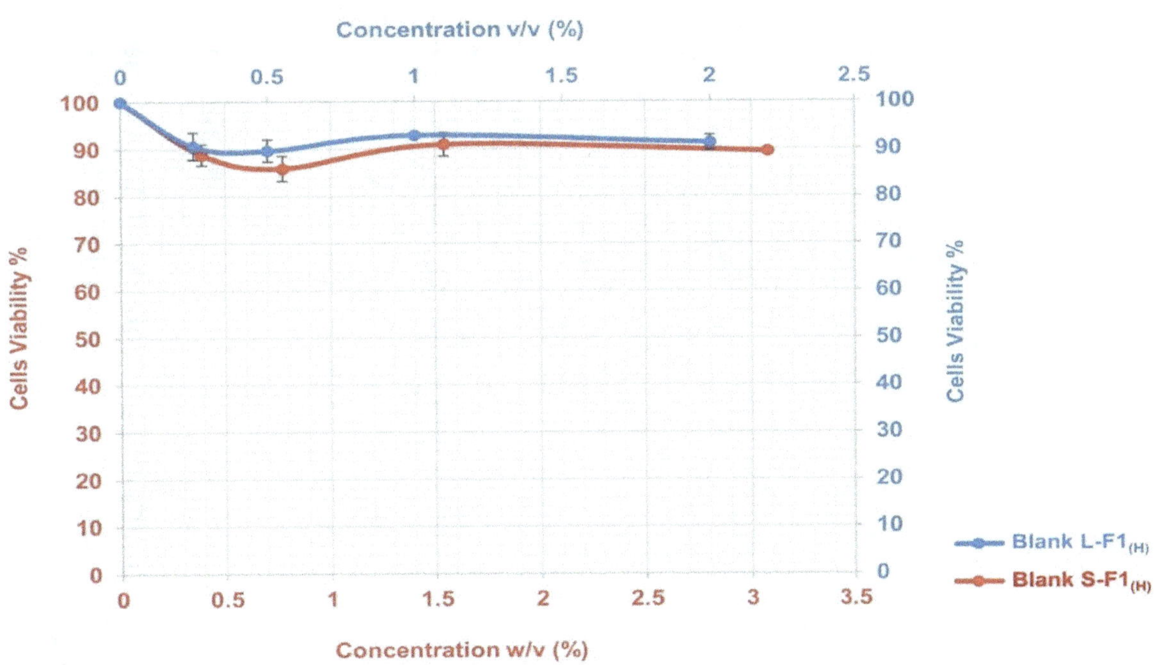

Figure 5. The cytotoxicity profile of Blank L-F1$_{(H)}$, and Blank S-F1$_{(H)}$ formulations at different concentrations. Mean ± SEM, n = 3.

3.7.2. Transepithelial Electrical Resistance Evaluation

The modulation of TJ is a potent strategy to improve hydrophobic drug delivery [131]; such modulations were related to the used formulations' excipients, mostly the surfactants [132–134] and some fatty acids [42]. In general, the opening of the TJ is associated with a decrease of transepithelial electrical resistance (TEER) [135,136]. The TEER evaluation study results are shown in Figure 6.

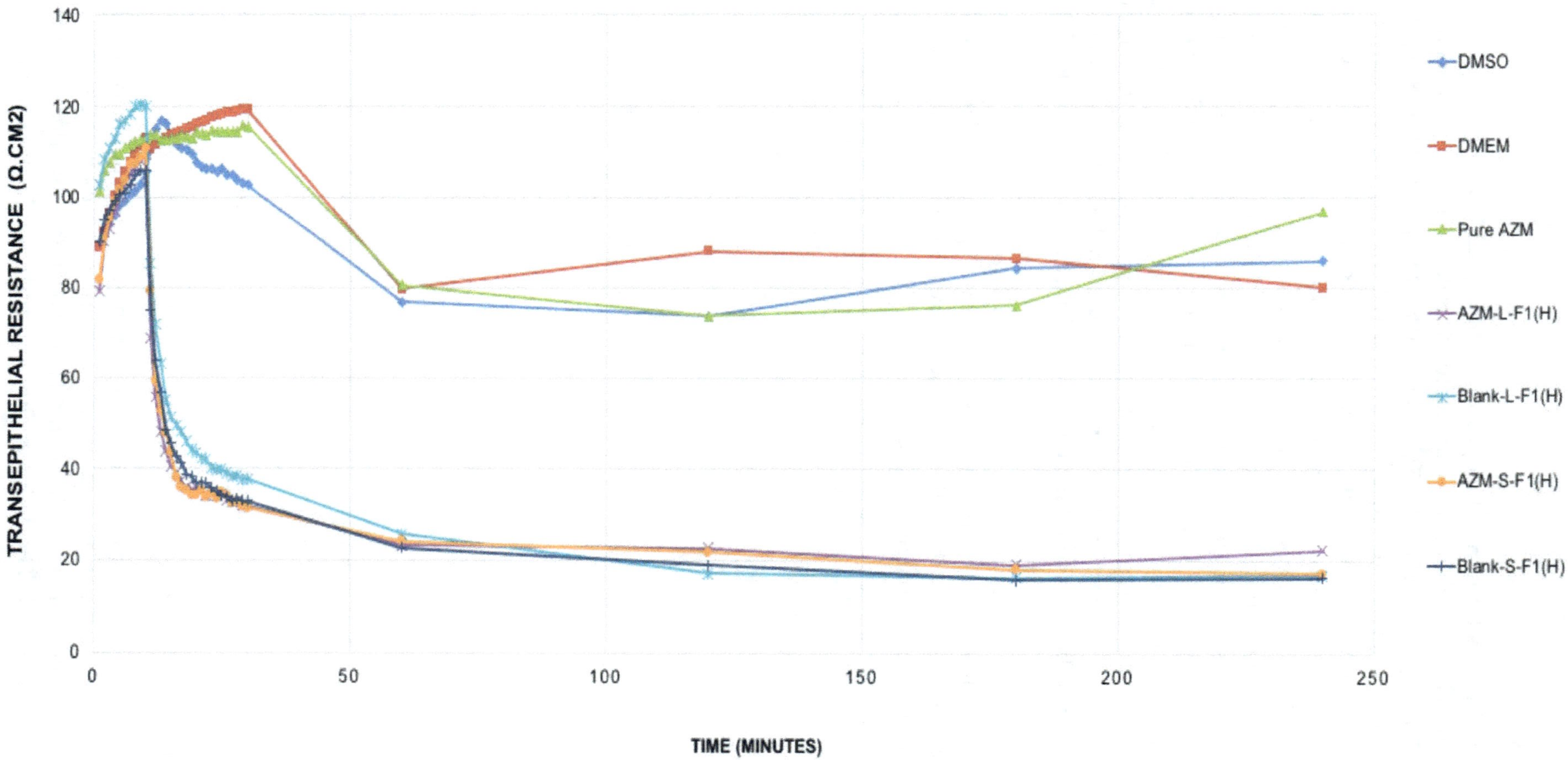

Figure 6. TEER resistance of the studied samples. Mean ± SEM, n = 3. DMSO: dimethyl sulfoxide, DMEM: Dulbecco's modified eagle's medium, AZM-L-$F1_{(H)}$: Azithromycin-loaded liquid SEDDs, Blank L-$F1_{(H)}$: Blank liquid SEDDS, Pure AZM: Pure Azithromycin, AZM-S-$F1_{(H)}$: Azithromycin-loaded solid SEDDs, Blank S-$F1_{(H)}$: Blank solid SEDDS.

It was revealed that pure AZM had no significant impact on TJ in the Caco-2 cell line model and within the studied period of 4 h. Such results are in contrast with previous studies that showed pure AZM could increase the TEER values in airway epithelial cells [21]. Such a difference in AZM behavior might be linked to the variations in cell lines' type, source, passage number, and culturing conditions. These results are suggesting the need for more studies to understand the exact cellular mechanisms of AZM permeation and its relation to its bioavailability using different cell lines and in vivo levels. Upon treating the cells with the set samples, and during the first 10 min of the measurement period, all samples (AZM, controls, blank and drug-loaded formulations) showed almost no significant changes in the TEER values. After that, only blank and drug-loaded formulations of L-SEDDs and S-SEDDs were able to decrease the TEER values sharply. These declines were significant ($p < 0.05$) in comparison to the TEER values of pure AZM, and could be linked to the ability of the optimized formulations to modulate the intestinal tight junction, possibly due to the presence of Capryol 90®, which has a proven ability to produce an appreciable reversible opening of TJ [33], which in turn might offer better delivery of AZM via paracellular pathways [137]

3.8. The In Vitro Release Studies

The in vitro release of AZM is usually conducted in a medium that mimics the intestinal pH such as phosphate buffer (pH = 6). This is because AZM is not sufficiently stable in acidic pH mediums such as simulated gastric fluids (SGF, pH = 1.2) [138]. Accordingly, three different release solutions were employed in this study including 0.1 mM HCl (pH = 4), DW (pH = 5.5), and SIF medium (pH = 6.8) [103,104,139]. Figure 7 represents the in vitro release profiles of AZM from AZM-L-$F1_{(H)}$ and AZM-S-$F1_{(H)}$ formulations, compared to the release of the pure AZM in the media of DW, 0.1 mM HCl, and SIF, respectively.

The liquid and solid SEDDs formulations were able to significantly ($p < 0.05$) increase the percentage of AZM release by 2.2-fold in DW, 1.9 and 1.8 folds in HCl, 1.7 and 1.6 folds in SIF, respectively in comparison with the pure AZM during the 4 h dissolution period.

The cumulative release percentages from the pure AZM were only 43.68 ± 0.84%, 50.57 ± 1.24% and 58.87 ± 2.23% in DW, HCl and SIF media respectively. In contrast, the AZM-L-$F1_{(H)}$ formulation released > 90% of the AZM within the first 5 min of the dissolution in all the studied dissolution media including 96.65 ± 1.77%, 96.21 ± 1.06%, 98.49 ± 0.77% in DW, HCl, and SIF, respectively. While the AZM-S-$F1_{(H)}$ formulation showed a slower release pattern whereby in 5 min, only 52.22%, 74.74%, and 70.01% were released in DW, HCL, and SIF, respectively. Unlike the L-SEDDs, S-SEDDs formulation needed 60 min, 30 min, and 15 min to reach > 90% of AZM in DW, HCL, and SIF. Such delay of AZM release from S-SEDDs formulation was in line with previous studies [34,140]. The researchers linked it to that the S-SEDDs formulation needed more step such as desorption of the adsorbed SEDDs from the Aerosol 200® during dissolution process [141]. Based on these results, the developed formulations were able to significantly enhance the dissolution rate of AZM in comparison to the pure drug powder.

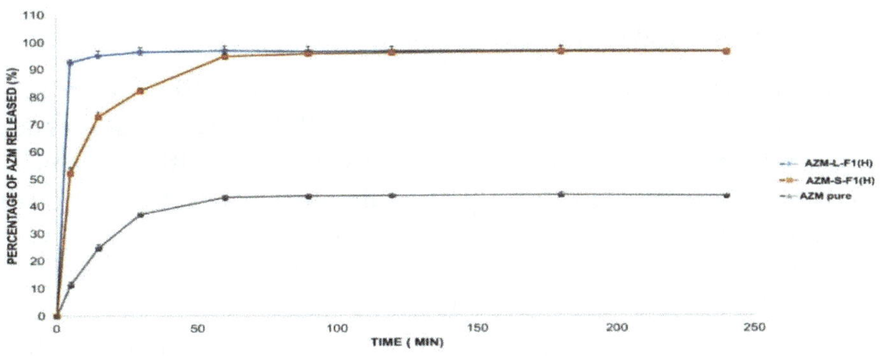

Figure 7. *Cont.*

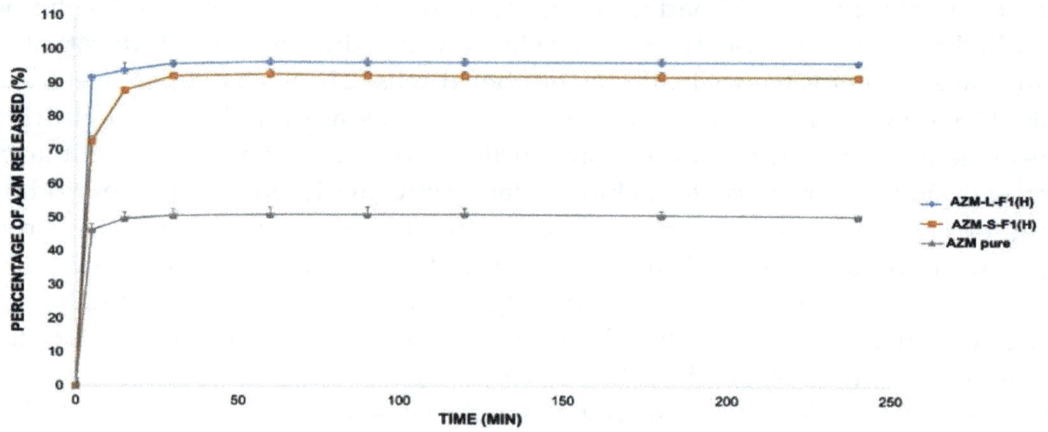

(**B**)

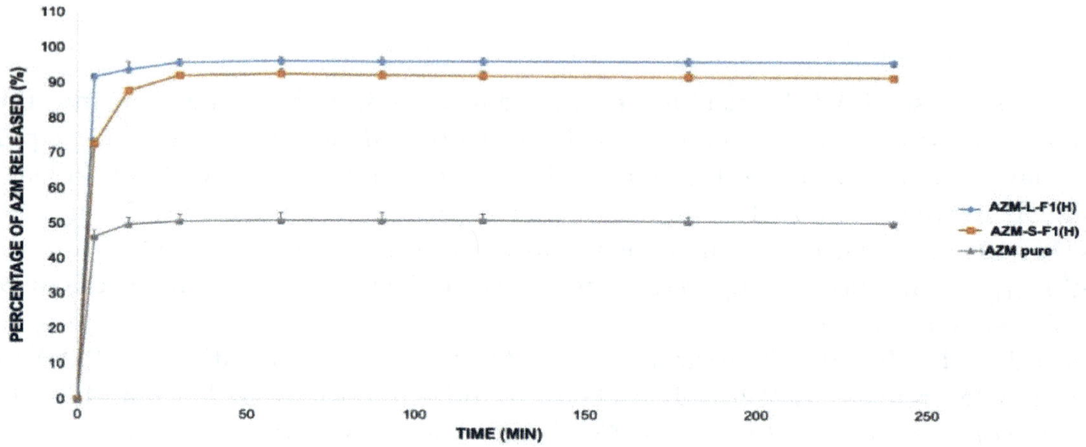

(**C**)

Figure 7. The in vitro release profile of AZM-L-F1$_{(H)}$, AZM-S-F1$_{(H)}$ formulations, and pure AZM in DW, HCl, and SIF, respectively. (**A**) The in vitro release profile in DW. (**B**) The in vitro release profile in 0.1 mM HCl (pH = 4). (**C**) The in vitro release profile in SIF pH = (6.8).

3.9. Stability Studies

3.9.1. Physical Stability

The physical appearance of AZM-L-F1$_{(H)}$ and AZM-S-F1$_{(H)}$ formulations were maintained unchanged during the 3 months of storage under the different conditions at the set different storage conditions.

3.9.2. Droplet Size, *Đ*, and Zeta Potential

The results of the stability studies of AZM-L-F1$_{(H)}$ and AZM-S-F1$_{(H)}$ formulations under the three different storage conditions are shown in Tables 8 and 9. Both formulations showed better stability in the refrigerator condition (4 ± 2 °C) when compared with the other studied storage conditions (i.e., room and humidity chamber conditions). For instance, after three months of storage in the refrigerator, the ZP values of both formulations were maintained unchanged, while there were slight but significant increases in DS of ~8 and 5 nm, respectively. The same increment patterns were seen in the *Đ* values of the AZM-L-F1$_{(H)}$ formulation at the three storage conditions. In contrast, there were no changes in the *Đ* values of the AZM-S-F1$_{(H)}$ formula under all the storage conditions during the three months period.

Table 8. Stability studies for AZM-L-$F1_{(H)}$ formulation under the three different storage conditions. Mean ± SD, n = 3.

Parameters	Time (Months)				
	0	0.5	1	2	3
Refrigerator (4 ± 2 °C)					
Physical stability					
DS (nm)	141.23 ± 0.38	141.6 ± 0.99	142 ± 1.15	146.87 ± 1.3	149.97 ± 1.16
Đ	0.528 ± 0.006	0.522 ± 0.01	0.534 ± 0.005	0.541 ± 0.009	0.56 ± 0.01
ZP (mV)	−26.78 ± 1.056	−27.43 ± 1.23	−26.73 ± 1.07	−25.69 ± 0.56	−26.3 ± 0.5
Chemical stability					
DC (%)	99.843 ± 0.353	99.79 ± 0.45	99.66 ± 0.162	99.37 ± 0.12	99.43 ± 0.22
Room condition (25 ± 2 °C/60 ± 5% RH)					
Physical stability					
DS (nm)	141.23 ± 0.38	142.03 ± 0.42	143.7 ± 1.31	148.23 ± 1.23	156.83 ± 1.5
Đ	0.528 ± 0.006	0.524 ± 0.04	0.53 ± 0.002	0.54 ± 0.003	0.552 ± 0.01
ZP (mV)	−26.78 ± 1.056	−26.7 ± 1.1	−26.37 ± 0.42	−25.73 ± 51	−25.47 ± 0.65
Chemical stability					
DC (%)	99.843 ± 0.353	99.65 ± 0.2	99.42 ± 0.14	99.241 ± 0.17	99.11 ± 0.12
Humidity chamber (40 ± 2 °C/75 ± 5% RH)					
Physical stability					
DS (nm)	141.23 ± 0.38	142.03 ± 1.16	147.55 ± 1.05	149.57 ± 1.37	166.63 ± 1.56
Đ	0.528 ± 0.006	0.529 ± 0.007	0.53 ± 0.003	0.542 ± 0.007	0.613 ± 0.05
ZP (mV)	−26.78 ± 1.056	−26.93 ± 0.15	−25.97 ± 0.7	−25.67 ± 0.32	−23.3 ± 0.56
Chemical stability					
DC (%)	99.843 ± 0.353	99.74 ± 0.13	99.12 ± 0.08	98.95 ± 0.1	98.58 ± 0.43

(DS, Droplet size; Đ, Dispersity; ZP, Zeta potential; DC%, Drug content percentage; RH, Relative humidity).

Table 9. Stability studies for AZM-S-$F1_{(H)}$ formulation under the three different storage conditions. Mean ± SD, n = 3.

Parameters	Time (Months)				
	0	0.5	1	2	3
Refrigerator (4 ± 3 °C)					
Physical stability					
DS (nm)	155.93 ± 1.39	155.13 ± 1.35	156.27 ± 1.19	157.33 ± 0.59	159.2 ± 0.78
Đ	0.64 ± 0.04	0.65 ± 0.015	0.64 ± 0.015	0.66 ± 0.021	0.66 ± 0.01
ZP (mV)	−19.28 ± 0.45	−19.23 ± 0.32	−19.27 ± 0.45	−18.97 ± 0.75	−18.49 ± 0.6
Chemical stability					
DC (%)	98.599 ± 0.32	98.52 ± 0.38	98.41 ± 0.57	98.37 ± 0.2	98.09 ± 0.5
Room condition (25 ± 2 °C/60 ± 5% RH)					
Physical stability					
DS (nm)	155.93 ± 1.39	155.8 ± 1.67	155.6 ± 1.25	158.3 ± 1.25	161.55 ± 1.1
Đ	0.64 ± 0.04	0.627 ± 0.025	0.65 ± 0.02	0.647 ± 0.03	0.68 ± 0.006
ZP (mV)	−19.28 ± 0.45	−19.15 ± 0.53	−18.97 ± 0.31	−18.77 ± 0.31	−16.27 ± 0.45

Table 9. *Cont.*

Parameters	Time (Months)				
	0	0.5	1	2	3
Chemical stability					
DC (%)	98.599 ± 0.32	98.42 ± 0.12	98.34 ± 0.36	98.06 ± 0.33	97.92 ± 0.43
Humidity chamber (40 ± 2 °C/75 ± 5% RH)					
Physical stability					
DS (nm)	155.93 ± 1.39	156.4 ± 0.6	158 ± 1	162.37 ± 1.1	164.1 ± 1.02
Đ	0.64 ± 0.04	0.65 ± 0.01	0.653 ± 0.015	0.657 ± 0.015	0.603 ± 0.006
ZP (mV)	−19.28 ± 0.45	−19.03 ± 0.4	−18.9 ± 0.3	−18.63 ± 0.42	−15.3 ± 0.56
Chemical stability					
DC (%)	98.599 ± 0.32	98.44 ± 0.28	98.014 ± 0.4	97.86 ± 0.37	97.48 ± 0.58

(DS, Droplet size; Đ, Dispersity; ZP, Zeta potential; DC%, Drug content percentage; RH, Relative humidity).

3.9.3. Chemical Stability

All formulations showed no statistically significant changes in DC% when stored in the refrigerator ($p < 0.05$). However, under the room storage condition (25 ± 2 °C/60 ± 5% RH), only AZM-S-F1$_{(H)}$ formulation was stable with no significant decreases in the DC% for the period of three months. On the other hand, decreases in DC% were observed in both formulations when stored at the humidity chamber (40 ± 2 °C/75 ± 5% RH).

4. Conclusions

Liquid and solid emulsifying SEDDS were successfully developed and optimized. The medium carbon chain triglycerides (MCT) were better than the long carbon chain triglycerides (LCT) as solubilizing agents for AZM. The hydrophobic solidifying agent (Aerosil 200®) was found to have the best solidification capacity among the studied solidifying agents to produce solid SEDDs. In this study, the main suggested reasons behind the low oral bioavailability of AZM were addressed, whereby both the liquid and solid SEDDs formulations improved the solubility and dissolution rate of the drug. However, more studies are required to specify the exact reasons that are responsible for the low oral bioavailability of this drug. The cytotoxicity study using MTT assay revealed that the AZM-SEDDs formulations had a low toxicity profile. Furthermore, the transepithelial electrical resistance (TEER) evaluations showed that both formulations had the abilities to open the tight epithelial junction. The formulations were relatively stable at the refrigerator storage condition for 3 months. Therefore, it is suggested that the developed liquid and solid self-emulsifying drug delivery systems are potential nanocarriers for the oral delivery of AZM.

Author Contributions: Conceptualization, R.A.A.; data curation, I.M.A. and S.M.A.; formal analysis, R.A.A., I.M.A., H.A.W., and S.M.A.; funding acquisition, C.S.Y., H.A.W., and Y.D.; methodology, R.A.A., I.M.A., T.S.M., C.S.Y., and Y.D.; project administration, T.S.M. and S.M.A.; resources, T.S.M., C.S.Y., H.A.W., S.M.A., and Y.D.; software, I.M.A.; supervision, T.S.M., H.A.W., and Y.D.; validation, R.A.A. and I.M.A.; visualization, C.S.Y. and Y.D.; writing—original draft, R.A.A.; writing—review and editing, I.M.A. and Y.D. All authors have read and agreed to the published version of the manuscript.

Acknowledgments: Reem Abou Assi and Ibrahim M. Abdulbaqi gratefully acknowledge Universiti Sains Malaysia (USM), the Institute of Postgraduate Studies (IPS), Penang, Malaysia for awarding of USM Fellowships.

References

1. Al-Achi, A.; Gupta, M.R.; Stagner, W.C. *Integrated Pharmaceutics: Applied Preformulation, Product Design, and Regulatory Science*; Wiley: Hoboken, NJ, USA, 2013; pp. 163–164.

2. Torne, S.R.; Sheela, A.; Sarada, N.C. A Review on Oral Liquid as an Emerging Technology in Controlled Drug Delivery System. *Curr. Pharm. Des.* **2018**, *24*, 1349–1356. [CrossRef] [PubMed]
3. Ghasemiyeh, P.; Mohammadi-Samani, S. Solid lipid nanoparticles and nanostructured lipid carriers as novel drug delivery systems: Applications, advantages and disadvantages. *Res. Pharm. Sci.* **2018**, *13*, 288–303. [CrossRef] [PubMed]
4. Laksitorini, M.; Prasasty, V.D.; Kiptoo, P.K.; Siahaan, T.J. Pathways and progress in improving drug delivery through the intestinal mucosa and blood-brain barriers. *Ther. Deliv.* **2014**, *5*, 1143–1163. [CrossRef] [PubMed]
5. *The United States Pharmacopoeia and National Formulary*, 38th ed.; The United States Pharmacopeial Convention: Rockville, MD, USA, 2015; Volume 39, p. 2339.
6. Imperi, F.; Leoni, L.; Visca, P. Antivirulence activity of azithromycin in Pseudomonas aeruginosa. *Front. Microbiol.* **2014**, *5*, 178. [CrossRef]
7. World Health Organization. WHO Model List of Essential Medicines. 2013. Available online: https://www.who.int/medicines/publications/essentialmedicines/en/ (accessed on 15 May 2020).
8. Peters, D.H.; Friedel, H.A.; McTavish, D. Azithromycin. A review of its antimicrobial activity, pharmacokinetic properties and clinical efficacy. *Drugs* **1992**, *44*, 750–799. [CrossRef]
9. Williams, J.D. Spectrum of Activity of Azithromycin. *Eur. J. Clin. Microbiol. Infect. Dis.* **1991**, *10*, 813–820. [CrossRef]
10. Gautret, P.; Lagier, J.-C.; Parola, P.; Hoang, V.T.; Meddeb, L.; Mailhe, M.; Doudier, B.; Courjon, J.; Giordanengo, V.; Vieira, V.E.; et al. Hydroxychloroquine and azithromycin as a treatment of COVID-19: Results of an open-label non-randomized clinical trial. *Int. J. Antimicrob. Agents* **2020**. [CrossRef]
11. Adeli, E.; Mortazavi, S.A. Design, formulation and evaluation of Azithromycin binary solid dispersions using Kolliphor series for the solubility and in vitro dissolution rate enhancement. *Int. J. Pharm. Investig.* **2014**, *44*, 119–131. [CrossRef]
12. Aucamp, M.; Odendaal, R.; Liebenberg, W.; Hamman, J. Amorphous azithromycin with improved aqueous solubility and intestinal membrane permeability. *Drug Dev. Ind. Pharm.* **2015**, *41*, 1100–1108. [CrossRef]
13. Adrjanowicz, K.; Zakowiecki, D.; Kaminski, K.; Hawelek, L.; Grzybowska, K.; Tarnacka, M.; Paluch, M.; Cal, K. Molecular dynamics in supercooled liquid and glassy states of antibiotics: Azithromycin, clarithromycin and roxithromycin studied by dielectric spectroscopy. Advantages given by the amorphous state. *Mol. Pharm.* **2012**, *9*, 1748–1763. [CrossRef]
14. Montejo-Bernardo, J.; García-Granda, S.; Bayod, M.; Llorente, I.; Llavona, L. An easy and general method for quantifying Azithromycin dihydrate in a matrix of amorphous Azithromycin. *Arkivoc* **2005**, *2005*, 321–331. [CrossRef]
15. Arora, S.C.; Sharma, P.K.; Irchhaiya, R.; Khatkar, A.; Singh, N.; Gagoria, J. Development, characterization and solubility study of solid dispersions of azithromycin dihydrate by solvent evaporation method. *J. Adv. Pharm. Technol.* **2010**, *1*, 221–228.
16. Tung, N.-T.; Tran, C.-S.; Nguyen, T.-L.; Hoang, T.; Trinh, T.-D.; Nguyen, T.-N. Formulation and biopharmaceutical evaluation of bitter taste masking microparticles containing azithromycin loaded in dispersible tablets. *Eur. J. Pharm. Biopharm.* **2018**, *126*, 187–200. [CrossRef] [PubMed]
17. Luke, D.R.; Foulds, G. Disposition of oral azithromycin in humans. *Clin. Pharmacol. Ther.* **1997**, *61*, 641–648. [CrossRef]
18. Garver, E.; Hugger, E.D.; Shearn, S.P.; Rao, A.; Dawson, P.A.; Davis, C.B.; Han, C. Involvement of intestinal uptake transporters in the absorption of azithromycin and clarithromycin in the rat. *Drug Metab. Dispos.* **2008**, *36*, 2492–2498. [CrossRef]
19. Nožinić, D.; Milić, A.; Mikac, L.; Ralić, J.; Padovan, J.; Antolović, R. Assessment of Macrolide Transport Using Pampa, Caco-2 and Mdckii-Hmdr1 assays. *Croat. Chem. Acta* **2010**, *83*, 323–331.
20. Fohner, A.E.; Sparreboom, A.; Altman, R.B.; Klein, T.E. PharmGKB summary: Macrolide antibiotic pathway, pharmacokinetics/pharmacodynamics. *Pharm. Genom.* **2017**, *27*, 164–167. [CrossRef]
21. Asgrimsson, V.; Gudjonsson, T.; Gudmundsson, G.H.; Baldursson, O. Novel Effects of Azithromycin on Tight Junction Proteins in Human Airway Epithelia. *Antimicrob. Agents Chemother.* **2006**, *50*, 1805–1812. [CrossRef]

22. Arason, A.J.; Joelsson, J.P.; Valdimarsdottir, B.; Sigurdsson, S.; Gudjonsson, A.; Halldorsson, S.; Johannsson, F.; Rolfsson, O.; Lehmann, F.; Ingthorsson, S.; et al. Azithromycin induces epidermal differentiation and multivesicular bodies in airway epithelia. *Respir. Res.* **2019**, *20*, 129. [CrossRef]
23. Salama, N.N.; Eddington, N.D.; Fasano, A. Tight junction modulation and its relationship to drug delivery. *Adv. Drug Deliv. Rev.* **2006**, *58*, 15–28. [CrossRef]
24. U.S. National Center for Biotechnology Information Database. Azithromycin. 2016. Available online: https://pubchem.ncbi.nlm.nih.gov/compound/Azithromycin (accessed on 15 May 2020).
25. Adeli, E. Preparation and evaluation of azithromycin binary solid dispersions using various polyethylene glycols for the improvement of the drug solubility and dissolution rate. *Braz. J. Pharm.* **2016**, *52*, 1–13. [CrossRef]
26. Hou, C.-D.; Wang, J.-X.; Le, Y.; Zou, H.-K.; Zhao, H. Preparation of azithromycin nanosuspensions by reactive precipitation method. *Drug Dev. Ind. Pharm.* **2012**, *38*, 848–854. [CrossRef] [PubMed]
27. Zhong, M.; Feng, Y.; Liao, H.; Hu, X.; Wan, S.; Zhu, B.; Zhang, M.; Xiong, H.; Zhou, Y.; Zhang, J. Azithromycin Cationic Non-Lecithoid Nano/Microparticles Improve Bioavailability and Targeting Efficiency. *Pharm. Res.* **2014**, *31*, 2857–2867. [CrossRef]
28. Pouton, C.W. Lipid formulations for oral administration of drugs: Non-emulsifying, self-emulsifying and 'self-microemulsifying' drug delivery systems. *Eur. J. Pharm. Sci.* **2000**, *11* (Suppl. 2), S93–S98. [CrossRef]
29. Pouton, C.W. Formulation of poorly water-soluble drugs for oral administration: Physicochemical and physiological issues and the lipid formulation classification system. *Eur. J. Pharm. Sci.* **2006**, *29*. [CrossRef] [PubMed]
30. Yakushiji, K.; Sato, H.; Ogino, M.; Suzuki, H.; Seto, Y.; Onoue, S. Self-Emulsifying Drug Delivery System of Celecoxib for Avoiding Delayed Oral Absorption in Rats with Impaired Gastric Motility. *AAPS PharmSciTech* **2020**, *21*, 135. [CrossRef] [PubMed]
31. Potharaju, S.; Mutyam, S.K.; Liu, M.; Green, C.; Frueh, L.; Nilsen, A.; Pou, S.; Winter, R.; Riscoe, M.K.; Shankar, G. Improving solubility and oral bioavailability of a novel antimalarial prodrug: Comparing spray-dried dispersions with self-emulsifying drug delivery systems. *Pharm. Dev. Technol.* **2020**, *25*, 625–639. [CrossRef]
32. Mazzeti, A.L.; Oliveira, L.T.; Gonçalves, K.R.; Schaun, G.C.; Mosqueira, V.C.F.; Bahia, M.T. Benznidazole self-emulsifying delivery system: A novel alternative dosage form for Chagas disease treatment. *Eur. J. Pharm. Sci.* **2020**, *145*, 105234. [CrossRef]
33. Ukai, H.; Iwasa, K.; Deguchi, T.; Morishita, M.; Katsumi, H.; Yamamoto, A. Enhanced Intestinal Absorption of Insulin by Capryol 90, a Novel Absorption Enhancer in Rats: Implications in Oral Insulin Delivery. *Pharmaceutics* **2020**, *12*, 462. [CrossRef]
34. Kamal, M.M.; Salawi, A.; Lam, M.; Nokhodchi, A.; Abu-Fayyad, A.; El Sayed, K.A.; Nazzal, S. Development and characterization of curcumin-loaded solid self-emulsifying drug delivery system (SEDDS) by spray drying using Soluplus® as solid carrier. *Powder Technol.* **2020**, *369*, 137–145. [CrossRef]
35. Tengshe, S.D.; Karande, K.M. A Review on Self Micro-Emulsifying Drug Delivery System: A Tool for Solubility Enhancement. *Int. J. Res. Anal. Rev.* **2020**, *7*, 101–114.
36. Aloisio, C.; Bueno, M.S.; Ponte, M.P.; Paredes, A.; Palma, S.D.; Longhi, M. Development of solid self-emulsifying drug delivery systems (SEDDS) to improve the solubility of resveratrol. *Ther. Deliv.* **2019**, *10*, 626–641. [CrossRef] [PubMed]
37. Assi, R.A.; Darwis, Y.; Abdulbaqi, I.M.; Asif, S.M. Development and validation of a stability-indicating RP-HPLC method for the detection and quantification of azithromycin in bulk, and selfemulsifying drug delivery system (SEDDs) formulation. *J. Appl. Pharm.* **2017**, *7*, 20–29.
38. Gurram, A.K.; Deshpande, P.B.; Kar, S.S.; Nayak, U.Y.; Udupa, N.; Reddy, M.S. Role of Components in the Formation of Self-microemulsifying Drug Delivery Systems. *Indian J. Pharm. Sci.* **2015**, *77*, 249–257.
39. Ye, J.; Wu, H.; Huang, C.; Lin, W.; Zhang, C.; Huang, B.; Lu, B.; Xu, H.; Li, X.; Long, X. Comparisons of in vitro Fick's first law, lipolysis, and in vivo rat models for oral absorption on BCS II drugs in SNEDDS. *Int. J. Nanomed.* **2019**, *14*, 5623–5636. [CrossRef]
40. Sobhani, H.; Tarighi, P.; Ostad, S.N.; Shafaati, A.; Nafissi-Varcheh, N.; Aboofazeli, R. Rapamycin-Loaded, Capryol(TM) 90 and Oleic Acid Mediated Nanoemulsions: Formulation Development, Characterization and Toxicity Assessment. *Iran. J. Pharm. Res.* **2018**, *17*, 830–850.
41. Nasr, A.M.; Qushawy, M.K.; Elkhoudary, M.M.; Gawish, A.Y.; Elhady, S.S.; Swidan, S.A. Quality by Design for the Development and Analysis of Enhanced In-Situ Forming Vesicles for the Improvement of the Bioavailability of Fexofenadine HCl in Vitro and in Vivo. *Pharmaceutics* **2020**, *12*, 409. [CrossRef]

42. Lindmark, T.; Kimura, Y.; Artursson, P. Absorption enhancement through intracellular regulation of tight junction permeability by medium chain fatty acids in Caco-2 cells. *J. Pharmacol. Exp. Ther.* **1998**, *284*, 362–369.
43. Suzuki, T. Regulation of the intestinal barrier by nutrients: The role of tight junctions. *Anim. Sci. J.* **2020**, *91*, e13357. [CrossRef] [PubMed]
44. Veeravalli, V.; Cheruvu, H.S.; Srivastava, P.; Vamsi Madgula, L.M. Three-dimensional aspects of formulation excipients in drug discovery: A critical assessment on orphan excipients, matrix effects and drug interactions. *J. Pharm. Anal.* **2020**. [CrossRef]
45. Zhao, G.; Huang, J.; Xue, K.; Si, L.; Li, G. Enhanced intestinal absorption of etoposide by self-microemulsifying drug delivery systems: Roles of P-glycoprotein and cytochrome P450 3A inhibition. *Eur. J. Pharm. Sci.* **2013**, *50*, 429–439. [CrossRef]
46. Shen, Y.; Lu, Y.; Jv, M.; Hu, J.; Li, Q.; Tu, J. Enhancing effect of Labrasol on the intestinal absorption of ganciclovir in rats. *Drug Dev. Ind. Pharm.* **2011**, *37*, 1415–1421. [CrossRef] [PubMed]
47. Gurjar, R.; Chan, C.Y.S.; Curley, P.; Sharp, J.; Chiong, J.; Rannard, S.; Siccardi, M.; Owen, A. Inhibitory Effects of Commonly Used Excipients on P-Glycoprotein in Vitro. *Mol. Pharm.* **2018**, *15*, 4835–4842. [CrossRef]
48. Yang, S.; Liu, J.; Chen, Y.; Jiang, J. Reversal effect of Tween-20 on multidrug resistance in tumor cells in vitro. *Biomed. Pharmacother.* **2012**, *66*, 187–194. [CrossRef] [PubMed]
49. Ma, R.; Li, G.; Wang, X.; Bi, Y.; Zhang, Y. Inhibitory effect of sixteen pharmaceutical excipients on six major organic cation and anion uptake transporters. *Xenobiotica* **2020**. [CrossRef]
50. Lin, H.; Gebhardt, M.; Bian, S.; Kwon, K.A.; Shim, C.K.; Chung, S.J.; Kim, D.D. Enhancing Effect of Surfactants on Fexofenadine Hcl Transport across the Human Nasal Epithelial Cell Monolayer. *Int. J. Pharm.* **2007**, *330*, 23–31. [CrossRef]
51. Zhang, H.; Yao, M.; Morrison, R.A.; Chong, S. Commonly used surfactant, Tween 80, improves absorption of P-glycoprotein substrate, digoxin, in rats. *Arch. Pharm. Res.* **2003**, *26*, 768–772. [CrossRef]
52. Prabhakar, K.; Afzal, S.M.; Surender, G.; Kishan, V. Tween 80 containing lipid nanoemulsions for delivery of indinavir to brain. *Acta Pharm. Sin. B* **2013**, *3*, 345–353. [CrossRef]
53. Yamagata, T.; Kusuhara, H.; Morishita, M.; Takayama, K.; Benameur, H.; Sugiyama, Y. Effect of excipients on breast cancer resistance protein substrate uptake activity. *J. Control. Release* **2007**, *124*, 1–5. [CrossRef] [PubMed]
54. Hong, J.Y.; Kim, J.K.; Song, Y.K.; Park, J.S.; Kim, C.K. A new self-emulsifying formulation of itraconazole with improved dissolution and oral absorption. *J. Control. Release* **2006**, *110*, 332–338. [CrossRef] [PubMed]
55. Khames, A. Formulation and Characterization of Eplerenone Nanoemulsion Liquisolids, An Oral Delivery System with Higher Release Rate and Improved Bioavailability. *Pharmaceutics* **2019**, *11*. [CrossRef] [PubMed]
56. Liu, J.; Hirschberg, C.; Fanø, M.; Mu, H.; Müllertz, A. Evaluation of self-emulsifying drug delivery systems for oral insulin delivery using an in vitro model simulating the intestinal proteolysis. *Eur. J. Pharm. Sci.* **2020**, *147*, 105272. [CrossRef] [PubMed]
57. Pal, S.; Mittapelly, N.; Husain, A.; Kushwaha, S.; Chattopadhyay, S.; Kumar, P.; Ramakrishna, E.; Kumar, S.; Maurya, R.; Sanyal, S.; et al. A butanolic fraction from the standardized stem extract of Cassia occidentalis L delivered by a self-emulsifying drug delivery system protects rats from glucocorticoid-induced osteopenia and muscle atrophy. *Sci. Rep.* **2020**, *10*, 195. [CrossRef] [PubMed]
58. Alghananim, A.; Özalp, Y.; Mesut, B.; Serakinci, N.; Özsoy, Y.; Güngör, S. A Solid Ultra Fine Self-Nanoemulsifying Drug Delivery System (S-SNEDDS) of Deferasirox for Improved Solubility: Optimization, Characterization, and In Vitro Cytotoxicity Studies. *Pharmaceuticals* **2020**, *13*, 162. [CrossRef]
59. Jianxian, C.; Saleem, K.; Ijaz, M.; Ur-Rehman, M.; Murtaza, G.; Asim, M.H. Development and in vitro Evaluation of Gastro-protective Aceclofenac-loaded Self-emulsifying Drug Delivery System. *Int. J. Nanomed.* **2020**, *15*, 5217–5226. [CrossRef]
60. Yeom, D.W.; Son, H.Y.; Kim, J.H.; Kim, S.R.; Lee, S.G.; Song, S.H.; Chae, B.R.; Choi, Y.W. Development of a solidified self-microemulsifying drug delivery system (S-SMEDDS) for atorvastatin calcium with improved dissolution and bioavailability. *Int. J. Pharm.* **2016**, *506*, 302–311. [CrossRef]
61. Janković, J.; Djekic, L.; Dobričić, V.; Primorac, M. Evaluation of critical formulation parameters in design and differentiation of self-microemulsifying drug delivery systems (SMEDDSs) for oral delivery of aciclovir. *Int. J. Pharm.* **2016**, *497*, 301–311. [CrossRef]
62. Singh, A.K.; Chaurasiya, A.; Singh, M.; Upadhyay, S.C.; Mukherjee, R.; Khar, R.K. Exemestane Loaded Self-Microemulsifying Drug Delivery System (SMEDDS): Development and Optimization. *AAPS PharmSciTech* **2008**, *9*, 628–634. [CrossRef]

63. Ostolska, I.; Wiśniewska, M. Application of the zeta potential measurements to explanation of colloidal $Cr_{(2)}O_{(3)}$ stability mechanism in the presence of the ionic polyamino acids. *Colloid Polym. Sci.* **2014**, *292*, 2453–2464. [CrossRef]
64. Hwang, C.J.; Na, Y.G.; Huh, H.W.; Kim, M.; Lee, H.K.; Cho, C.W. The Effect of Pharmaceutical Excipients for Applying to Spray-Dried Omega-3 Powder. *Appl. Sci.* **2019**, *9*, 1–11.
65. Tan, A.; Rao, S.; Prestidge, C.A. Transforming Lipid-Based Oral Drug Delivery Systems into Solid Dosage Forms: An Overview of Solid Carriers, Physicochemical Properties, and Biopharmaceutical Performance. *Pharm. Res.* **2013**, *30*, 2993–3017. [CrossRef] [PubMed]
66. Katteboina, S.; Chandrasekhar, P.; Balaji, S. Approaches for the development of solid self-emulsifying drug delivery systems and dosage forms. *Asian J. Pharm. Sci.* **2009**, *4*, 240–253.
67. Beg, S.; Katare, O.P.; Saini, S.; Garg, B.; Khurana, R.K.; Singh, B. Solid self-nanoemulsifying systems of olmesartan medoxomil: Formulation development, micromeritic characterization, in vitro and in vivo evaluation. *Powder Technol.* **2016**, *294*, 93–104. [CrossRef]
68. Kasturi, M.; Agrawal, S.; Janga, K.Y. Development and Characterization of Ramipril Loaded Solid self Nanoemulsifying Drug Delivery System (SNEDDS) for Improved Oral Delivery of Lipophilic Drugs. *Int. J. Pharm. Biol. Sci. Arch.* **2015**, *6*, 10–17.
69. Bhagwat, D.A.; Souza, J.I.D. Formulation and evaluation of solid self micro emulsifying drug delivery system using aerosil 200 as solid carrier. *Int. Curr. Pharm.* **2012**, *1*, 414–419. [CrossRef]
70. Hauptstein Sabine, P.F.; Andreas, B.S. Self-nanoemulsifying drug delivery systems as novel approach for pDNA drug delivery. *Int. J. Pharm.* **2015**, *487*, 25–31. [CrossRef] [PubMed]
71. Watari, A.; Hashegawa, M.; Yagi, K.; Kondoh, M. Homoharringtonine increases intestinal epithelial permeability by modulating specific claudin isoforms in Caco-2 cell monolayers. *Eur. J. Pharm. Biopharm.* **2015**, *89*, 232–238. [CrossRef]
72. Bandivadekar, M.; Pancholi, S.; Kaul-Ghanekar, R.; Choudhari, A.; Koppikar, S. Single non-ionic surfactant based self-nanoemulsifying drug delivery systems: Formulation, characterization, cytotoxicity and permeability enhancement study. *Drug Dev. Ind. Pharm.* **2013**, *39*, 696–703. [CrossRef]
73. Ujhelyi, Z.; Kalantari, A.; Vecsernyés, M.; Róka, E.; Fenyvesi, F.; Póka, R.; Kozma, B.; Bácskay, I. The enhanced inhibitory effect of different antitumor agents in self-microemulsifying drug delivery systems on human cervical cancer HeLa cells. *Molecules* **2015**, *20*, 13226–13239. [CrossRef]
74. Zhang, Q.; He, N.; Zhang, L.; Zhu, F.; Chen, Q.; Qin, Y.; Zhang, Z.; Zhang, Q.; Wang, S.; He, Q. The in vitro and in vivo study on self-nanoemulsifying drug delivery system (SNEDDS) based on insulin-phospholipid complex. *J. Biomed. Nanotechnol.* **2012**, *8*, 90–97. [CrossRef]
75. Srinivasan, B.; Kolli, A.R.; Esch, M.B.; Abaci, H.E.; Shuler, M.L.; Hickman, J.J. TEER measurement techniques for in vitro barrier model systems. *J. Lab. Autom.* **2015**, *20*, 107–126. [CrossRef] [PubMed]
76. Mine, Y.; Zhang, J.W. Surfactants enhance the tight-junction permeability of food allergens in human intestinal epithelial Caco-2 cells. *Int. Arch. Allergy Immunol.* **2003**, *130*, 135–142. [CrossRef]
77. Lea, T. Epithelial Cell Models; General Introduction. In *The Impact of Food Bioactives on Health: In Vitro and Ex Vivo Models*; Verhoeckx, K., Cotter, P., López-Expósito, I., Kleiveland, C., Lea, T., Mackie, A., Requena, T., Swiatecka, D., Wichers, H., Eds.; Springer International Publishing: Cham, Switzerland, 2015; pp. 95–102. [CrossRef]
78. USFDA. Guidance for Industry: Dissolution Methods of Azithromycin Pharmaceutical Forms. 2006. Available online: https://www.accessdata.fda.gov/scripts/cder/dissolution/ (accessed on 18 May 2020).
79. Yeom, D.W.; Song, Y.S.; Kim, S.R.; Lee, S.G.; Kang, M.H.; Lee, S.; Choi, Y.W. Development and optimization of a self-microemulsifying drug delivery system for ator vastatin calcium by using d-optimal mixture design. *Int. J. Nanomed.* **2015**, *10*, 3865–3878. [CrossRef]
80. Sun, L.; Zhang, W.; Liu, X.; Sun, J. Preparation and evaluation of sustained-release azithromycin tablets in vitro and in vivo. *Asian J. Pharm. Sci.* **2014**, *9*, 155–161. [CrossRef]
81. Izgelov, D.; Shmoeli, E.; Domb, A.J.; Hoffman, A. The effect of medium chain and long chain triglycerides incorporated in self-nano emulsifying drug delivery systems on oral absorption of cannabinoids in rats. *Int. J. Pharm.* **2020**, *580*, 119201. [CrossRef]
82. Grove, M.; Pedersen, G.P.; Nielsen, J.L.; Müllertz, A. Bioavailability of seocalcitol I: Relating solubility in biorelevant media with oral bioavailability in rats—Effect of medium and long chain triglycerides. *J. Pharm. Sci.* **2005**, *94*, 1830–1838. [CrossRef] [PubMed]

83. Grove, M.; Müllertz, A.; Nielsen, J.L.; Pedersen, G.P. Bioavailability of seocalcitol: II: Development and characterisation of self-microemulsifying drug delivery systems (SMEDDS) for oral administration containing medium and long chain triglycerides. *Eur. J. Pharm. Sci.* **2006**, *28*, 233–242. [CrossRef]
84. Patel, A.R.; Vavia, P.R. Preparation and in vivo evaluation of SMEDDS (Self-microemulsifying drug delivery system) containing fenofibrate. *AAPS J.* **2007**, *9*, E344–E352. [CrossRef]
85. Bhandari, V.; Avachat, A. Formulation and characterization of self emulsifing pellets of carvedilol. *Braz. J. Pharm.* **2015**, *51*, 663–671. [CrossRef]
86. Behrens, D.; Fricker, R.; Bodoky, A.; Drewe, J.; Harder, F.; Heberer, M. Comparison of Cyclosporin A Absorption from LCT and MCT Solutions following Intrajejunal Administration in Conscious Dogs. *J. Pharm. Sci.* **1996**, *85*, 666–668. [CrossRef]
87. Porter, C.J.H.; Kaukonen, A.M.; Boyd, B.J.; Edwards, G.A.; Charman, W.N. Susceptibility to Lipase-Mediated Digestion Reduces the Oral Bioavailability of Danazol After Administration as a Medium-Chain Lipid-Based Microemulsion Formulation. *Pharm. Res.* **2004**, *21*, 1405–1412. [CrossRef] [PubMed]
88. Persson, L.C.; Porter, C.J.H.; Charman, W.N.; Bergström, C.A.S. Computational Prediction of Drug Solubility in Lipid Based Formulation Excipients. *Pharm. Res.* **2013**, *30*, 3225–3237. [CrossRef] [PubMed]
89. Kaukonen, A.M.; Boyd, B.J.; Porter, C.J.; Charman, W.N. Drug solubilization behavior during in vitro digestion of simple triglyceride lipid solution formulations. *Pharm. Res.* **2004**, *21*, 245–253. [CrossRef] [PubMed]
90. Kollipara, S.; Gandhi, R.K. Pharmacokinetic aspects and in vitro–in vivo correlation potential for lipid-based formulations. *Acta Pharm. Sin. B* **2014**, *4*, 333–349. [CrossRef] [PubMed]
91. Zhang, X.; Wei, Y.; Cao, Z.; Xu, Y.; Lu, C.; Zhao, M.; Gou, J.; Yin, T.; Zhang, Y.; He, H.; et al. Aprepitant Intravenous Emulsion Based on Ion Pairing/Phospholipid Complex for Improving Physical and Chemical Stability During Thermal Sterilization. *AAPS PharmSciTech* **2020**, *21*, 75. [CrossRef] [PubMed]
92. Kalepu, S.; Manthina, M.; Padavala, V. Oral lipid-based drug delivery systems—An overview. *Acta Pharm. Sin. B* **2013**, *3*, 361–372. [CrossRef]
93. Pouton, C.W. Formulation of self-emulsifying drug delivery systems. *Adv. Drug Deliv. Rev.* **1997**, *25*, 47–58. [CrossRef]
94. Gupta, S.; Kesarla, R.; Omri, A. Formulation Strategies to Improve the Bioavailability of Poorly Absorbed Drugs with Special Emphasis on Self-Emulsifying Systems. *ISRN Pharm.* **2013**, *2013*, 848043. [CrossRef]
95. Agrawal, S.; Giri, T.K.; Tripathi, D.K.; Alexander, A. A Review on Novel Therapeutic Strategies for the Enhancement of Solubility for Hydrophobic Drugs through Lipid and Surfactant Based Self Micro Emulsifying Drug Delivery System: A Novel Approach. *Am. J. Drug Discov. Devel.* **2012**, *2*, 143–183. [CrossRef]
96. Yan, B.; Ma, Y.; Guo, J.; Wang, Y. Self-microemulsifying delivery system for improving bioavailability of water insoluble drugs. *J. Nanopart. Res.* **2020**, *22*, 18. [CrossRef]
97. Chatterjee, B.; Hamed Almurisi, S.; Ahmed Mahdi Dukhan, A.; Mandal, U.K.; Sengupta, P. Controversies with self-emulsifying drug delivery system from pharmacokinetic point of view. *Drug Deliv.* **2016**, *23*, 3639–3652. [CrossRef]
98. Akula, S.; Gurram, A.K.; Devireddy, S.R. Self-Microemulsifying Drug Delivery Systems: An Attractive Strategy for Enhanced Therapeutic Profile. *Int. Sch. Res. Not.* **2014**, *2014*, 11. [CrossRef]
99. Zhang, L.; Chen, Z.; Mao, J.; Wang, S.; Zheng, Y. Quantitative evaluation of inclusion homogeneity in composites and the applications. *J. Mater. Res. Technol.* **2020**, *9*, 6790–6807. [CrossRef]
100. Pouton, C.W. Self-emulsifying drug delivery systems: Assessment of the efficiency of emulsification. *Int. J. Pharm.* **1985**, *27*, 335–348. [CrossRef]
101. Madan, J.R.; Patil, K.; Awasthi, R.; Dua, K. Formulation and evaluation of solid self-microemulsifying drug delivery system for azilsartan medoxomil. *Int. J. Polym. Mater.* **2019**, 1–17. [CrossRef]
102. Gupta, S.; Chavhan, S.; Sawant, K.K. Self-nanoemulsifying drug delivery system for adefovir dipivoxil: Design, characterization, in vitro and ex vivo evaluation. *Colloids Surf. A Physicochem. Eng. Asp.* **2011**, *392*, 145–155. [CrossRef]
103. Kohli, K.; Chopra, S.; Dhar, D.; Arora, S.; Khar, R.K. Self-emulsifying drug delivery systems: An approach to enhance oral bioavailability. *Drug Discov. Today* **2010**, *15*, 958–965. [CrossRef]
104. Buya, A.B.; Ucakar, B.; Beloqui, A.; Memvanga, P.B.; Préat, V. Design and evaluation of self-nanoemulsifying drug delivery systems (SNEDDSs) for senicapoc. *Int. J. Pharm.* **2020**, *580*, 119180. [CrossRef] [PubMed]
105. Constantinides, P.P. Lipid Microemulsions for Improving Drug Dissolution and Oral Absorption: Physical and Biopharmaceutical Aspects. *Pharm. Res.* **1995**, *12*, 1561–1572. [CrossRef]

106. Azman, N.A.Z.; Raman, I.A.; Jantan, I.; Derawi, D. Formulation Screening of Palm-based Nanoemulsion for an OralDrug Vehicle of Phyllanthin. *Malays. J. Chem.* **2019**, *21*, 43–49.
107. Singh, K.; Sharma, M.; Gandhi, K. Recent approaches in self emulsifying drug delivery system. *Int. J. Pharm. Sci. Res.* **2012**, *3*, 4192–4201.
108. Zaichik, S.; Steinbring, C.; Caliskan, C.; Bernkop-Schnürch, A. Development and in vitro evaluation of a self-emulsifying drug delivery system (SEDDS) for oral vancomycin administration. *Int. J. Pharm.* **2019**, *554*, 125–133. [CrossRef] [PubMed]
109. Zhang, P.; Liu, Y.; Feng, N.; Xu, J. Preparation and evaluation of self-microemulsifying drug delivery system of oridonin. *Int. J. Pharm.* **2008**, *355*, 269–276. [CrossRef]
110. Parmar, B.; Patel, U.; Bhimani, B.; Sanghavi, K.; Patel, G.; Daslaniya, D. SMEDDS: A Dominant Dosage Form Which Improve Bioavailability. *Am. J. PharmTech Res.* **2012**, *2*, 54–72.
111. Almeida, S.R.D.; Tippavajhala, V.K. A Rundown Through Various Methods Used in the Formulation of Solid Self-Emulsifying Drug Delivery Systems (S-SEDDS). *AAPS PharmSciTech* **2019**, *20*, 323. [CrossRef]
112. Mantry, S.; Majumder, D. Development of Liquid and Solid Self-Emulsifying Drug Delivery System of Silymarin. *J. Drug Deliv. Ther.* **2019**, *9*, 54–61.
113. Dash, R.N.; Mohammed, H.; Humaira, T.; Ramesh, D. Design, optimization and evaluation of glipizide solid self-nanoemulsifying drug delivery for enhanced solubility and dissolution. *Saudi Pharm. J.* **2015**, *23*, 528–540. [CrossRef]
114. Kim, D.W.; Kwon, M.S.; Yousaf, A.M.; Balakrishnan, P.; Park, J.H.; Kim, D.S.; Lee, B.-J.; Park, Y.J.; Yong, C.S.; Kim, J.O.; et al. Comparison of a solid SMEDDS and solid dispersion for enhanced stability and bioavailability of clopidogrel napadisilate. *Carbohydr. Polym.* **2014**, *114*, 365–374. [CrossRef]
115. Cho, W.; Kim, M.-S.; Kim, J.-S.; Park, J.; Park, H.J.; Cha, K.-H.; Park, J.-S.; Hwang, S.-J. Optimized formulation of solid self-microemulsifying sirolimus delivery systems. *Int. J. Nanomed.* **2013**, *8*, 1673–1682. [CrossRef]
116. Dixit, R.P.; Nagarsenker, M.S. Self-nanoemulsifying granules of ezetimibe: Design, optimization and evaluation. *Eur. J. Pharm. Sci.* **2008**, *35*, 183–192. [CrossRef]
117. Guan, Q.; Zhang, G.; Sun, S.; Fan, H.; Sun, C.; Zhang, S. Enhanced Oral Bioavailability of Pueraria Flavones by a Novel Solid Self-microemulsifying Drug Delivery System (SMEDDS) Dropping Pills. *Biol. Pharm. Bull.* **2016**, *39*, 762–769. [CrossRef] [PubMed]
118. Man, N.; Wang, Q.; Li, H.; Adu-Frimpong, M.; Sun, C.; Zhang, K.; Yang, Q.; Wei, Q.; Ji, H.; Toreniyazov, E.; et al. Improved oral bioavailability of myricitrin by liquid self-microemulsifying drug delivery systems. *J. Drug Deliv. Sci. Technol.* **2019**, *52*, 597–606. [CrossRef]
119. Sha, X.; Wu, J.; Chen, Y.; Fang, X. Self-microemulsifying drug-delivery system for improved oral bioavailability of probucol: Preparation and evaluation. *Int. J. Nanomed.* **2012**, *7*, 705–712. [CrossRef]
120. Ameeduzzafar; El-Bagory, I.; Alruwaili, N.K.; Elkomy, M.H.; Ahmad, J.; Afzal, M.; Ahmad, N.; Elmowafy, M.; Alharbi, K.S.; Md Shoaib, A. Development of novel dapagliflozin loaded solid self-nanoemulsifying oral delivery system: Physiochemical characterization and in vivo antidiabetic activity. *J. Drug Deliv. Sci. Technol.* **2019**, *54*, 101279. [CrossRef]
121. Wei, Y.; Ye, X.; Shang, X.; Peng, X.; Bao, Q.; Liu, M.; Guo, M.; Li, F. Enhanced oral bioavailability of silybin by a supersaturatable self-emulsifying drug delivery system (S-SEDDS). *Colloids Surf. A Physicochem. Eng. Asp.* **2012**, *396*, 22–28. [CrossRef]
122. Mencucci, R.; Pellegrini-Giampietro, D.E.; Paladini, I.; Favuzza, E.; Menchini, U.; Scartabelli, T. Azithromycin: Assessment of intrinsic cytotoxic effects on corneal epithelial cell cultures. *Clin. Ophthalmol.* **2013**, *7*, 965–971. [CrossRef]
123. Schögler, A.; Kopf, B.S.; Edwards, M.R.; Johnston, S.L.; Casaulta, C.; Kieninger, E.; Jung, A.; Moeller, A.; Geiser, T.; Regamey, N.; et al. Novel antiviral properties of azithromycin in cystic fibrosis airway epithelial cells. *Eur. Respir. J.* **2015**, *45*, 428–439. [CrossRef] [PubMed]
124. Sullivan, D.W., Jr.; Gad, S.C.; Julien, M. A review of the nonclinical safety of Transcutol®, a highly purified form of diethylene glycol monoethyl ether (DEGEE) used as a pharmaceutical excipient. *Food Chem. Toxicol.* **2014**, *72*, 40–50. [CrossRef] [PubMed]
125. Cox, S.; Sandall, A.; Smith, L.; Rossi, M.; Whelan, K. Food additive emulsifiers: A review of their role in foods, legislation and classifications, presence in food supply, dietary exposure, and safety assessment. *Nutr. Rev.* **2020**. [CrossRef]

126. USFDA. Center for Drug Evaluation and Research. Application Number 209394orig1s000. Non-clinical Review(s). Available online: https://www.accessdata.fda.gov/drugsatfda_docs/nda/2017/209394Orig1s000PharmR.pdf (accessed on 30 August 2020).
127. Larregieu, C.A.; Benet, L.Z. Drug discovery and regulatory considerations for improving in silico and in vitro predictions that use Caco-2 as a surrogate for human intestinal permeability measurements. *AAPS J.* **2013**, *15*, 483–497. [CrossRef]
128. Shah, P.; Jogani, V.; Bagchi, T.; Misra, A. Role of Caco-2 Cell Monolayers in Prediction of Intestinal Drug Absorption. *Biotechnol. Prog.* **2006**, *22*, 186–198. [CrossRef]
129. Li, W.; Zhou, J.; Xu, Y. Study of the in vitro cytotoxicity testing of medical devices (Review). *Biomed. Rep.* **2015**, *3*, 617–620. [CrossRef] [PubMed]
130. Berridge, M.V.; Herst, P.M.; Tan, A.S. Tetrazolium dyes as tools in cell biology: New insights into their cellular reduction. *Biotechnol. Annu. Rev.* **2005**, *11*, 127–152. [CrossRef] [PubMed]
131. Tscheik, C.; Blasig, I.E.; Winkler, L. Trends in drug delivery through tissue barriers containing tight junctions. *Tissue Barriers* **2013**, *1*, e24565. [CrossRef]
132. Sha, X.; Yan, G.; Wu, Y.; Li, J.; Fang, X. Effect of self-microemulsifying drug delivery systems containing Labrasol on tight junctions in Caco-2 cells. *Eur. J. Pharm. Sci.* **2005**, *24*, 477–486. [CrossRef]
133. Deli, M.A. Potential use of tight junction modulators to reversibly open membranous barriers and improve drug delivery. *BBA-Bioenergetics* **2009**, *1788*, 892–910. [CrossRef]
134. Dimitrijevic, D.; Shaw, A.J.; Florence, A.T. Effects of some non-ionic surfactants on transepithelial permeability in Caco-2 cells. *J. Pharm. Pharmacol.* **2000**, *52*, 157–162. [CrossRef]
135. Gopalakrishnan, S.; Durai, M.; Kitchens, K.; Tamiz, A.P.; Somerville, R.; Ginski, M.; Paterson, B.M.; Murray, J.A.; Verdu, E.F.; Alkan, S.S.; et al. Larazotide acetate regulates epithelial tight junctions in vitro and in vivo. *Peptides* **2012**, *35*, 86–94. [CrossRef]
136. Mariano, C.; Sasaki, H.; Brites, D.; Brito, M.A. A look at tricellulin and its role in tight junction formation and maintenance. *Eur. J. Cell Biol.* **2011**, *90*, 787–796. [CrossRef]
137. Liu, Y.; Chiu, G.N.C. Dual-Functionalized PAMAM Dendrimers with Improved P-Glycoprotein Inhibition and Tight Junction Modulating Effect. *Biomacromolecules* **2013**, *14*, 4226–4235. [CrossRef]
138. USFDA. Centre for Drug Evaluation and Research Approval Package for: Application Number 50-784. Clinical Pharmacology and Biopharmaceutics Review. 2002. Available online: www.accessdata.fda.gov (accessed on 25 May 2020).
139. USFDA. Zithromax® (Azithromycin Tablets and Azithromycin for Oral Suspension). Reference ID: 3141345; 2012; pp. 1–22. Available online: https://www.accessdata.fda.gov/drugsatfda_docs/label/2013/050710s039,050711s036,050784s023lbl.pdf (accessed on 30 August 2020).
140. Czajkowska-Kosnik, A.; Szekalska, M.; Amelian, A.; Szymanska, E.; Winnicka, K. Development and Evaluation of Liquid and Solid Self-Emulsifying Drug Delivery Systems for Atorvastatin. *Molecules* **2015**, *20*, 21010–21022. [CrossRef]
141. Mohd, A.B.; Sanka, K.; Bandi, S.; Diwan, P.V.; Shastri, N. Solid self-nanoemulsifying drug delivery system (S-SNEDDS) for oral delivery of glimepiride: Development and antidiabetic activity in albino rabbits. *Drug Deliv.* **2015**, *22*, 499–508. [CrossRef]

3

MRI of the Colon in the Pharmaceutical Field: The Future Before us

Sarah Sulaiman and Luca Marciani *

Nottingham Digestive Diseases Centre and National Institute for Health Research (NIHR) Nottingham Biomedical Research Centre, Nottingham University Hospitals NHS Trust and University of Nottingham, Nottingham NG7 2UH, UK; msxss56@nottingham.ac.uk

* Correspondence: luca.marciani@nottingham.ac.uk

Abstract: Oral solid drug formulation is the most common route for administration and it is vital to increase knowledge of the gastrointestinal physiological environment to understand dissolution and absorption processes and to develop reliable biorelevant in vitro tools. In particular, colon targeted drug formulations have raised the attention of pharmaceutical scientists because of the great potential of colonic drug delivery. However, the distal bowel is still a relatively understudied part of the gastrointestinal tract. Recently, magnetic resonance imaging (MRI) has been gaining an emerging role in studying the colon. This article provides a comprehensive; contemporary review of the literature on luminal MRI of the colonic environment of the last 15 years with specific focus on colon physiological dimensions; motility; chyme and fluids; transit and luminal flow. The work reviewed provides novel physiological insight that will have a profound impact on our understanding of the colonic environment for drug delivery and absorption and will ultimately help to raise the in vitro/in vivo relevance of computer simulations and bench models.

Keywords: magnetic resonance imaging; MRI; large intestine; gut; large bowel; volume; transit; motility; flow

---

1. Introduction

Oral solid formulations are the most popular way of drug manufacturing [1] and their dissolution in the gastrointestinal (GI) environment is a determinant process of drug absorption [2]. Therefore, it is key to improve understanding of GI dissolution processes as well as the factors that affect them to enhance the efficiency of oral pharmaceutical forms. These factors are related to drug properties (e.g., dose, pKa, solubility, diffusion coefficient, crystal form, permeability, particle size) and also to the gastrointestinal conditions as well such as anatomical and physiological (liquid and non-liquid contents, buffer capacity, pH, bile salts, flow, motility, transit, and membrane) characteristics [2,3]. It is known that these characteristics continuously change throughout the GI tract, with some becoming less favorable more distally except for pH, which generally rises [4].

Current animal models as well as in vitro and in silico biorelevant models predict inadequately drug bioavailability because there are still "uncharted waters" in the field of drug absorption in the GI tract [5,6]. Since the majority of the new drugs approved are delivered per os there is a need of creating reliable predictive in vitro tools that not only reflect the complexity of the in vivo conditions but that can also be applied throughout the whole manufacturing procedure of oral formulations [7].

The latest approach on improving drug manufacturing procedures and performance includes designing and using biorelevant in vitro predictive techniques based on data acquired from in vivo measurements. These techniques are believed to be the future for assessing drug absorption because they are expected to cover the needs for a toolkit that prevents inaccurate discarding of drugs in the preclinical phase, reduces the use of animals and human subjects and offers realistic evaluation of new, old, and controlled dosage forms during their development and quality control. To fulfil all these requirements, the toolkit has to reflect the diversity and the complexity of the in vivo conditions [1,2]. Currently, despite all the previously developed biorelevant models there still exists a huge gap, and therefore a potential, between the in vitro and in vivo correlations [3]. When it comes to oral modified release formulations, the design of one representative predictive model that combines all the determining in vivo conditions becomes even more challenging, due to the lack of knowledge of the lower GI tract physiology. Formulations evaluation may remain inaccurate because of the compromises that are made when existing tools are used [1–3]. It is proposed that the enhanced evaluation of modified release formulations is going to derive from a toolkit that is going to reflect the in vivo conditions that determine drug release [2].

The colon forms the distal part of the human gastrointestinal tract [4]. Colonic length and diameter are estimated to be around 150 cm and 5 cm respectively [5]. Its absorbing surface area is about 0.05 m^2 and there are no villi. The anatomical regions from proximal to distal consist of the cecum, the ascending colon, the transverse colon, the descending colon and the sigmoid colon [5]. As the rest of the GI tract, it is formed by an inner mucosal layer, where absorption and secretion occur, the submucosal layer where nerves, lymphatics, and connective tissue are located, a smooth muscle layer divided in the longitudinal and circular muscle and the outer serosal area [4]. Mucus is formed in two layers in the colon and the inner one is 50–200 μm thick and strongly attached to the epithelium compared to the outer one which is easily removable [6].

The colon's primary function is to ferment food components and absorb water, vitamins and electrolytes [4] whilst transforming the discarded material into faeces. Only little secretory activity occurs [7]. Colon secretion concerns mostly potassium, water and bicarbonate [7]. Nerves exert a significant role in controlling the colonic environment. Colonic activity is determined by the enteric nervous system (ENS) which controls the smooth muscle and the mucosa, has autonomy, and is responsible for transmitting colonic information to the rest of the body with its sensory and motor neurons. Apart from the ENS, the colon is regulated by external nerves that belong to the parasympathetic and sympathetic system and that are transmitters, too. Abnormal motor regulation of the colon can also happen on abnormal epithelial permeability due to injuries, inflammation and modified gene expression [4]. It naturally hosts the biggest part of human microbiota and therefore has a huge role in the immune system and pathophysiology mostly by balancing host and microbiota interaction with the mucosal barrier [8]. The GI tract, colon included, is a rather complex area to study because of its multiple role (irregular motility, movement of the contents, and secretion) that interplay with each other [9]. Understanding colonic physiology is pivotal for drug development because of its role in both functional and non-functional diseases [8,9]. MRI is an attractive tool to explore the colonic environment because of the absence of invasiveness and therefore the more biorelevant insights that it can provide on undisturbed colonic physiology and pathology. In healthy and diseased subjects, MRI is applied for the evaluation of gut motility, transit, and dislocation of its contents (liquid, non-liquid, gaseous) which can be quantified during the same study session, thereby reducing the number of possible appointments required and providing added value [9].

Pharmaceutical formulations that deliver the integrated drugs specifically to the site of the colon are considered not only for the treatment of colonic diseases but also for alternative ways of delivering active substances. The latter originates from the low enzymic and proteolytic activity of the site, which allows the intact absorption of proteins and peptides, the higher local residence times and the increased effectiveness of absorption enhancers in the large intestine. It is important though that the colon-targeting oral formulations can protect the active substances until they reach the colon for the delivery to occur and therefore it is vital to gain a better understanding of the physiology of the GI tract [4,8]. Conditions in the colon differ significantly from the rest of the GI tract and colon-targeted oral forms should be designed and tested on tools that reflect in vivo conditions, e.g., colon residence time which can be more than 24 h. In the early phase of drug assessment, colon-targeted drug formulations should be developed also using in vitro and in silico techniques designed on relevant in vivo data, and for this to happen deeper knowledge of colon physiology is needed. These tools could provide enhanced accuracy and reduce costs. So far, the applied in vitro tests are conventional and exclude important characteristics such as colon volumes and hydrodynamics [1,10].

Whilst knowledge of the upper GI tract is improving, the lower GI tract remains much less explored, partly because of the difficulty of access under physiological, undisturbed (unprepared) conditions [7]. Imaging techniques have the potential to enrich the current knowledge by providing new non-invasive insights on the undisturbed GI tract, with the real-time assessment of the physiological environment surrounding drug products until they reach the blood or lymphatic stream [6,9].

The most common imaging techniques in the medical field are based on X-rays (e.g., computed tomography), ultrasound and radionuclides (gamma scintigraphy), endoscopy, and magnetic resonance imaging (MRI) [6]. Computed tomography and gamma scintigraphy provide a radiation dose, which is undesirable and endoscopy is invasive and requires unphysiological bowel preparation [6,10,11]. The application of ultrasound techniques in the in vivo assessment of oral dosage forms is not common because of the small field of view and the adverse effect of the presence of gas on ultrasound waves propagation [6]. MRI has been emerging as a unique alternative to the limitations of the imaging methods mentioned above [9] and has been gaining increasing attention in the pharmaceutical field [11–20]. MRI is non-invasive and based on radio frequency waves, therefore it does not provide an ionizing radiation dose. It offers good image quality with excellent soft tissue contrast. Multiple parameters can be acquired during the same study day using a variety of techniques (for example cine, dynamic, tagging). MRI also carries limitations, such as the unsuitability for subjects who may have metal implants such as cardiac pacemakers or infusion pumps [11], has a high cost of instrumentation (though the cost of a scan is limited compared to other invasive techniques), it is motion-sensitive and carries a burden of data processing [6,12,19,21–26].

MRI has been applied for the study of functional GI diseases (irritable bowel syndrome, functional dyspepsia) and also other bowel diseases such as Crohn's, scleroderma and colorectal cancer. One limitation is the need to standardize the methods and compare against gold standards [1]. More specifically, MRI has been used as an additional tool to assess the impact of mesalazine administration in the treatment of diarrhoea-predominant irritable bowel syndrome by quantifying the small bowel water content and using these data as an indicator for intestinal tone [12]. In the case of Crohn's disease, MRI has been suggested as a tool for the follow-up of the disease while antibody to tumour necrosis factor (anti-TNF) is administered to patients [13,14]. MRI has been validated against endoscopy with good correlation between the two techniques and is considered to be reliable to assess the effect of anti-TNF on the disease state [14]. MRI has been also considered and tested in colon cancer assessment [15–17]. MRI application in staging of advanced colorectal cancer was evaluated against histopathological staging and it was found to be reliable in assessing T3-T4 colorectal cancer [15]. MRI has gained a role also in the assessment of liver and hepatic metastases from colorectal cancer as well as for the colon mucosal layers, including the potential for colon cancer staging [16,17].

Over the past 15 years, MRI has become an emerging tool for pharmaceutical sciences and it is timely to review its contribution to investigate the most unexplored area of the gastrointestinal tract. This review is a comprehensive summary of MRI of colon function in terms of dimensions, chyme and fluid characteristics, motility, transit and flow, and it highlights the application of MRI in understanding these key factors of the large intestine that determine oral drug bioavailability.

2. Colon Anatomy and Physical Dimensions

The data on colon organ geometric, physical dimension is scarce and mostly based on prepared bowel or post-mortem measurements [18]. MRI is uniquely suited to measure body organ three-dimensional shape and dimensions. These investigations can be very helpful to understand better the space to which drug products are delivered.

The segmental diameters of the colon were measured in 12 healthy volunteers as part of a study assessing the effects of administration of senna tea and erythromycin on the gut environment [19]. The minimum ascending colon diameter in response to senna tea and erythromycin was 3.48 cm and 3.4 cm respectively whereas the maximum one was 3.83 cm and 3.74 cm respectively. In the segment of the transverse colon the minimum values were 3.38 cm and 3.31 cm while the maximum ones were 3.49 cm and 3.48 cm respectively. Lastly, the minimum respective results for the descending colon were 2.83 cm and 2.77 cm while the maximum ones were 2.93 cm and 2.89 cm respectively.

Food effects can change the volume of this organ substantially. Ascending and transverse colon diameters were also measured by MRI in 16 healthy subjects who were fed 40 g of either glucose, fructose or inulin diluted in 500 mL of water or a mixture of 40 g of glucose and 40 g of fructose [20]. Fructose is malabsorbed in the bowel and was expected to increase fluid inflow to the colon; inulin ferments in the colon and was predicted to increase colonic gas volume. Indeed, colonic gas rose up to higher levels (as assessed by calculating the AUC from the volume versus time plots, yielding mean (95% CI) values of 33 (20) L·min) on inulin consumption rather than glucose and glucose-fructose scheme (both $p < 0.05$). At t = 255 min after fructose administration compared to glucose caused a larger diameter increase in the transverse colon (30% (43%) and 8% (21%) respectively). This effect was more evident in this segment rather than in the ascending colon where the biggest change took place at t = 75 min (18% (20%) and 4% (26%) respectively).

The role of lactulose ingestion (10 g diluted in 200 mL of water) on the intestinal environment was evaluated in healthy participants ($n = 16$) and patients with irritable bowel syndrome (IBS, $n = 52$ in total) in fasted and fed conditions [21]. During the study, MRI was used to assess the diameter of the large intestine as well. Overall, this study concluded that lactulose decreased the diameter of the ascending colon possibly due to the dysfunctional ileocecal region of IBS patients. Lactulose ingestion decreased significantly the ascending and transverse colon diameter of the diarrhoea predominant IBS (IBS-D) subjects compared to the healthy ones ($p = 0.020$ and 0.045 respectively). At the same time, it caused a distension in the descending colon of all groups (all IBS $p = 0.014$, IBS-D $p = 0.03$, constipation predominant IBS or IBS-C $p = 0.006$ and healthy $p = 0.014$) except for the mixed IBS or IBS-M subgroup where it reduced its diameter ($p = 0.043$).

A different study estimated the length of the lower intestine and rectum [22] using a novel tracking system (Motilis Medica SA, Lausanne, Switzerland) which consists of electromagnetic capsules that can be detected while they travel through the gastrointestinal tract and compared this to the findings from MRI scanning, which could not be performed at the same time. The length of the whole organ was assessed in 25 healthy subjects. The length was 95 (75–153) cm as measured by the electromagnetic capsule tracking system method and 99 (77–147) cm as measured by MRI, $p = 0.15$ (CV% = 7.8%). The MRI-measured length of the cecum/ascending colon was found 26% ($p = 0.002$) smaller than for the capsules method possibly to higher retention times of the capsules in this segment but this was the only significant difference between the two techniques (all $p > 0.05$). More specifically, MRI assessed the length of ascending, transverse, descending and rectosigmoid colon as 16 ± 23.5 cm, 27.8 ± 5.4 cm, 23.7 ± 4.1 cm, and 27.8 ± 11.2 cm respectively and electromagnetic capsule findings were 22.0 ± 7.5 cm, 28.4 ± 4.7 cm, 24.0 ± 7.4 cm, and 24.7 ± 8.7 cm respectively. Figure 1 displays an image of the whole abdomen for colonic length determination acquired by MRI.

3. Colonic Motility

Motility in the colon is erratic. Inter-individual and intra-individual variability can also affect the residence times in each segment of the colon, which in turn could influence oral drug bioavailability. Applications of MRI to study the colonic motility patterns are recent and expanding. MRI has the advantage of requiring no unphysiological bowel cleansing, which is instead required for manometric studies.

The bowel motility response to senna tea and erythromycin were measured in 12 healthy subjects by identifying the intestinal diameter of the various segments [19]. Senna generated a significant rise in the peristalsis of the ascending and descending colon. Specifically, senna caused, on average, 71.6% significant modifications in the ascending colon, 80% in the transverse colon, and 55% in the descending colon whereas erythromycin caused 60%, 46.67%, and 60% respectively. The mean difference of the percentage of the significant modifications was 13.31%.

The intestinal motion activity was also studied by the application of multi-nuclear ^{19}F and ^{1}H MRI in two healthy subjects who were administered one ^{19}F capsule on study day 1 and two others with 300 mL of water on study day 2 and each time a meal and a commercial fibre drink was used for bowel distension [23]. On study day 1, the investigators identified high local bowel motion. The estimated forward velocity for subject A was 0.27 mm/s and for subject B 0.38 mm/s and the mean capsule velocity was 1.0 mm/s and 1.0 mm/s respectively for a total travel length of 3.15 m and 2.34 m respectively. On study day 2, the dual system allowed the identification of three different pendular types of motility at the first 10 min. These kinds were described as slow pendular (duration of 0–2.5 min, frequency of $1/20 \pm 5$ s), quiescence period (2.5–5 min) and a mixture of fast and slow pendular movements.

A different study used 10 mg of bisacodyl in order to create high amplitude propagated pressure waves (HAPPWs) in 10 healthy volunteers and assess them by manometry and cine-MRI at the same time over 24 min [24]. Overall, 11 HAPPWs were assessed by both techniques mostly 9–16 min following bisacodyl stimuli with a mean value of 63.5 mmHg. There was the case of three subjects were MRI identified three contractions which were not visible by manometry ('negative contractions'). The authors suggested that the technique of cine-MRI is capable of bowel motility measurements and these measurements were in accordance with pressure changes assessed by the manometry.

The effect of ingestion of PEG electrolyte on the intestinal movements was studied in 24 healthy subjects [25]. They were divided into two equal groups who ingested a split dose of either 1 L the day before the MRI study day and the other 1 L on the MRI study day or a single dose of 2 L on the MRI scanning day. This study revealed that both dosing regimens had positive results but the single larger dose ascending colon movements caused twofold compared to the split dose ($p = 0.0103$). The positive changes in motion were correlated with ascending colon volumes (Spearman's $r = 0.53$, $p = 0.0128$).

In a different study, a cine-MRI technique was developed for intestinal motility assessment and applied to four healthy subjects and eight possible IBD patients before and after intravenous injection of butylscopolamine [26]. In healthy volunteers, butylscopolamine reduced intestinal motion by (mean) 59% ($p\ 1/4 = 0.171$). Specifically, before the butylscopolamine injection, the mean score of the motility assessment in each volunteer was 910, 1605, 1860, and 5492 (mean 2467) and after the injection 524, 1057, 885, and 1557 (mean 1006). Mean difference was estimated to be 1461. Regarding the IBD patients, the investigators were able to identify the inflamed parts of the gut because of their reduced activity. The mean motility values of the maximum map were 15914, 4546, 5574, 9005, 8379, 8552, 7013, and 7637 and the respective ones of the mean map 5958, 1867, 2041, 3381, 3281, 3359, 2678, and 3385.

In another study, the impact of the laxative Moviprep on gut motion was assessed in 48 subjects (24 subjects with functional constipation or FC and 24 with IBS-C) [27]. The ascending colon motility index for subjects with FC was (mean (SD)) 0.055 (0.044) significantly lower than the one for IBS-C patients which was 0.107 (0.070) (line analysis 0.5 mm/s index), $p < 0.01$. After the Moviprep administration to the FC group, the required time for the first intestinal movement was (median (interquartile range)) 295 (116–526) min bigger than that for the IBS-C group which was 84 (49–111) min, $p < 0.01$. This first intestinal movement time was associated with the volume level in the ascending colon at that time (2 h) (higher volumes in the ascending colon caused delayed first bowel movements). Patients were considered to suffer from FC and not IBS-C when the required minutes for the first intestinal movement are above 230 (cut-off point, 55% sensitivity but 95% specificity). Considering the impact of Moviprep on intestinal movements, the FC group experienced a smaller intestinal activity for the first 24 h than the lower standard limit (6 movements) with the average number being 2–5 compared to the IBS-C average movement number which was 6–10, $p < 0.01$.

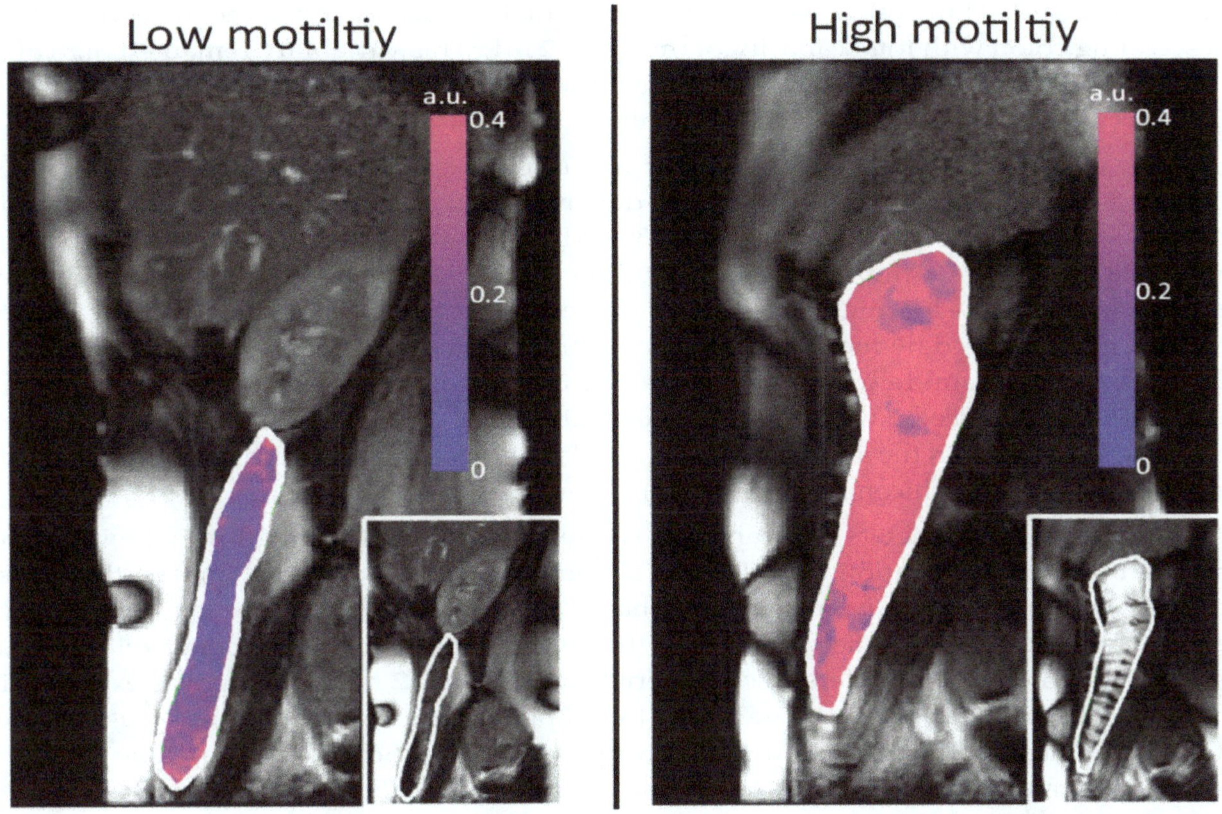

Figure 1. Motility assessment by the cine MRI technique. The figure depicts overlay (red/blue) of standard deviation of Jacobian. Reproduced from [28], Blackwell Publishing LTD, 2015 with permission.

The motion of the ascending colon wall was also evaluated by MRI in 23 healthy subjects before and after a laxative stimulus [28]. The stimulus was provided by two different types of macrogol drinks. Eleven subjects ingested 1 L of macrogol whereas the remaining twelve drank 2 L. The team was able to identify the following five types of contractions—segmental antegrade, segmental retrograde, whole ascending colon antegrade and retrograde, and large amplitude contractions—and display them as a movie as they come from a cine database. The large amplitude contractions were simultaneous (<20 s on average) but affected the diameter of the whole gut. In most of the cases, these movements were followed by distension as well. A representative image of the motility assessment of this study is shown in Figure 1.

4. Colonic Chyme and Fluid

The appraisal of chyme characteristics and of water volumes in the colonic region has been a difficult task. This organ is poorly accessible in the physiological unprepared state but water distribution is a key determinant for oral drug absorption. Since standard MRI images are based on water hydrogen proton imaging, MRI could provide unique insights in the colonic undisturbed physiological chime and fluid state. MRI sequences typically used for cholangiopancreatography studies collect high signal from freely mobile fluids, which have long transverse relaxation time T2. T2 is one of the standard time constants of the MRI phenomenon and it is linked to water mobility. These MRI sequences are ideal to identify pockets of fluid in the body though signal from less fluid ('thick') components such as mucous are lost.

In a landmark study, the intestinal water distribution was estimated in 12 healthy subjects who consumed non-disintegrating capsules in fasting and fed conditions [29]. It was concluded that food ingestion had minimum effect on colonic water volumes (13 ± 12 mL) but increased the number of colonic pockets from 4 to 6 ($p < 0.005$). More specifically fasting inter-subject variability of colonic volumes was high (1–44 mL) and water pockets were mainly located in the cecum, ascending colon and descending colon with total capacity of (median) 2 mL. This variability remained high after the meal consumption too (2–97 mL) which caused increase in the number of water pockets ($p < 0.005$) but did not affect their volume capacity ((mean) 1 mL).

The intestinal freely mobile water content was also assessed in 18 healthy subjects who were administered mannitol as a model of secretory diarrhoea and capsules of placebo or loperamide or loperamide and simethicone at the same time [30]. MRI following the placebo intervention showed an increase in the water distribution in the ascending colon 45 min following the mannitol ingestion. On the contrary, at first (0–135 min) the other two active interventions caused the ascending colon water distribution to be reduced by more than 40% ($p < 0.004$). Later on (135–270 min), placebo behaved the same way as loperamide whereas, at the same time, loperamide combined with simethicone decreased the ascending colon water. MRI images of the placebo administration showed the presence of 6.9 $\pm$ 1.3 mL of water in the ascending colon similar to loperamide administration (6.8 $\pm$ 1.5 mL) and loperamide plus simethicone (4.5 $\pm$ 0.9 mL).

Additional MRI parameters that can be measured by MRI are the longitudinal relaxation time T1 and the transverse relaxation time T2. As already mentioned above, the relaxation times are fundamental time constants of the magnetic resonance environment of the water in the chyme, and are related to water mobility and the thickness of the colonic chime, whereby longer relaxation times generally relate to more liquid, less thick material. Use of the T2 relaxometry was explored in the mannitol/loperamide study mentioned above [30]. Loperamide and loperamide plus simethicone resulted in significantly lower T2 values than for placebo. Specifically, at a magnetic field of 1.5 T, at t = 90 min T2 values were 79 $\pm$ 4 ms, 67 $\pm$ 6 ms vs. 144 $\pm$ 28 ms (both $p = 0.001$) respectively and at t = 180 min loperamide plus simethicone resulted in T2 values of 130 $\pm$ 22 ms vs. 82 $\pm$ 6 ms for the placebo ($p = 0.01$). T1 and T2 relaxation time were also used in a study of ispaghula supplementation [31]. In the group of the healthy volunteers, again at a magnetic field of 1.5 T, T1 of the ascending colon was 720 (572–904) ms, 690 (594–911) ms, and 966 (67–1093) ms on maltodextrin, psyllium 10.5 g/d and psyllium 21 g/d intervention respectively. T1 of the descending colon was 440 (352–884) ms, 570 (473–700) ms, and 763 (575–985) ms respectively. T1 constant of the ascending colon of patients was 509 (472–670) ms and 890 (478–1030) ms on maltodextrin and on psyllium intervention while T1 of the descending colon was 213 (176–420) ms and 590 (446–1338) ms respectively. Respectively the T2 values in the ascending colon of the healthy group were 70 (56–72) ms, 73 (62–86) ms, and 83 (67–88) ms and T2 in the descending colon were 53 (40–67) ms, 54 (45–70) ms, and 74 (56–80) ms. The T2 of the patients' ascending colon was 58 (42–73) ms on maltodextrin and 72 (51–105) ms on psyllium, while the respective values for the descending colon were 42 (34–52) ms and 66 (54–86) ms. Also, in a study of kiwifruit supplementation [32], the AUC (in seconds$\times$minute units of measure) of the T1 constant of the ascending colon was 356 $\pm$ 109 on kiwifruit intervention and 291 $\pm$ 110 on control at time = 0–420 min whereas the AUC of the T1 from 240 to 420 min was 137 $\pm$ 39 and 108 $\pm$ 40, respectively. For the descending colon, the respective values were 216 $\pm$ 120 and 203 $\pm$ 114 from 0–420 min and 96 $\pm$ 50 and 87 $\pm$ 52 from 240–420 min. This initial body of work shows the absolutely unique ability of relaxation times measurements to detect changes in the properties of the colonic chyme in response to intervention without using invasive procedures.

The effect of per os PEG electrolyte in two dosing regimens (single of 2 L and split of 1 L twice) on colonic expansion was evaluated in 12 healthy volunteers [25]. They found out that the larger single dose had a higher positive impact in the total volume of the large intestine (102 $\pm$ 27%, range: 9–289%) than the split dose (35 $\pm$ 8%, range: 0–81%), $p = 0.0332$. The formulation affected mostly the ascending (single dose caused a greater increase, $p = 0.0099$) and the transverse colon rather than the descending colon (because of the defecation of the subjects the researchers assumed that it had passed through that region). The effect of the PEG dosing scheme on colonic water content is shown in Figure 2.

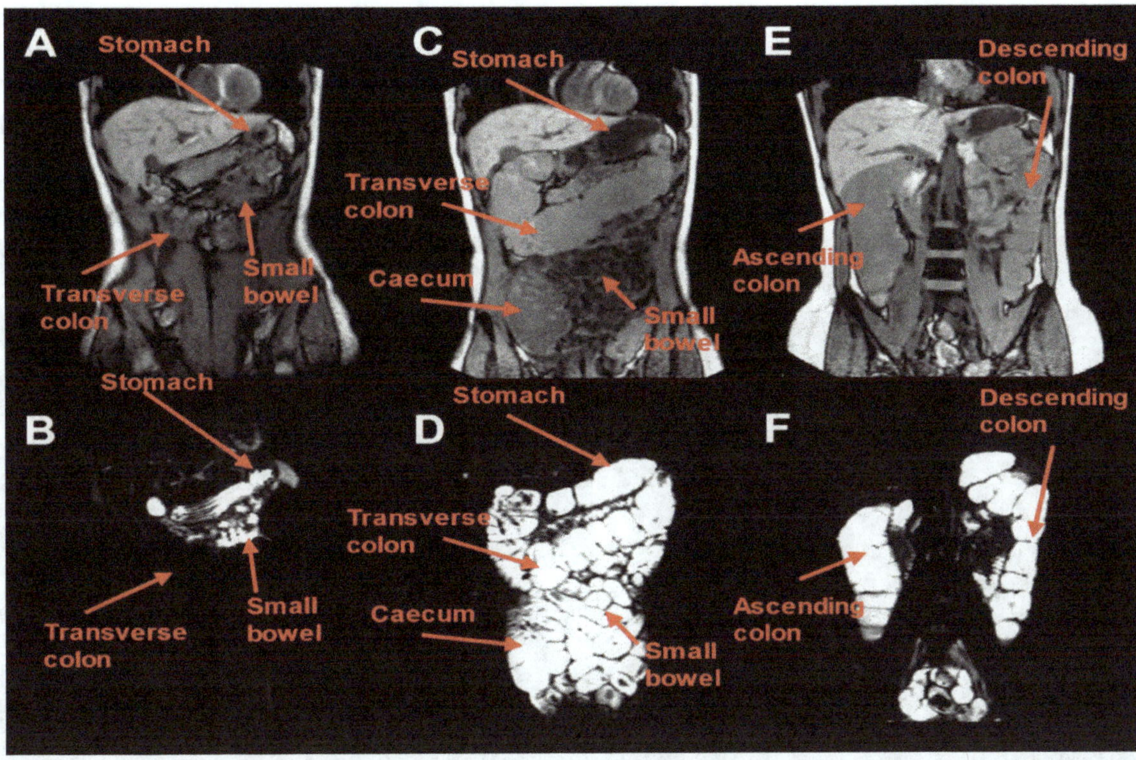

Figure 2. MRI quantification of water colonic content of one volunteer after ingestion of a single 2 L PEG electrolyte scheme. (**A**,**B**) concern fasting baseline conditions. White colour stands for water presence and black colour for water absence. In (**B**), water was found in the small bowel and the stomach (limited resting fluid) but not in the transverse colon. (**C**–**F**) conditions appear immediately after the ingestion of the 2 L PEG dose and therefore in (**D**) water was found in the stomach, the cecum and the transverse colon while (**F**) is a posterior image and represents water appearance in the ascending and descending colon. Reproduced from [25], Blackwell Publishing LTD, 2014 with permission.

A different study quantified the gut segmental liquid presence in 25 IBS-D patients and 75 healthy volunteers in the fasted and in the fed (rice pudding) state [33]. The team found out that the fasted segmental volume in both groups was similar and specifically in healthy control group ascending colon volume was estimated 203 ± 75 mL, transverse colon volume 198 ± 79 mL and descending colon volume 160 ± 86 mL while from IBS-D patients 205 ± 69 mL, 232 ± 100 mL and 151 ± 71 mL respectively. On the contrary, food effect was not the same for the two study groups. As far as the healthy group is concerned, post feeding, through a higher ileo-colonic activity 10% expansion of the ascending colon content occurred and later (90–240 min) the last parts of the meal induced a smaller expansion in the same region. In the case of the IBS-D patients, feeding resulted in a smaller increase of the ascending colon volume and later (t = 90 min) a greater transverse one. A detailed MRI image of the colonic anatomy can be found in Figure 3.

The segmental and whole intestinal chyme content were studied in 25 healthy subjects [34]. This study also assessed variability between different study days. In addition, they also performed MRI in another seven healthy volunteers before and after defecation as they used stool volumes as a mean to validate the changes in colon volumes. Regarding the intestinal volumes on the two different scanning days, no significant overall or segmental change was detected (p>0.05) as overall volume was reported to be 760 mL (662–858) and 757 mL (649–865) on each observation. More specifically, on scanning day A the volume in the cecum/ascending colon was 177 mL (147–208) while on scanning day B 186 mL (159–212). In the same way, in the transverse colon it was estimated 192 mL (159–226) and 197 mL (155–240), in the descending colon 133 mL (110–157) and 193 mL (111–168) and in the rectosigmoid colon 257 mL (213–302) and 235 mL (193–277) respectively. The impact of defecation on regional volume distribution was only significant in the case of the rectosigmoid colon with 329 mL

(248–409) before and 183 mL (130–236) after faecal excretion. In each other case, water volume in the cecum/ascending colon was 208 mL (167–248) and 198 mL (154–242), in the transverse colon 171 mL (100–242) and 173 mL (109–237) and finally, in the descending colon 185 mL (153–217) and 171 mL (129–212). Total intestinal water volume was reported 892 mL (723–1062) and 726 mL (635–816) prior and after defecation.

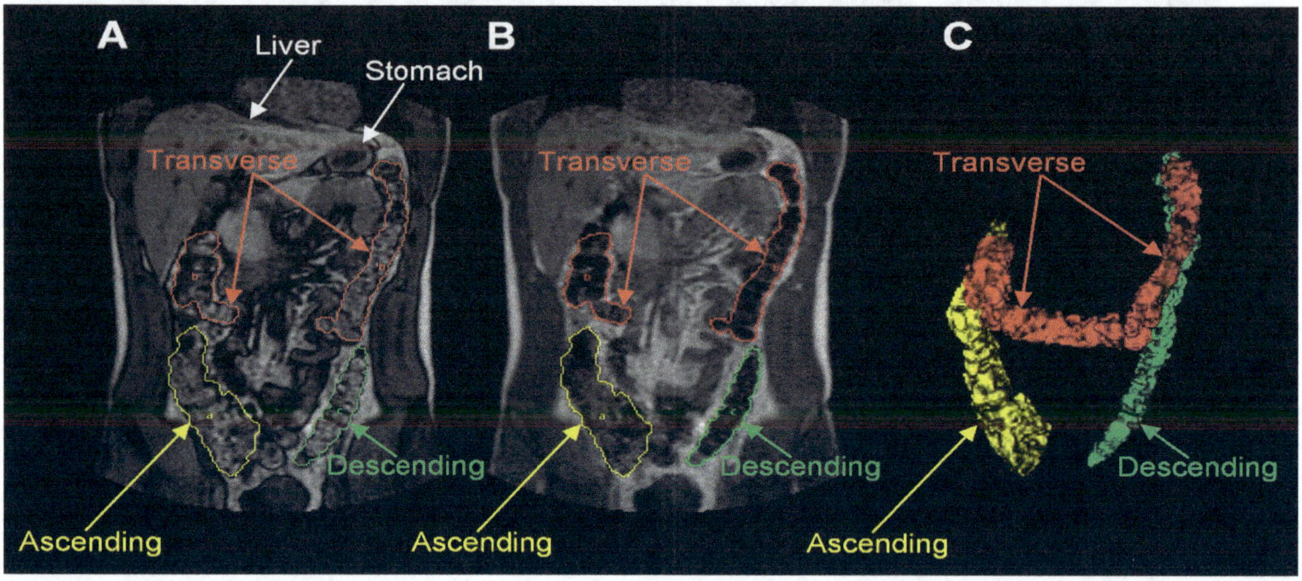

Figure 3. MRI images for colonic anatomy. (**A**,**B**) are different out of phase and in phase water and fat dual-echo imaging and (**C**) is a 3D reconstruction. Reproduced from [33], Blackwell Publishing LTD, 2013 with permission.

A different study of gut water quantification in 18 healthy volunteers focused on the effect of stress caused by IV administration of corticotrophin releasing hormone (CRH) and cold water hand immersion on the intestinal environment [35]. The volunteers were divided in two groups and were fed a standard test meal (rice pudding). After the comparison of the saline and the CRH arms of the study, it was found that CRH injection expanded the intestinal water presence from (mean AUC (SD)) 46,227 (10,927) to 49,817 (10,770), ANOVA $p = 0.002$. Comparison of ice water immersion to warm water immersion revealed no differences with the corresponding values being 48,991 (17,501) and 48,964 (16,950) respectively, $p = 0.730$. The consumption of the meal did not increase significantly the ascending colon water volume (t = 0–45 min) only on CRH injection (15 (32) mL, $p = 0.3$). On saline injection, warm immersion and ice immersion water volume increased significantly (16 (32) mL, $p = 0.040$, 33 (51) mL, $p = 0.020$, 22 (27) mL, $p = 0.005$ respectively). Transverse water volumes were only significantly affected (decreased) only on water immersion ($p = 0.0107$). Water distribution in the descending colon was unaffected in any case.

The regional colonic water was studied in four healthy subjects finding that the median (interquartile range) of total colon volume was 819 mL (687–898.5). Regarding each segment, the volume of the ascending colon was determined as 200 mL (169.5–260), the volume of the transverse 200.5 mL (113.5–242.5), the descending 148 mL (121.5–178.5) and in the final part of the colon (sigmoid-rectum) 277 mL (192–345) [36].

A different study investigated how gluten affects the colonic volume and gas in 12 healthy subjects [37]. Fasted colonic volume in total after gluten-free bread (GFB) diet was (mean ± SEM) 748 ± 258 mL, after normal gluten content bread (NGCB) 659 ± 291 mL and after added gluten content bread (AGCB) 576 ± 252 mL. Segmental respective volumes were estimated as following: ascending colon 250 ± 119 mL, 256 ± 149 mL, 224 ± 128 mL, transverse colon 289 ± 95 mL, 212 ± 73 mL, 178 ± 86 mL, and descending colon 209 ± 73 mL,187 ± 92 mL, and 172 ± 77 mL. Statistical differences were only detected in the case of the volume of the transverse colon which was higher after the GFB diet compared to NGCB and AGCB diets ($p = 0.02$).

The effect of a laxative PEG electrolyte formulation on gut volumes was studied in 24 patients with functional constipation and 24 with IBS-C [27]. Baseline measurements in the fasted state revealed higher ascending colon content in the FC group (mean (SD) 314 (101) mL) when compared to the IBS-C group (226 (71) mL, $p < 0.001$). The same applied to the overall colonic volumes which were 847 (280) mL and 662 (240) mL, respectively ($p = 0.03$). Similar differences existed in the volumes of the ascending colon 120 min after the PEG electrolyte ingestion which were 597 (170) mL and 389 (169) mL respectively ($p < 0.01$) and the total large intestinal volumes 1505 (387) mL and 1039 (418) mL respectively ($p < 0.01$) at the same time.

The impact of the co-administration of fructose and corticotropin-releasing factor (CRF) or saline on the intestinal water was studied in a healthy group of 11 male and 10 female volunteers [38]. On the CRF arm of the study, the baseline of the ascending colon water volume was 210 ± 77 mL (t = −45 min) and after the administration of the fructose meal the volume rose to 270 ± 109 mL. This increase was more intense (29%) compared to the saline effect (12% rise) where the volume was measured 226 ± 74 mL and 252 ± 83 mL respectively. The study showed higher ascending colon water in men than in women only in the case of CRF administration.

The effect of oxycodone administration on the regional gut water distribution of healthy subjects was also characterised [39]. The researchers evaluated the segmental intestinal volumes in two arms (oxycodone and placebo) and in two different days (day 1 and day 5). On oxycodone, there was a volume rise in caecum/ascending colon mean (95% confidence interval) from day 1 (177 (147–208) mL) to day 5 (249 (209–291) mL), $p = 0.005$ (statistically significant), in transverse colon from 192 (159–226) mL to 230 (190–270) mL, $p = 0.005$ (statistically significant) respectively and in descending colon from 133 (110–157) mL to 153 (132–175) mL ($p = 0.08$) respectively. On the contrary, there was a non-significant decrease in the rectosigmoid colonic volume from 257 (213–302) mL to 249 (213–284) mL respectively ($p = 0.64$) but overall oxycodone affected positively the total large intestinal volume (760 (662–858) mL to 881 (783–979) mL respectively, $p = 0.008$ (statistically significant)). The placebo ingestion lead to a rise in the caecum/ascending colon volume from 186 (159–212) mL in day 1 to 211 (184–238) mL in day 5 ($p = 0.03$, statistically significant) and in rectosigmoid colon volume from 235 (193–277) mL to 244 (200–288) mL respectively ($p = 0.06$). At the same time there was a decrease both in transverse colon volume from 197 (155–240) mL to 183 (152–213) mL respectively ($p = 0.57$) and in descending colon volume from 139 (111–168) mL to 121 (101–142) mL respectively ($p = 0.07$). Overall, the placebo administration scheme did not affect significantly the total large intestinal volume (757 (649–856) mL to 759 (670–848) mL respectively, $p = 0.26$).

The intestinal liquid and non-liquid content was also evaluated in 10 healthy volunteers in regards with high- and low-residue diets, meals and faecal output [40]. Low-residue diet affected positively the non-gaseous content in the right region of the colon which climbed up to 41 ± 11 mL 4 h following the meal ingestion compared to fasted state (−15 ± 8 mL; $p = 0.006$ vs. fed). A significant reduction on the non-gaseous content caused by the faecal output was only present in the distal intestine. As far as the meal effect on the colonic contents is examined, non-gaseous colonic content had escalated only in the proximal intestine (by 37% ± 14%, $p = 0.007$) in the case where subjects underwent a fasting scan and a second scan 4 h following the meal ingestion. Generally, the gas content had risen (by 31% ± 14%, $p = 0.064$). In the fasted state, there was no reduction in the non-gaseous content 4 h after the first scan (−29% ± 11%, $p = 0.040$).

The administration of the meal (fed state) had a statistically significant effect (increase) only in the volume of chyme excluding gas ($p = 0.006$ vs. fed). Faecal output lowered the gas volume as well as the non-gaseous ($p < 0.001$) in the whole intestine and the biggest change was in the pelvic colon. This output consisted the 38% ± 5% of the chyme, excluding gas.

The segmental water volumes were also measured as a part of a study of 34 healthy subjects and 30 patients with IBS-D, 16 with IBS-C and 11 with IBS-M in the fasted and the fed state (using a rice pudding, strawberry jam, wheat bran, and orange juice test meal) [41]. At t = 45 min, in the fasted state, colonic volume of the ascending solon was estimated (median (interquartile range)) 194 (150–234) mL in the healthy group, 217 (191–268) mL in the IBS-C group and 209 (147–248) mL in the non-constipated IBS or IBS-nonC group respectively. Respectively, the transverse colonic volume was 165 (117–255) mL, 253 (200–329) mL, and 198 (106–248) mL and the reduced volumes in the IBS-C group were the only ones to be considered as statistically significant ($p = 0.02$). For the descending colon, the respective values were (mean (SD)) 143 (61) mL, 153 (47) mL and 114 (52) mL when the overall intestinal volume was found 513 (174) mL, 644 (148) mL, and 498 (175) mL respectively. Postprandially, at t = 0, the volumes in the ascending colon increased slightly in every group apart from the IBS-D group but not significantly and then decreased in all groups. When transverse colon is concerned, volume were unchanged at first but increased at t = 180 min reaching a significant high state at t = 405 min (compared to the healthy group, $p = 0.04$) but generally unaffected compared to fasting transverse volumes at t = −45 min of IBS-C and IBS-nonC group. Overall, the intestinal volumes were higher in IBS-C than in IBS-nonC.

The effect of consuming glucose, fructose and inulin on intestinal water volumes was evaluated in 29 healthy volunteers and 29 IBS patients [42]. In the healthy group, glucose ingestion caused a reduction in the total colonic volume (mean (±SEM)) of 20.9 (15.7) mL whereas fructose and inulin increased it about 50.8 (16.2) mL and 136.8 (17.6) mL on average respectively. Regarding the patients' group, glucose affected the gut volume the least causing a slight rise of 3.8 (11.4) mL while fructose and inulin caused a bigger rise of 58.5 (20.3) mL and 129.6 (19.9) mL respectively. The researchers concluded that intestinal volume was primarily affected by fructose and inulin rather than glucose in both groups.

A different study estimated the timeline of total and segmental unbound water in terms of volume and number of liquid pockets (Figure 4) in the large intestine of 12 healthy volunteers after the administration of 240 mL of water being the first team to conduct this kind of study [43]. They found that the number of bound colonic water pockets water in the fasted state were 11 ± 5 mL and each of them contained approximately 2 ± 1 mL in total. 30 min after the water ingestion the colonic liquid reached the peak of 7 ± 4 mL divided in 17 ± 7 pockets. By time, the number of the liquid pockets and their volumes decreased but, one hour later, only the amount of the colonic pockets peaked again (17 ± 7) while their volumes remained in lower levels (3–4 mL). The team reported that there was a high variability regarding the number of the pockets (0 to 89) and the total unbound colonic water (0 to 49 mL). They also reported that the main site of the freely liquid was the ascending colon.

The colonic water distribution was also evaluated as part of a study of the effect of macrogol on large bowel flow of 11 healthy and 11 constipated volunteers [44]. Baseline scanning revealed very little water content and no significant differences between the healthy and the constipated subjects (2 (0–7) mL and 11 (1–29) mL respectively, $p = 0.16$). At t = 60 min, macrogol boosted significantly the water volumes in both healthy (140 (104–347) mL, $p = 0.001$) and constipated (228 (91–259) mL, $p = 0.0039$, (Wilcoxon ranked pairs test)). 120 min following the macrogol administration, the ascending colon unbound water content was still significantly high in both groups (healthy: $p = 0.002$ and constipated: $p = 0.0039$) but it had decreased in the patient group where it was found 84 (3–195) mL compared to control group [146 (32–227) mL].

The regional and total bowel water was assessed in 9 healthy subjects and 20 constipated patients on maltodextrin (placebo), 10.5 g and 21 g of psyllium [31]. In both groups, in the fasting state colonic volumes were risen from (median (interquartile range)) 372 (284–601) mL to 578 (510–882) mL in healthy controls and from 831 (745–934) mL to 1104 (847–1316) mL in patients by the administration of 7 g of psyllium ($p < 0.05$). The ascending colon water was (median (interquartile range)) 0.2 (0.1–0.6) mL in the maltodextrin intervention, 4.0 (2.4–7.0) mL and 7.4 (2.8–16.5) mL in the 10.5 g/d and 21 g/day psyllium intervention respectively in the healthy group whereas in patients group it was estimated 0.13 (0.01–0.66) mL on maltodextrin administration and 3.41 (0.10–7.69) mL on 21 g/day psyllium administration. Segmentally, significant differences occurred while on the placebo intervention in the colonic volumes of the fasted state between patients and healthy subjects (745 (455–844) mL and 372 (284–601) mL respectively, $p < 0.5$). The cause of these differences were mainly because of higher volumes in the ascending and transverse region of the intestine.

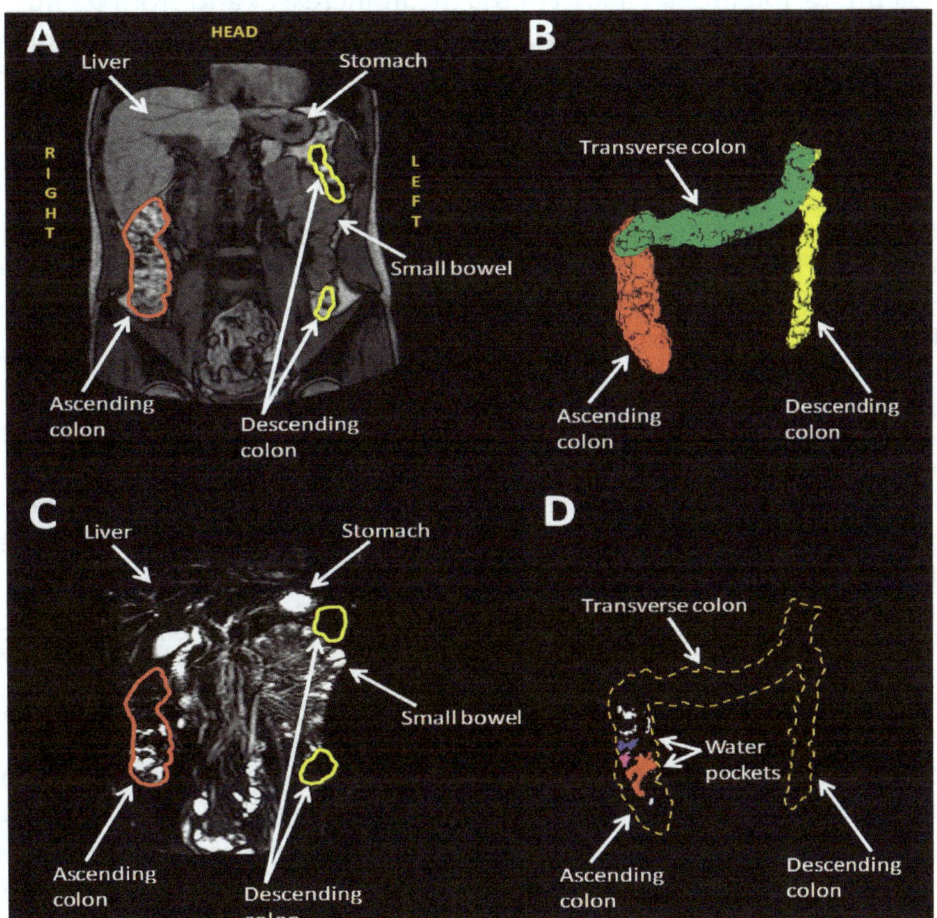

Figure 4. (**A**) MRI bowel image. (**B**) 3D reconstruction of the bowel. Red, green, and yellow stand for ascending, transverse and descending colon respectively. (**C**) Highly T2 weighted image with the same angle of (**A**). Unbound liquid appears white whereas bound and less mobile liquid seem darker. (**D**) Unbound liquid of the colon. Reproduced from [43], American Chemical Society, 2017 with permission.

The effect of oxycodone plus macrogol and prolonged-release (PR) naloxone and oxycodone on the segmental gut water of 20 healthy subjects was evaluated [45]. The comparison of baseline and day 5 scanning of PR naloxone intervention showed that regional intestinal volumes increased in the cecum/ascending colonic volume (mean (±SD)) from 220 ± 25 mL to 257 ± 41 mL ($p = 0.156$), the transverse colonic volume from 258 ± 42 mL to 295 ± 47 mL ($p = 0.161$), the descending colonic volume from 187 ± 32 mL to 210 ± 51 mL ($p = 0.384$) and the total from 941 ± 108 mL to 1036 ± 176 mL

(p = 0.087) respectively. The volume also increased from 276 ± 60 mL to 273 ± 71 mL (p = 0.904) in the rectosigmoid colon. The same comparison of the macrogol intervention caused a volume rise in each intestinal region and more specifically in the ascending colon where volumes rose from 216 ± 39 mL to 277 ± 53 mL (p = 0.005), in the transverse colon from 270 ± 59 mL to 328 ± 51 mL (p = 0.006), in the descending colon from 184 ± 55 mL to 231 ± 44 mL (p = 0.022), in the rectosigmoid colon from 242 ± 55 mL to 287 ± 52 mL (p = 0.026) and in total from 912 ± 158 mL to 1123 ± 145 mL ($p < 0.001$). The results showed that the macrogol administration increased the volume significantly in every segment. Significant volume rise in the whole intestine occurred only on macrogol administration.

The role of a low fermentable oligo-, di-, mono-saccharides and polyols or FODMAP regimen with the administration of either oligofructose or maltodextrin on the intestinal water volumes was investigated in 37 healthy volunteers [46]. MRI analysis revealed that both oligofructose and maltodextrin exerted a positive effect on the intestinal volume since it was increased on average from 110 mL, 95% CI 30 mL to 190 mL, p = 0.01 (19.6% mean increase) and from 90 mL, 95% CI 6 mL to 175 mL, p = 0.04 (15.5% mean increase) respectively. When it comes to segmental colonic volumes only oligofructose was capable to rise the volumes' values in the ascending (mean 35 mL, 95% CI 9 mL to 61 mL, p = 0.01), transverse (mean 44 mL, 95% CI 4 mL to 84 mL p = 0.03) and distal colon (mean 26 mL, 95% CI 0 mL to 52 mL, p = 0.05). It was also noted that there was no significant difference when the results from the two substances were compared to each other.

The role of foods in modulating gut water content of 15 subjects and either a bread meal, a rhubarb meal, or a lettuce meal [47]. The bread meal created an AUC (area under the curve) (mean (SEM)) of 78 (43) mL whereas the rhubarb and the lettuce meal created a much higher rise of 291 (89) mL ($p < 0.01$ Wilcoxon) and 409 (231) mL respectively.

5. Colon Transit and Luminal Flow

Transit times of oral dosage forms exert a significant role on their efficacy. Modified release oral formulations and colon-targeted drugs have to release their active substance in the colon. Therefore, changes in the transit and flow patterns may affect drug release. MRI has been increasingly used to study the transit times as summarised in Table 1.

Tagging is a MRI method commonly used to assess motion in the heart in cardiac imaging. It has been used previously in the stomach environment and is now finding new applications to assess colonic luminal motion of the chyme [44]. Pritchard et al. evaluated the application of MRI tagging to study the ascending colonic flow in 11 healthy and 11 constipated volunteers on magrocol administration. Analysis of the baseline scanning revealed weak flow procedures regardless volunteer group (healthy 20% (14–23), constipated 12% (11–20), p = 0.1). 60 min after macrogol administration, dislocation of the tags could be observed mainly in the healthy group (30% (26–35), p = 0.002, Wilcoxon test) rather than the constipated one (17% (13–230, p = 0.57, Wilcoxon test). This dislocation was characterized as forward and backward and took place at the same time and region of the ascending colon (central). Moreover, there was a fast (>4.8 cm) retrograde central 'jet' and a decrease in the tag intensity as well. Results from all the scanning allowed the observation of higher central motion in the ascending colon rather membrane motion which was weaker but still detectable at t = 120 min mainly in the healthy large intestine (25% (18–360), p = 0.002) and not in so much in the constipated (13% (12–180), p = 0.76). The researchers concluded that there were significant differences in the %COV in each time point between the two conditions (60 min (p = 0.0020), 120 min (p = 0.003), Mann–Whitney rank sum test).

Table 1. Colonic transit of contents with various MRI techniques.

Reference	Aims	Methods	Outcomes
[29]	Assessment of the intestinal transit by MRI	12 healthy volunteers were scanned in fasted and fed state and after consumption of gel-filled capsules	Location of the capsules was affected by food consumption (in the large intestine: fasted vs. fed state was 3 vs. 17 capsules respectively, $p < 0.01$)
[48]	Assessment of new MRI technique of estimating intestinal transit with per os capsules containing gadolinium-saline solution	7 females and 8 males (all healthy) consumed 5 capsules	Mean transit time for female and male volunteers was 41 ± 9 h and 31 ± 10 h respectively
[23]	Application of ^{19}F and ^{1}H MRI on intestinal transit	2 healthy subjects consumed perfluoro-[15]-crown-5-ether capsules: 1 each on scanning day 1 and 2 each on scanning day 2	Single capsule tracking: total transit lasted 27 h and 32 h for subjects A and B respectively (mean capsule velocity was 1.0 mm/s and 1.0 mm/s respectively). Capsule found outside the stomach 170 min and 220 min respectively Dual capsule tracking: capsules located out of the stomach 210 min after ingestion
[49]	Validate MRI technique towards OCTT[3] and WGT[1] measurements	21 healthy subjects OCTT[3] estimated by the arrival of the head of the meal into the beginning of the large bowel with MRI and by LUBT[4] WGT[1] estimated by MRI marker capsules and ROMs[5]	MRI measurement of OCTT[3] was (median(IQR)) 225 (180–270) min and of WGT[1] was 28 (4–50) h
[25]	Investigation of the effect of oral PEG electrolyte in two dosing regimens on colonic motility	12 healthy subjects consumed the split dose (1 L before the first scanning day and 1 L on the scanning day) and the other 12 healthy volunteers the single dose (2 L on the first scanning day) Each volunteer ingested MRI marker pills the day before the MRI transit scan (days 8, 14, 28)	No differences due to dosing regimens as Mean position score of split vs. single dose at Day 8: 6.2 ± 0.4 vs. 5.4 ± 0.6, $p = 0.2527$, Day 14: 5.8 ± 0.4 vs. 5.5 ± 0.5, $p = 0.6076$, Day 28: 6.1 ± 0.5 vs. 6.6 ± 0.3, $p = 0.3327$ No differences between the days regardless dosing: Day 8 vs. 14: $p = 0.7750$ Day 8 vs. 28: $p = 0.2350$
[50]	Evaluation of MRI techniques of OCTT[3] assessment towards LHBT[6] in healthy volunteers	28 healthy volunteers were recruited OCTT[3] was assessed by the arrival of the head of the lactulose ingestion (10 g/125 mL)	OCTT[3] by MRI measurements was (median (IQR)) 135 (120–150) min
[27]	MRI investigation of the effect of PEG electrolyte as a laxative on the colonic environment	24 patients with functional constipation and 24 with IBS-C participated in this study. They has to consume 5 MRI marker pills before the scanning day and 1 L of PEG electrolyte after the baseline scan on the study day	WAPS[2] for FC (3.6 (2.5–4.2)) was higher than the IBS-C (2.0 (1.5–3.2)), $p = 0.01$
[41]	Distinguish subgroups of IBS based on MRI markers	91 volunteers took part (34 healthy, 30 with IBS-D, 16 with IBS-C, and 11 IBS-M as mixed. IBS-M and IBS-D were listed as IBS-nonC)	WGT[1] for IBS-C, healthy volunteers and IBS-D was 69 (51–111) h, 34 (4–63) h and 34 (17–78) h respectively and OCTT[3] was 203 (154–266) min, 188 (135–262) min and 165 (116–244) min respectively
[44]	Study the ascending colonic transit in healthy and constipated subjects	11 healthy and 11 constipated subjects were scanned fasted and after ingestion of 500 mL of macrogol and consumption MR markers	WAPS[2] between healthy and patients was (median (IQR)) 0.6 (0–1) and 2.6 (1.4–3.6) respectively, $p = 0.0011$
[51]	Evaluation of the applicability of gadolinium filled MRI capsules towards radio-opaque markers (ROMs[5]) on colon transit time (CTT)	7 constipated and 9 healthy subjects ingested 5 gadolinium-based capsules as MRI markers and 20 ROMs[5]	MRI measurements revealed that CTTs in healthy and constipated were 30.9 ± 15.9 h and 74.1 ± 7.2 h respectively, $p < 0.05$ Patients had higher CTTs than the healthy ones
[52]	Establishment of an MRI technique for bowel motion and transit assessment	Baseline and fed state MRI scanning of 15 healthy subjects Meal: chicken or mushroom soup Each subject consumed 5 MRI capsules of Gadoteric acid the day before the study day	WAPS[2] (24 h) = 1.0 (0–3.8) WGT[1] (hours) = 33 hr
[31]	Evaluation of psyllium consumption on colonic environment of healthy and constipated volunteers	9 healthy subjects received maltodextrin (placebo) and psyllium 10.5 g and 21 g for 6 days randomly and 20 constipated subjects ingested maltodextrin and 21 g of psyllium in the same way On treatment day 5, each volunteer ingested 5 MRI marker capsules with gadoteric acid	WGT[1] was higher in healthy than patients ($p < 0.05$) Controls: WAPS[2]24 showed no differences as (median (IQR)) it was 1.0 (0.1–2.2) on maltodextrin, 1.4 (0.2–2.1) on 10.5 g of psyllium and 0.6 (0–1.9) on 21 g of psyllium Patients decreased from 4.2 (3.2–5.3) on maltodextrin to 2.0 (1.5–4.0) on psyllium ($p = 0.067$)
[32]	Evaluation of intestinal volumes and function on kiwifruit consumption	2 kiwifruits or maltodextrin (control) 2 times per day for 3 days in the fasted and fed state	WGT for kiwifruit was (median (IQR)) 0.8 (0–1.4) and for control 1.0 (0.5–3.1), $p = 0.11$

WGT[1]: whole gut transit WAPS[2]: median average weighted position score OCTT[3]: orocecal transit time LUBT[4]: lactose ureide breath test ROMs[5]: radio-opaque markers LHBT[6]: lactulose hydrogen breath test.

6. Conclusions and Future Outlook

Recent developments in MRI imaging techniques have opened up the possibility to expand knowledge of the colonic environment providing unprecedented insights on colonic dimensions, chyme and fluid characteristics, motility, transit, and flow. These physiological parameters will, in turn, have profound impact on drug dissolution and absorption. New knowledge of colonic parameters can also increase the in vivo relevance of in vitro models. Colonic motility has yet to be fully included in the biorelevant in vitro modelling [43]. MRI has the potential to become the modality of choice for early phase assessment of new colonic-targeted drugs' functionality confirming their proof of concept and helping to explain mode of action [11,31]. This is of great regulatory value. The future of MRI of the abdomen includes ultra-high-field (7 T and above) scanners [53] and developments in the design of open magnets that have the advantage of imaging volunteers in the sitting position [11,54]. Also, susceptibility differences and air-tissue interfaces can be responsible for generating artifacts, some of which may be difficult to remove though some could potentially be eliminated by using diamagnetic elements to improve the quality and reliability of the images and data acquired [55]. Another great advantage of MRI is its non-ionizing nature [56]. This can help to extend the studies of gut physiology to children, a group where knowledge of the physiological GI parameters is particularly scanty. Furthermore, one of the latest advancements in the MRI field is the use of ultrashort echo time (UTE) MRI, which has been applied for abdominal imaging purposes [57,58]. The UTE abdominal MRI has not been established and standardized yet but is has great potential since it allows imaging areas whose signal decay fast [58]. Lastly, another common method to minimize abdominal motion artifacts is the application of respiratory gating techniques and this practice could reduce the needs for breath holds or allow for longer sequences [55].

However, there exist some limitations regarding the imaging of the colon and regional drug behaviour. The colon is a large organ and current imaging of the whole colon at once is not of high temporal quality and therefore development of 4D MRI imaging could be helpful [9]. Modified release solid formulations deliver the active substance 6–24 h after administration and for this reason MRI should be applied on the large intestine for longer than the usual 2 h [43]. The bore of the magnet may feel small to claustrophobic participants and can limit studies in clinically obese subjects [11]. In the case of very young children, sedation might be suggested [55]. When it comes to reduction of motion artifacts and bowel movement, antiperistaltic drugs and gating correction techniques could be of use to reduce artifacts [55]. MRI cannot provide luminal pressure data which are of interest too. Specifically, motility is not periodical with large time intervals of relative quiescence between larger contractions [9]. Further studies are needed to analyse the potential of MRI for the exploration of the interactions between the mixing and transportation of contents with meal type. Analysis of flow types such as antegrade and retrograde can reveal the ascending colon's ability of mixing and propelling its contents. Breath hold imaging techniques can help to remove respiratory artifacts and develop MRI as a tool [44]. Furthermore, carrying out MRI experiments is still perceived as expensive compared to well-established techniques in the pharmaceutical field such as gamma-scintigraphy when, on the same time, it yet needs to be optimized and validated towards them [11,31], though costs are decreasing. A comprehensive MRI study day provides a large amount of data, which requires extended image processing time. Practices vary between labs and therefore there is increasing need of standardisation and image analysis automation [11].

In conclusion, MRI of the colon has developed substantially over the recent period considered in this review, and further exciting developments can be expected. The novel physiological insight will no doubt have a profound impact on our understanding of the colonic environment for drug delivery and absorption and will ultimately help to increase the in vitro/in vivo relevance of computer simulations and bench models.

References

1. Reppas, C.; Karatza, E.; Goumas, C.; Markopoulos, C.; Vertzoni, M. Characterization of Contents of Distal Ileum and Cecum to Which Drugs/Drug Products are Exposed During Bioavailability/Bioequivalence Studies in Healthy Adults. *Pharm. Res.* **2015**, *32*, 3338–3349. [CrossRef]

2. Kostewicz, E.S.; Abrahamsson, B.; Brewster, M.; Brouwers, J.; Butler, J.; Carlert, S.; Dickinson, P.A.; Dressman, J.; Holm, R.; Klein, S.; et al. In vitro models for the prediction of in vivo performance of oral dosage forms. *Eur. J. Pharm. Sci.* **2014**, *57*, 342–366. [CrossRef]
3. Lennernas, H.; Aarons, L.; Augustijns, P.; Beato, S.; Bolger, M.; Box, K.; Brewster, M.; Butler, J.; Dressman, J.; Holm, R.; et al. Oral biopharmaceutics tools—Time for a new initiative—An introduction to the IMI project OrBiTo. *Eur. J. Pharm. Sci.* **2014**, *57*, 292–299. [CrossRef]
4. Van Meerveld, B.G.; Johnson, A.C.; Grundy, D. Gastrointestinal Physiology and Function. *Handb. Exp. Pharmacol.* **2017**, *239*, 1–16. [CrossRef]
5. Kararli, T.T. Comparison of the gastrointestinal anatomy, physiology, and biochemistry of humans and commonly used laboratory animals. *Biopharm. Drug Dispos.* **1995**, *16*, 351–380. [CrossRef] [PubMed]
6. Hansson, G.C. Role of mucus layers in gut infection and inflammation. *Curr. Opin. Microbiol.* **2012**, *15*, 57–62. [CrossRef] [PubMed]
7. Phillips, S.F. Absorption and secretion by the colon. *Gastroenterology* **1969**, *56*, 966–971. [CrossRef] [PubMed]
8. Sellers, R.S.; Morton, D. The colon: From banal to brilliant. *Toxicol. Pathol.* **2014**, *42*, 67–81. [CrossRef]
9. Hoad, C.; Clarke, C.; Marciani, L.; Graves, M.J.; Corsetti, M. Will MRI of gastrointestinal function parallel the clinical success of cine cardiac MRI? *Br. J. Radiol.* **2018**, *91*, 20180433. [CrossRef]
10. Tannergren, C.; Bergendal, A.; Lennernas, H.; Abrahamsson, B. Toward an increased understanding of the barriers to colonic drug absorption in humans: Implications for early controlled release candidate assessment. *Mol. Pharm.* **2009**, *6*, 60–73. [CrossRef] [PubMed]
11. Marciani, L. Assessment of gastrointestinal motor functions by MRI: A comprehensive review. *Neurogastroenterol. Motil.* **2011**, *23*, 399–407. [CrossRef] [PubMed]
12. Leighton, M.P.; Lam, C.; Mehta, S.; Spiller, R.C. Efficacy and mode of action of mesalazine in the treatment of diarrhoea-predominant irritable bowel syndrome (IBS-D): Study protocol for a randomised controlled trial. *Trials* **2013**, *14*, 10. [CrossRef] [PubMed]
13. Tozer, P.; Ng, S.C.; Siddiqui, M.R.; Plamondon, S.; Burling, D.; Gupta, A.; Swatton, A.; Tripoli, S.; Vaizey, C.J.; Kamm, M.A.; et al. Long-term MRI-guided combined anti-TNF-alpha and thiopurine therapy for Crohn's perianal fistulas. *Inflamm. Bowel Dis.* **2012**, *18*, 1825–1834. [CrossRef] [PubMed]
14. Stoppino, L.P.; Della Valle, N.; Rizzi, S.; Cleopazzo, E.; Centola, A.; Iamele, D.; Bristogiannis, C.; Stoppino, G.; Vinci, R.; Macarini, L. Magnetic resonance enterography changes after antibody to tumor necrosis factor (anti-TNF) alpha therapy in Crohn's disease: Correlation with SES-CD and clinical-biological markers. *BMC Med. Imaging* **2016**, *16*, 37. [CrossRef]
15. Inoue, A.; Ohta, S.; Nitta, N.; Yoshimura, M.; Shimizu, T.; Tani, M.; Kushima, R.; Murata, K. MRI can be used to assess advanced T-stage colon carcinoma as well as rectal carcinoma. *Jpn. J. Radiol.* **2016**, *34*, 809–819. [CrossRef]
16. Nerad, E.; Lambregts, D.M.; Kersten, E.L.; Maas, M.; Bakers, F.C.; van den Bosch, H.C.; Grabsch, H.I.; Beets-Tan, R.G.; Lahaye, M.J. MRI for Local Staging of Colon Cancer: Can MRI Become the Optimal Staging Modality for Patients With Colon Cancer? *Dis. Colon Rectum* **2017**, *60*, 385–392. [CrossRef] [PubMed]
17. Koh, F.H.X.; Tan, K.K.; Teo, L.L.S.; Ang, B.W.L.; Thian, Y.L. Prospective comparison between magnetic resonance imaging and computed tomography in colorectal cancer staging. *Anz. J. Surg.* **2018**, *88*, E498–E502. [CrossRef]
18. Helander, H.F.; Fändriks, L. Surface area of the digestive tract—Revisited. *Scand. J. Gastroenterol.* **2014**, *49*, 681–689. [CrossRef]
19. Buhmann, S.; Kirchhoff, C.; Wielage, C.; Mussack, T.; Reiser, M.F.; Lienemann, A. Assessment of large bowel motility by cine magnetic resonance imaging using two different prokinetic agents: A feasibility study. *Investig. Radiol.* **2005**, *40*, 689–694. [CrossRef]
20. Murray, K.; Wilkinson-Smith, V.; Hoad, C.; Costigan, C.; Cox, E.; Lam, C.; Marciani, L.; Gowland, P.; Spiller, R.C. Differential effects of FODMAPs (fermentable oligo-, di-, mono-saccharides and polyols) on small and large intestinal contents in healthy subjects shown by MRI. *Am. J. Gastroenterol.* **2014**, *109*, 110–119. [CrossRef] [PubMed]
21. Undseth, R.; Berstad, A.; Klow, N.E.; Arnljot, K.; Moi, K.S.; Valeur, J. Abnormal accumulation of intestinal fluid following ingestion of an unabsorbable carbohydrate in patients with irritable bowel syndrome: An MRI study. *Neurogastroenterol. Motil.* **2014**, *26*, 1686–1693. [CrossRef]

22. Mark, E.B.; Poulsen, J.L.; Haase, A.M.; Frokjaer, J.B.; Schlageter, V.; Scott, S.M.; Krogh, K.; Drewes, A.M. Assessment of colorectal length using the electromagnetic capsule tracking system: A comparative validation study in healthy subjects. *Colorectal Dis.* **2017**, *19*, O350–O357. [CrossRef]
23. Hahn, T.; Kozerke, S.; Schwizer, W.; Fried, M.; Boesiger, P.; Steingoetter, A. Visualization and quantification of intestinal transit and motor function by real-time tracking of 19F labeled capsules in humans. *Magn. Reson. Med.* **2011**, *66*, 812–820. [CrossRef] [PubMed]
24. Kirchhoff, S.; Nicolaus, M.; Schirra, J.; Reiser, M.F.; Goke, B.; Lienemann, A. Assessment of colon motility using simultaneous manometric and functional cine-MRI analysis: Preliminary results. *Abdom. Imaging* **2011**, *36*, 24–30. [CrossRef] [PubMed]
25. Marciani, L.; Garsed, K.C.; Hoad, C.L.; Fields, A.; Fordham, I.; Pritchard, S.E.; Placidi, E.; Murray, K.; Chaddock, G.; Costigan, C.; et al. Stimulation of colonic motility by oral PEG electrolyte bowel preparation assessed by MRI: Comparison of split vs. single dose. *Neurogastroenterol. Motil.* **2014**, *26*, 1426–1436. [CrossRef]
26. Hahnemann, M.L.; Nensa, F.; Kinner, S.; Gerken, G.; Lauenstein, T.C. Motility mapping as evaluation tool for bowel motility: Initial results on the development of an automated color-coding algorithm in cine MRI. *J. Magn. Reson. Imaging* **2015**, *41*, 354–360. [CrossRef]
27. Lam, C.; Chaddock, G.; Marciani, L.; Costigan, C.; Paul, J.; Cox, E.; Hoad, C.; Menys, A.; Pritchard, S.; Garsed, K.; et al. Colonic response to laxative ingestion as assessed by MRI differs in constipated irritable bowel syndrome compared to functional constipation. *Neurogastroenterol. Motil.* **2016**, *28*, 861–870. [CrossRef]
28. Hoad, C.L.; Menys, A.; Garsed, K.; Marciani, L.; Hamy, V.; Murray, K.; Costigan, C.; Atkinson, D.; Major, G.; Spiller, R.C.; et al. Colon wall motility: Comparison of novel quantitative semi-automatic measurements using cine MRI. *Neurogastroenterol. Motil.* **2016**, *28*, 327–335. [CrossRef]
29. Schiller, C.; Frohlich, C.P.; Giessmann, T.; Siegmund, W.; Monnikes, H.; Hosten, N.; Weitschies, W. Intestinal fluid volumes and transit of dosage forms as assessed by magnetic resonance imaging. *Aliment. Pharmacol. Ther.* **2005**, *22*, 971–979. [CrossRef] [PubMed]
30. Placidi, E.; Marciani, L.; Hoad, C.L.; Napolitano, A.; Garsed, K.C.; Pritchard, S.E.; Cox, E.F.; Costigan, C.; Spiller, R.C.; Gowland, P.A. The effects of loperamide, or loperamide plus simethicone, on the distribution of gut water as assessed by MRI in a mannitol model of secretory diarrhoea. *Aliment. Pharmacol. Ther.* **2012**, *36*, 64–73. [CrossRef] [PubMed]
31. Major, G.; Murray, K.; Singh, G.; Nowak, A.; Hoad, C.L.; Marciani, L.; Silos-Santiago, A.; Kurtz, C.B.; Johnston, J.M.; Gowland, P.; et al. Demonstration of differences in colonic volumes, transit, chyme consistency, and response to psyllium between healthy and constipated subjects using magnetic resonance imaging. *Neurogastroenterol. Motil.* **2018**, *30*, e13400. [CrossRef] [PubMed]
32. Wilkinson-Smith, V.; Dellschaft, N.; Ansell, J.; Hoad, C.; Marciani, L.; Gowland, P.; Spiller, R. Mechanisms underlying effects of kiwifruit on intestinal function shown by MRI in healthy volunteers. *Aliment. Pharmacol. Ther.* **2019**. [CrossRef] [PubMed]
33. Pritchard, S.E.; Marciani, L.; Garsed, K.C.; Hoad, C.L.; Thongborisute, W.; Roberts, E.; Gowland, P.A.; Spiller, R.C. Fasting and postprandial volumes of the undisturbed colon: Normal values and changes in diarrhea-predominant irritable bowel syndrome measured using serial MRI. *Neurogastroenterol. Motil.* **2014**, *26*, 124–130. [CrossRef] [PubMed]
34. Nilsson, M.; Sandberg, T.H.; Poulsen, J.L.; Gram, M.; Frokjaer, J.B.; Ostergaard, L.R.; Krogh, K.; Brock, C.; Drewes, A.M. Quantification and variability in colonic volume with a novel magnetic resonance imaging method. *Neurogastroenterol. Motil.* **2015**, *27*, 1755–1763. [CrossRef] [PubMed]
35. Pritchard, S.E.; Garsed, K.C.; Hoad, C.L.; Lingaya, M.; Banwait, R.; Thongborisute, W.; Roberts, E.; Costigan, C.; Marciani, L.; Gowland, P.A.; et al. Effect of experimental stress on the small bowel and colon in healthy humans. *Neurogastroenterol. Motil.* **2015**, *27*, 542–549. [CrossRef] [PubMed]
36. Sandberg, T.H.; Nilsson, M.; Poulsen, J.L.; Gram, M.; Frokjaer, J.B.; Ostergaard, L.R.; Drewes, A.M. A novel semi-automatic segmentation method for volumetric assessment of the colon based on magnetic resonance imaging. *Abdom. Imaging* **2015**, *40*, 2232–2241. [CrossRef] [PubMed]
37. Coletta, M.; Gates, F.K.; Marciani, L.; Shiwani, H.; Major, G.; Hoad, C.L.; Chaddock, G.; Gowland, P.A.; Spiller, R.C. Effect of bread gluten content on gastrointestinal function: A crossover MRI study on healthy humans. *Br. J. Nutr.* **2016**, *115*, 55–61. [CrossRef] [PubMed]

38. Murray, K.A.; Lam, C.; Rehman, S.; Marciani, L.; Costigan, C.; Hoad, C.L.; Lingaya, M.R.; Banwait, R.; Bawden, S.J.; Gowland, P.A.; et al. Corticotropin-releasing factor increases ascending colon volume after a fructose test meal in healthy humans: A randomized controlled trial. *Am. J. Clin. Nutr.* **2016**, *103*, 1318–1326. [CrossRef] [PubMed]
39. Nilsson, M.; Poulsen, J.L.; Brock, C.; Sandberg, T.H.; Gram, M.; Frokjaer, J.B.; Krogh, K.; Drewes, A.M. Opioid-induced bowel dysfunction in healthy volunteers assessed with questionnaires and MRI. *Eur. J. Gastroenterol. Hepatol.* **2016**, *28*, 514–524. [CrossRef] [PubMed]
40. Bendezu, R.A.; Mego, M.; Monclus, E.; Merino, X.; Accarino, A.; Malagelada, J.R.; Navazo, I.; Azpiroz, F. Colonic content: Effect of diet, meals, and defecation. *Neurogastroenterol. Motil.* **2017**, 29. [CrossRef]
41. Lam, C.; Chaddock, G.; Marciani Laurea, L.; Costigan, C.; Cox, E.; Hoad, C.; Pritchard, S.; Gowland, P.; Spiller, R. Distinct Abnormalities of Small Bowel and Regional Colonic Volumes in Subtypes of Irritable Bowel Syndrome Revealed by MRI. *Am. J. Gastroenterol.* **2017**, *112*, 346–355. [CrossRef]
42. Major, G.; Pritchard, S.; Murray, K.; Alappadan, J.P.; Hoad, C.L.; Marciani, L.; Gowland, P.; Spiller, R. Colon Hypersensitivity to Distension, Rather Than Excessive Gas Production, Produces Carbohydrate-Related Symptoms in Individuals With Irritable Bowel Syndrome. *Gastroenterology* **2017**, *152*, 124–133. [CrossRef] [PubMed]
43. Murray, K.; Hoad, C.L.; Mudie, D.M.; Wright, J.; Heissam, K.; Abrehart, N.; Pritchard, S.E.; Al Atwah, S.; Gowland, P.A.; Garnett, M.C.; et al. Magnetic Resonance Imaging Quantification of Fasted State Colonic Liquid Pockets in Healthy Humans. *Mol. Pharm.* **2017**, *14*, 2629–2638. [CrossRef] [PubMed]
44. Pritchard, S.E.; Paul, J.; Major, G.; Marciani, L.; Gowland, P.A.; Spiller, R.C.; Hoad, C.L. Assessment of motion of colonic contents in the human colon using MRI tagging. *Neurogastroenterol. Motil.* **2017**, 29. [CrossRef]
45. Poulsen, J.L.; Mark, E.B.; Brock, C.; Frokjaer, J.B.; Krogh, K.; Drewes, A.M. Colorectal Transit and Volume During Treatment with Prolonged-release Oxycodone/Naloxone Versus Oxycodone Plus Macrogol 3350. *J. Neurogastroenterol. Motil.* **2018**, *24*, 119–127. [CrossRef]
46. Sloan, T.J.; Jalanka, J.; Major, G.A.D.; Krishnasamy, S.; Pritchard, S.; Abdelrazig, S.; Korpela, K.; Singh, G.; Mulvenna, C.; Hoad, C.L.; et al. A low FODMAP diet is associated with changes in the microbiota and reduction in breath hydrogen but not colonic volume in healthy subjects. *PLoS ONE* **2018**, *13*, e0201410. [CrossRef] [PubMed]
47. Wilkinson-Smith, V.C.; Major, G.; Ashleigh, L.; Murray, K.; Hoad, C.L.; Marciani, L.; Gowland, P.A.; Spiller, R.C. Insights Into the Different Effects of Food on Intestinal Secretion Using Magnetic Resonance Imaging. *J. Parenter. Enter. Nutr.* **2018**, *42*, 1342–1348. [CrossRef]
48. Buhmann, S.; Kirchhoff, C.; Ladurner, R.; Mussack, T.; Reiser, M.F.; Lienemann, A. Assessment of colonic transit time using MRI: A feasibility study. *Eur. Radiol.* **2007**, *17*, 669–674. [CrossRef] [PubMed]
49. Chaddock, G.; Lam, C.; Hoad, C.L.; Costigan, C.; Cox, E.F.; Placidi, E.; Thexton, I.; Wright, J.; Blackshaw, P.E.; Perkins, A.C.; et al. Novel MRI tests of orocecal transit time and whole gut transit time: Studies in normal subjects. *Neurogastroenterol. Motil.* **2014**, *26*, 205–214. [CrossRef] [PubMed]
50. Savarino, E.; Savarino, V.; Fox, M.; Di Leo, G.; Furnari, M.; Marabotto, E.; Gemignani, L.; Bruzzone, L.; Moscatelli, A.; De Cassan, C.; et al. Measurement of oro-caecal transit time by magnetic resonance imaging. *Eur. Radiol.* **2015**, *25*, 1579–1587. [CrossRef] [PubMed]
51. Zhi, M.; Zhou, Z.; Chen, H.; Xiong, F.; Huang, J.; He, H.; Zhang, M.; Su, M.; Gao, X.; Hu, P. Clinical application of a gadolinium-based capsule as an MRI contrast agent in slow transit constipation diagnostics. *Neurogastroenterol. Motil.* **2017**, 29. [CrossRef] [PubMed]
52. Khalaf, A.; Hoad, C.L.; Menys, A.; Nowak, A.; Taylor, S.A.; Paparo, S.; Lingaya, M.; Falcone, Y.; Singh, G.; Spiller, R.C.; et al. MRI assessment of the postprandial gastrointestinal motility and peptide response in healthy humans. *Neurogastroenterol. Motil.* **2018**. [CrossRef]
53. Roth, C.G.; Marzio, D.H.-D.; Guglielmo, F.F. Contributions of Magnetic Resonance Imaging to Gastroenterological Practice: MRIs for GIs. *Dig. Dis. Sci.* **2018**, *63*, 1102–1122. [CrossRef]
54. Camilleri, M. New imaging in neurogastroenterology: An overview. *Neurogastroenterol. Motil.* **2006**, *18*, 805–812. [CrossRef] [PubMed]
55. Yang, R.K.; Roth, C.G.; Ward, R.J.; deJesus, J.O.; Mitchell, D.G. Optimizing Abdominal MR Imaging: Approaches to Common Problems. *RadioGraphics* **2010**, *30*, 185–199. [CrossRef]

56. Anupindi, S.A.; Podberesky, D.J.; Towbin, A.J.; Courtier, J.; Gee, M.S.; Darge, K.; Dillman, J.R. Pediatric inflammatory bowel disease: Imaging issues with targeted solutions. *Abdom. Imaging* **2015**, *40*, 975–992. [CrossRef]
57. Roh, A.T.; Xiao, Z.; Cheng, J.Y.; Vasanawala, S.S.; Loening, A.M. Conical ultrashort echo time (UTE) MRI in the evaluation of pediatric acute appendicitis. *Abdom. Radiol.* **2019**, *44*, 22–30. [CrossRef] [PubMed]
58. Ibrahim, E.-S.H.; Cernigliaro, J.G.; Pooley, R.A.; Bridges, M.D.; Giesbrandt, J.G.; Williams, J.C.; Haley, W.E. Detection of different kidney stone types: An ex vivo comparison of ultrashort echo time MRI to reference standard CT. *Clin. Imaging* **2016**, *40*, 90–95. [CrossRef] [PubMed]

4

Intestinal Permeability and Drug Absorption: Predictive Experimental, Computational and In Vivo Approaches

David Dahlgren and Hans Lennernäs *

Department of Pharmacy, Uppsala University, Box 580 SE-751 23 Uppsala, Sweden
* Correspondence: hans.lennernas@farmaci.uu.se

Abstract: The main objective of this review is to discuss recent advancements in the overall investigation and in vivo prediction of drug absorption. The intestinal permeability of an orally administered drug (given the value P_{eff}) has been widely used to determine the rate and extent of the drug's intestinal absorption (F_{abs}) in humans. Preclinical gastrointestinal (GI) absorption models are currently in demand for the pharmaceutical development of novel dosage forms and new drug products. However, there is a strong need to improve our understanding of the interplay between pharmaceutical, biopharmaceutical, biochemical, and physiological factors when predicting F_{abs} and bioavailability. Currently, our knowledge of GI secretion, GI motility, and regional intestinal permeability, in both healthy subjects and patients with GI diseases, is limited by the relative inaccessibility of some intestinal segments of the human GI tract. In particular, our understanding of the complex and highly dynamic physiology of the region from the mid-jejunum to the sigmoid colon could be significantly improved. One approach to the assessment of intestinal permeability is to use animal models that allow these intestinal regions to be investigated in detail and then to compare the results with those from simple human permeability models such as cell cultures. Investigation of intestinal drug permeation processes is a crucial biopharmaceutical step in the development of oral pharmaceutical products. The determination of the intestinal P_{eff} for a specific drug is dependent on the technique, model, and conditions applied, and is influenced by multiple interactions between the drug molecule and the biological membranes.

Keywords: intestinal permeability; intestinal drug absorption; experimental and computational permeability methods

---

1. Introduction

Bioavailability is a key pharmacokinetic parameter that represents the fraction of an orally administered drug that reaches the systemic circulation in an uncharged molecular form (Equation (1)):

$$F = F_{abs} \times (1 - E_G) \times (1 - E_H) \tag{1}$$

where F is the bioavailability, and E_G and E_H are the fractions extracted in the gut wall and liver, respectively. The fraction of the dose that is absorbed (F_{abs}) and its absorption rate are largely determined by the following biopharmaceutical factors: the dissolution, solubility, luminal stability (chemical and/or enzymatic), intestinal transit time, and intestinal permeability of the active pharmaceutical ingredient (API). In order to achieve a sufficiently high systemic bioavailability, most drug products require pharmaceutical development to produce a plasma concentration-time profile that provides the optimal pharmacodynamic response and acceptable side effects. This is especially important for modified-release (MR) products, which are designed to improve the pharmacodynamic response. In general, oral products with poor bioavailability (F below 25%–35%) are recognized as having wider intra- and interindividual variability in plasma exposure (C.V. > 60%–120%) [1]. In 1996, Hellriegel et al. reported an inverse association between the bioavailability of oral drug products and the total variability of the bioavailability parameter. Now, more than two decades later, we know a little more about the reasons for poor and highly variable bioavailability values for oral pharmaceutical products. However, we still need to understand significantly more about the interactions between advanced oral dosage forms and the complex and dynamic gastrointestinal (GI) physiology of both healthy subjects and patients at all ages, from new-born to elderly, before these dynamic processes can be considered to be sufficiently understood [2]. It is crucial to obtain this knowledge so that it can be incorporated into sophisticated software that can then be applied in decision-making in drug development and regulatory work.

To accomplish high bioavailability and low variability for oral pharmaceutical products, the API needs to be dissolvable and stable in the GI lumen, and also sufficiently absorbed at relevant sites in the small and large intestine. The regional intestinal effective permeability (P_{eff}) is a key biopharmaceutical parameter that determines the absorption potential of the API from any dosage form [3]. Knowledge of the extent of drug absorption from the human large intestine is especially important for accurately predicting the manufacturing potential of a dosage form. The colon, as the final major organ in the GI tract, plays a key role in regulating diarrhea, constipation and the microflora composition, as well as delivery of drugs that are intended for prolonged release and administered once daily [4]. Although the regional intestinal P_{eff} is an important biopharmaceutical parameter, the final drug absorption profile for a drug in the intestinal tract is determined by the interplay of various processes such as motility, transit, solubility, dissolution, precipitation and stability. The Biopharmaceutics Classification System (BCS) of drugs provides information relevant to understanding and predicting GI drug absorption and bioavailability in general that is also relevant to the absorption potential for the colon [5,6].

There are many GI absorption models that investigate transport mechanisms, determine the P_{eff} and predict the plasma pharmacokinetic profile throughout the drug discovery/development process [7]. These models are often applied in the following order: in silico, in vitro, in situ and, most importantly, in vivo (Figure 1). In silico simulation of the absorption process from the GI tract has recently been used to optimize the API release rate, dose and dose distribution from the various release fractions in MR dosage forms. The accurate, reliable in silico prediction of GI absorption data for novel APIs and their dosage forms, vital for drug discovery and pharmaceutical product development, is a major challenge. Establishing an in vitro-in vivo link is also important, as emphasized in a recent report on patient-centric drug development from a product quality perspective [8]. Modeling and simulation approaches are used to characterize this in vitro-in vivo link with respect to the influence and clinical relevance of disease. Recently, eleven large pharmaceutical companies responded to a questionnaire regarding their use of in vitro and in silico biopharmaceutics tools for predicting in vivo outcomes. The companies are using these predictive models at various drug development stages, during regulatory contact for, for example, scientific advice, and for drug applications of various kinds [9]. Biorelevant dissolution-absorption physiologically based pharmacokinetic (PBPK) modeling and simulation were used by 88% of the responding companies in early drug development processes. The biopharmaceutical models were especially useful for investigating the impact of API particle size on intestinal drug absorption and for investigating different pharmaceutical dosage forms.

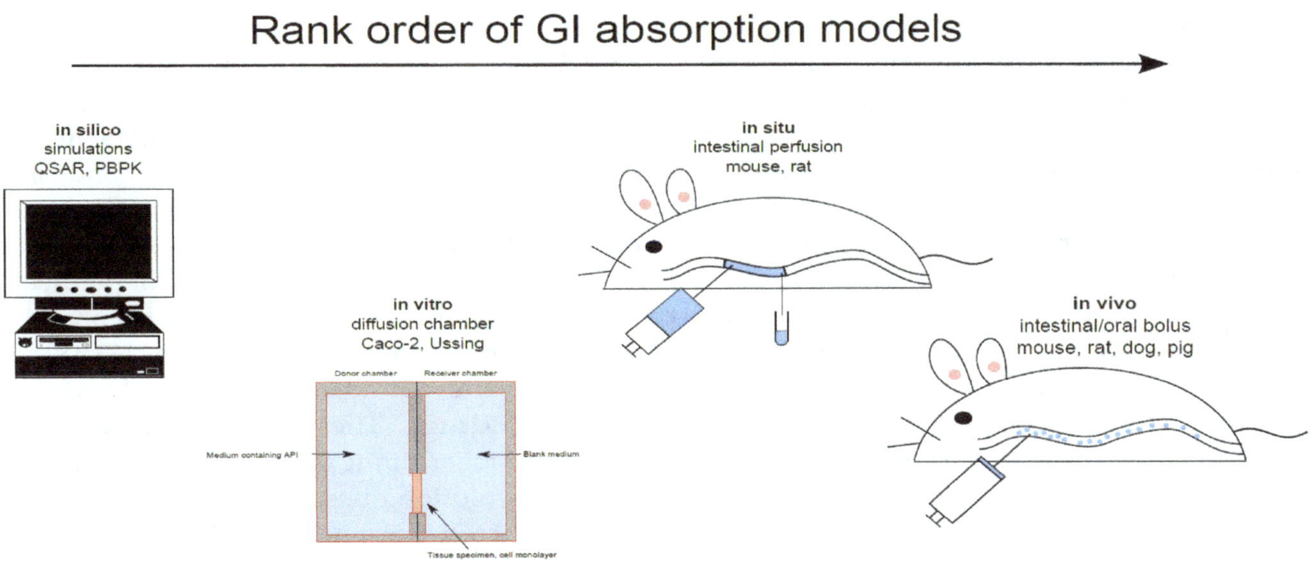

Figure 1. Gastrointestinal (GI) non-clinical absorption models ranked according to the order of their use in the drug discovery/development process for investigating transport mechanisms, determining intestinal permeability, and predicting plasma pharmacokinetic profiles. API = active pharmaceutical ingredient; PBPK = physiologically based pharmacokinetics; QSAR = quantitative structure-activity relationships.

Extensive early human research has established that a good correlation exists between P_{eff} determined using the SPIP model and the F_{abs} from an immediate-release, dosage form [10]. Pharmacokinetic/mass-balance clinical studies are the best way of determining the fraction absorbed for an orally administered drug. However, these mass balance studies are very complex and expensive, as they require the API to be radiolabeled to enable validation of the drug and metabolite recovery [11]. Since the Food and Drug Administration (FDA) and European Medicines Agency bioequivalence guidelines use the F_{abs} to classify the permeation of drugs through the intestine in the BCS, the FDA BCS guidance committee have suggested using F_{abs} as a surrogate for P_{eff} [12].

The main objective of this review is to discuss recent advancements in the overall investigation and in vivo prediction of GI drug absorption. Intestinal P_{eff} has been widely used to determine the rate and extent of the intestinal absorption of orally administered drugs in humans. Among the various biopharmaceutical processes discussed, the focus of the review will be on intestinal permeability at different sites along the intestine.

2. In Silico Gastrointestinal Absorption Predictions

In silico methods are now becoming widely used by the pharmaceutical industry and regulatory agencies to support decisions regarding dosage form development, bioequivalence and other bridging development processes. Pharmaceutical characteristics such as the particle size of the API and the coating layer, which affect the dissolution and subsequent intestinal absorption of the drug, and the plasma drug concentration-time profile are often applied [8]. Another common application for theoretical predictive software is to establish intestinal permeability and the quantitative structure-activity relationship (QSAR). These computer programs relate various molecular descriptors and physicochemical properties of the drug molecule (e.g., lipophilicity, the logarithmic acid dissociation constant pKa, hydrogen bonds, molecular mass) to crucial biopharmaceutical processes [13]. The success of a computational approach in predicting membrane permeability in the early high-throughput drug discovery phase is dependent on the statistical approach, the choice of molecular descriptors, and the quality of the experimental permeability data. The QSAR approach is consequently of limited use in the drug development process; it is primarily used for excluding molecules with obvious permeability limitations [14]. However, because of the increase in computer power, studies of drug permeation can now be performed using complex molecular simulations. These models can simulate the interaction between a molecule and a biological membrane, and thereby improve our mechanistic understanding of membrane transport [15,16]. Pharmaceutical scientists interested in developing MR dosage forms have focused their efforts on optimization of drug transport across biological membranes in the small and large intestines. For instance, the formation of intramolecular hydrogen bonds in the lipid bilayer, charge neutralization, and formation of zwitterions have been investigated for optimizing oral drug delivery through lipid bilayers. Alternatively, specific transporter proteins may be targeted by developing structural adaptations or by using a prodrug. In silica software programs for permeation models and hydrodynamic flow models based on chemical engineering approaches have been valuable in optimizing structure-activity relationships to retain key biopharmaceutical properties [17,18].

More complex in silico models are used to predict overall GI absorption and plasma drug concentration-time profiles following oral administration of drugs. These simulations depend on API-specific physiochemical properties, such as solubility and logarithmic distribution coefficient (log D), and other drug parameters, such as disintegration and dissolution rates, physiological parameters (e.g., intestinal pH, transit times, and morphology), flow characteristics, and the drug first-pass effects in gut and liver, as well as subsequent disposition in vivo [19]. Computer simulations should ideally integrate experimental in vitro and in vivo data to increase their accuracy [20]. However, the accuracy of these models in predicting the fraction absorbed from well characterized physicochemical and biopharmaceutical factors is currently too low to compete with experimental in vitro and in vivo studies in drug development [21]. Nonetheless, a validated in silico model could be useful for evaluating, for instance, the impact of changes in drug formulation or drug-drug and food-drug interactions, which could help guide the design of both preclinical studies (for instance, toxicokinetic studies for safety evaluation) and clinical studies [22].

The full results of the survey by Flanagan et al. in 2016 revealed that biorelevant dissolution testing in simulated media and physiologically based dissolution and PBPK studies are widely used for oral drug product development by the European Federation of Pharmaceutical Industries and Associations (EFPIA) participants in the Innovative Tools for Oral Biopharmaceutics (OrBiTo) project, to investigate the interplay between various biopharmaceutics factors [23]. When in vitro dissolution investigation is introduced in the projects, 80% of the companies use biorelevant dissolution media (SGF, FaSSIF, FeSSIF) in the first step, prior to using simplified buffers for BCS class II and IV APIs. In addition, the survey indicated that these data are seldom presented to regulators. Approximately 70% of companies seldom or never submit these biorelevant dissolution data at the investigational new drug stage, and the corresponding fraction at the new drug application/marketing authorization application stage is 60%. The potential usefulness of in vitro dissolution studies performed in biorelevant media for quality control release testing was also considered. Three PBPK software packages (GI-Sim, Simcyp® Simulator, and GastroPlus™) were tested and compared within the OrBiTo project during a blinded "bottom-up" study of human pharmacokinetics. It was found that the bioavailability of orally administered APIs that permeated the intestine poorly was underpredicted, probably because accurate and physiologically relevant estimates of the intestinal surface area, the absorption properties from the large intestine, and/or the role and importance of transport-mediated intestinal permeation were not available [24–26]. The bioavailability of APIs with acidic pKa was underpredicted, possibly because of underestimation of intestinal permeation (role of ionization and transport-mediated absorption) and/or underestimation of the luminal solubilization of weak acids as a result of less-than-optimal intestinal pH settings or underestimation of the bile micelle contribution. The bioavailability of weak bases was overpredicted, suggesting inadequate models of luminal precipitation or absence of in vitro precipitation information. The relative bioavailability of both highly hydrophobic compounds and poorly aqueous-soluble APIs was underpredicted, suggesting inadequate models of solubility/dissolution, underperforming bile dissolution enhancement models and/or lack of biorelevant solubility measurements. These results clearly identify areas for improvement in theoretically based software, modeling strategies, and production of relevant experimental input data.

One emerging area in the in silico prediction of fraction absorbed and bioavailability that has gained regulatory interest and is being prioritized to justify product specifications or formulation/process changes is the use of integrated in silico PBPK absorption models in combination with high quality biopharmaceutical in vitro data [19,27]. For instance, the in silico approach may be useful for demonstrating the bioequivalence of different formulation concepts, defining the API and formulation design space and manufacturing controls, anticipating post-approval manufacturing changes and obtaining biowaivers.

3. Gastrointestinal Experimental Absorption Models

Preclinical GI absorption models are currently in demand for the pharmaceutical development of novel dosage forms and new drug products. However, we need to improve our understanding of the interplay between pharmaceutical, biopharmaceutical, biochemical and physiological factors in determining the fraction absorbed and bioavailability before reliable models can be developed. Currently, our knowledge of GI secretion, GI motility and regional intestinal permeability, in both healthy subjects and patients with GI disease, is limited by the relative inaccessibility of some intestinal segments of the human GI tract [28]. Conventional clinical approaches of exploring and collecting GI content remain invasive, resource intensive, and often unable to capture all the information contained in these heterogeneous GI samples. A new class of GI sampling capsules is available, which is based on an intra-luminal technique that offers the possibilities of the spatial and temporal information of the GI samples [29]. The future use of these clinical techniques in oral biopharmaceutics expects to improve our understanding of the GI processes involved in oral drug delivery. Our understanding of the complex and highly dynamic physiology of the region from mid-jejunum to the sigmoid colon in particular could be significantly improved. One approach to the assessment of intestinal permeability is to use animal models that allow these intestinal regions to be investigated in detail and then to compare the results with those from simple human permeability models such as cell cultures.

3.1. *In Situ*

The various in situ models for determining P_{eff} are often based on disappearance of the drug from a defined perfused intestinal segment. The selected intestinal segment may be continuously perfused, as in the single-pass intestinal perfusion (SPIP) model, or be closed off, as in the closed-loop Doluisio model [30]. Intestinal P_{eff} is calculated in different ways depending on the hydrodynamics in the specific model.

The SPIP model is generally used after the drug discovery phase and in the early formulation development stage of drug development, when more relevant biopharmaceutical data are needed. One major advantage of the SPIP model is that it enables relevant mechanistic investigations of drug absorption and anticipates the effects of various physiological processes. Some of the advantages of the SPIP model over in vitro models are the intact intestinal morphology, the presence of blood flow, the presence of neural and hormonal feed-back mechanisms and the possibility to control luminal conditions [31].

The rat SPIP model is commonly used to investigate GI physiology, membrane drug transport, and the potential for a new drug candidate to be formulated in an oral MR dosage form. The potentially negative effects of abdominal surgery in this model are reduced by concomitant treatment of the rats with parecoxib, a selective cyclo-oxygenase-2 inhibitor that has been shown to positively affect some intestinal functions such as GI motility, epithelial permeability, fluid flux, and ion transport [32–34]. However, in a recent SPIP study, treatment with parecoxib had only minimal effects on membrane permeability and water flux [35]. It was also established that the permeability of the intestine to poorly permeating drugs is best determined on the basis of the appearance of the parent drug in plasma rather than the disappearance of the drug from the perfused intestinal segment (Figure 2) [35]. A study by Dahlgren et al. in 2019 also clearly showed that when the intestinal P_{eff} is estimated using luminal disappearance, it should include negative values in the calculation to increase the accuracy of the final P_{eff} [35].

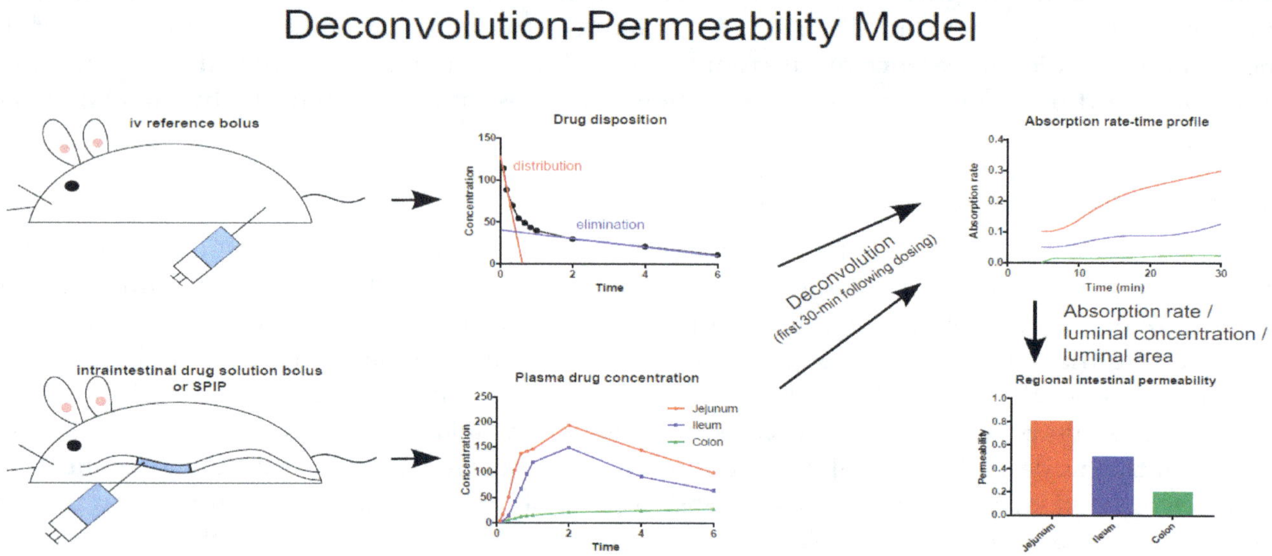

Figure 2. Schematic illustration of the deconvolution-permeability model, which can be used to determine the regional intestinal permeability of model drugs based on their appearance in the plasma following intravenous and intraintestinal administration of the drug in solution [36]. The method has been successfully applied to determination of intestinal permeability in rats, dogs, and humans [3,31,33,35,37,38]. SPIP = single-pass intestinal perfusion.

3.2. *In Vivo*

Classical in vivo single-dose pharmacokinetic models in which drug solutions or formulations are administered orally, or directly into the stomach or intestine in suitable animal species, may also be used to investigate the P_{eff}, the fraction absorbed and the bioavailability. In such studies, the value for the fraction absorbed includes the impact of other biopharmaceutical processes such as dissolution, precipitation, transit, etc. [37]. These in vivo animal models are the most clinically relevant because physiological factors, such as gastric emptying time, luminal water content and drug degradation, and post-absorption first-pass metabolism affect the determined parameters and the predicted outcome. These types of models are obviously less applicable for mechanistic studies of intestinal absorption, as the relative impact of the different factors can be difficult to assess in detail.

When using these in vivo GI models, motility is defined as movements of the GI tract that cause mixing and transit of luminal chyme above the absorptive and secretary intestinal surface. These mixing and transit processes are located both in the lumen and in the area adjacent to the intestinal epithelium, and are coordinated and regulated through a complex circuitous interaction between a number of physiological systems including, but not limited to, the enteric, autonomic, and central nervous systems. It has been suggested that long-distance and short-distance motor activities in the GI tract could interact to propel undigested luminal chyme along the tract, where regional mixing promotes intestinal absorption [39]. If disturbances occur in any of these systems, it could disrupt the coordination of the propulsive peristalsis, potentially leading to dysmotility and ultimately various GI-specific symptoms. The relevance of these motility patterns to the intestinal absorption of drugs and nutrients is an important research topic for the future.

It is also crucial to consider the effects that these GI digestive processes may have on the intestinal absorption of drugs from different formulations and the local effects of some drugs with targets in the lumen (luminal enzymes such as lipases and α-amylases) or receptors on the luminal side of the epithelium. When isolated from the central nervous system, the gut is the only organ that has integrative neuronal activity. This activity may be stimulated by luminal contents that act as specific sensory transducers on certain specific epithelial cells, such as enterochromaffin cells, which release 5-hydroxytryptamine. 5-hydroxytryptamine stimulate intrinsic and extrinsic primary afferent neurons that are present in both the submucosal and myenteric plexuses. The role of integrative neuronal and local endocrine effects on intestinal absorption needs to be better understood.

3.3. *In Vitro*

Common in vitro models for studying membrane permeability include monolayers of cells grown on cell culture filters (e.g., Caco-2 cells), and excised intestinal tissue samples mounted in a diffusion (Ussing) chamber. The apparent permeability (P_{app}) is calculated by relating the mass of the drug appearing in the receiver chamber at multiple time points (dM/dt) to the area of the barrier (A), and the drug concentration in the donor chamber (C_{donor}) [40–42]. The intestinal P_{app} is an intrinsic constant associated with a molecule that relates the flux to the concentration gradient; it can therefore be used to predict drug transport over any type of biological cell barrier by adjusting for, for instance, area, hydrodynamics and the pH of the medium. In addition, the controlled aqueous conditions in a cell-based in vitro system offer the possibility of performing mechanistic transport investigations if the expression and function of the involved proteins are accurate [43,44]. The Ussing chamber system enables regional intestinal permeability [7]. Limitations associated with these models include the high inter- and intra-laboratory variability, and sensitivity of the cell/tissue to the preparation setup and chamber media. For permeability investigations in drug discovery, it is therefore recommended that relative P_{app} values (compared to reference standards) be used, instead of absolute P_{app} values [45]. The BCS can also be used to predict in vivo drug absorption based on in vitro drug dissolution data [6]. It is also well established that these systems are more sensitive for pharmaceutical excipients and enhancers with intended absorption-modifying properties.

One recent and exciting advancement of an in vitro intestinal absorption models is intestinal organoids [46]. Organoid technology from various species bridges the gap between conventional two-dimensional cell line culture and in vivo models [47–49]. One of the objective with this in vitro approach is to improve organ development and accordingly improve the in vivo relevance. Intestinal organoids is expected to become a useful drug development technology for various biopharmaceutical and pharmacokinetic analysis and in vivo predictions.

4. Intestinal Membrane Transport

The movement of ions, transmitter compounds, nutrients and other endogenous substances across various biological membranes is a central dynamic molecular process that is essential for life in mammals. Selective permeability is a key feature of biological membranes and is determined by the physicochemical properties of the lipid bilayer and the channel-forming membrane proteins together with the physicochemical properties and molecular structure of the drug molecules. These transport processes across biological membranes with a diverse composition occur via direct and indirect energy-demanding carrier-mediated (CM) mechanisms even against a concentration gradient. Facilitated membrane diffusion, passive membrane diffusion and paracellular diffusion occur along a concentration gradient. Biological membranes encapsulate cells and their contents to optimize the various functions that cells are responsible for in a living organism. At the core of any biological membrane is a lipid bilayer, which in vivo can be composed of hundreds of different types of lipid molecules. Membrane lipids have amphiphilic molecular properties with a polar head group and a non-polar tail comprising esterified fatty acids. These lipid molecules vary widely in terms of size, chemical structure and polarity and can be combined and assembled to provide a wide variety of physical properties and functions.

Movement of drugs across various membranes is essential for many pharmacokinetic and pharmacodynamic processes. The basic nature of drug transport is divided into transcellular and paracellular processes, where the transcellular route is the most common (Figure 3). Transcellular transport, either passive diffusion or CM, occurs across the intestinal cell (enterocyte), through both the apical and basolateral membranes. Paracellular transport occurs between the epithelial cells. During the last decade, a large number of published articles have discussed the existence and role of passive diffusion across biological membranes as a relevant mechanism [50–53]. The overall conclusion is that passive transcellular diffusion is the predominant mechanism for transfer of drug substances, but that this co-exists with CM trans-membrane processes.

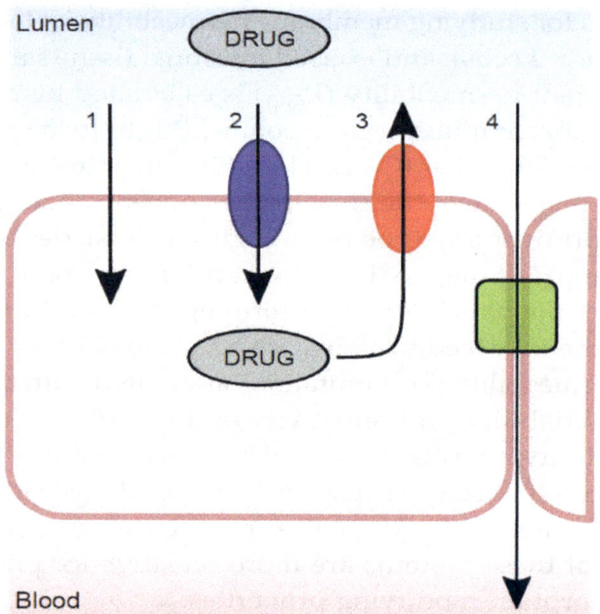

Figure 3. The transport mechanisms from the lumen across the intestinal epithelium, which determine the net permeability of a luminally dissolved drug molecule. (**1**) Passive transcellular diffusion; (**2**) absorptive carrier-mediated transport; (**3**) efflux carrier-mediated transport; and (**4**) passive paracellular diffusion.

The pH partitioning theory states that the charged species of a weak acid or base do not contribute to passive lipoidal diffusion across the cell lipid bilayer, as they do not partition into octanol [54]. The permeation of these molecules is highly dependent on the pH at the surface of the lipid cell membrane and the pKa of the drug [20]. This has been experimentally illustrated in the Caco-2 cell monolayer model, where the transport of alfentanil and cimetidine was linearly correlated to the un-ionized fraction (i.e., the pH) [55]. The pH also affects the transport of propranolol in Caco-2 cells, MDCK cells, and the rat Ussing chamber; reducing the pH from 7.4 to 6.5 in the donor compartment reduces the transport of this low molecular mass (259.3) basic drug [56].

The concept of the pH partitioning theory for predicting passive membrane transport of drugs and other xenobiotics is, however, not that straightforward [54]. This is illustrated by the permeation of a charged species across cell barriers in the water-filled paracellular pores, a process which is typically faster for smaller (molecular mass less than approximately 250) and longer molecules [57,58]. These paracellular pores can also have different charge-selectivity, based on the claudin proteins (a large family of proteins that modulate paracellular permeability [59,60]. More research is required on the mechanisms that underlie differences in paracellular absorption for drugs of different sizes (g/mol), both within and between species (Figure 4A,B) [58,61]. Although we have some information on the roles of individual claudins, some of which are thought to form charge- and size-selective tight-junction pores for smaller molecules, relatively little is known about their interactions [62]. Further, the permeation of charged anions through the lipoidal membrane can be many times more rapid than expected, controlling membrane transport at all in vivo-relevant pHs [54]. This must be taken into consideration to avoid overestimation of the fraction of a compound that is transported across the paracellular route [63]. Two extensively permeating compounds, ketoprofen and metoprolol, are, for example, rapidly absorbed across human and rat intestinal mucosal barriers, where the pH is between 6.5 and 7.4 and only about 0.1 to 1% is in the neutral form [3,64]. This is despite the pH-dependent decrease in ketoprofen permeation observed when increasing pHs in a parallel artificial membrane permeability assay [65]. In addition, quaternary ammonium compounds also permeate lipoidal membranes to different degrees, despite their permanent charge [65,66].

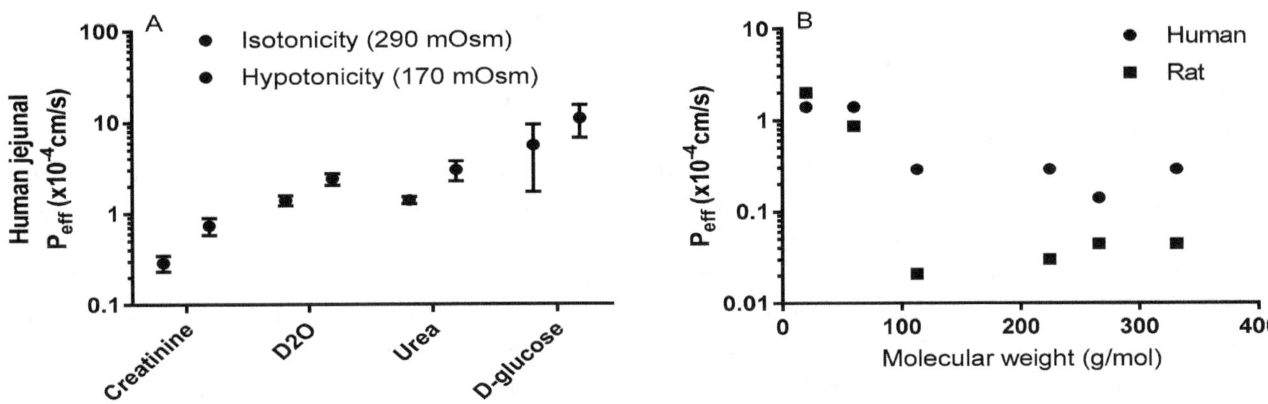

Figure 4. (**A**) The influence of luminal tonicity on the effective permeability (P_{eff}) of human jejunum to four model compounds with different molecular masses: D_2O 20 g/mol, urea 60 g/mol, creatinine 113 g/mol, and D-glucose 180 g/mol [58]; (**B**) The influence of the molecular mass of six passively absorbed compounds on the human and rat jejunal P_{eff} values: D_2O 20 g/mol, urea 60 g/mol, creatinine 113 g/mol, terbutaline 225 g/mol, atenolol 266 g/mol, furosemide 331 g/mol [58]. Figures are remade based on historical data.

Hence, it is obvious that the pH partitioning theory alone cannot be used to predict the passive lipoidal diffusion of compounds. Several non-CM transcellular transport mechanisms have consequently been proposed to account for the transport of charged and/or hydrophilic drug molecules (as well as other xenobiotics) across the lipoidal membrane. Two mechanisms, based on molecular simulations and membrane experiments, propose the creation of water pores, or lipid head-group pores [67]. Water pores are thought to exist because water has been shown to be present in the assumed water-free membrane core [68]. This water reduces the energy cost of a hydrophilic drug dissolving in the lipoidal membrane, as the need for molecular dehydration is reduced. The total cost for a drug dissolving in the lipid membrane is hence lower than would be expected. Lipid head-group pores are assumed to be formed by an interaction of ions or the drug doxorubicin with the lipid head groups [69,70]. These head-group pores would then facilitate the transport of charged and hydrophilic compounds.

An additional theory is that transmembrane transporter proteins increase the transport of small hydrophilic molecules by facilitating transport along the exterior [71]. This would not, however, explain the substantial transport of charged molecules over protein-free lipoidal membranes. The transport of charged molecules by co-permeation with a counter ion is also a possibility [72,73]. However, given the rapid transport of, for instance, ketoprofen in vivo, and the limited effect of ion pairing with non-organic ions, ion pairing seems a less likely mechanism behind the substantial absorption of some charged drugs in vivo [3,73,74].

Among the molecular descriptors evaluated by Lipinski (e.g., polar surface area, hydrogen bond donors (HBDs)/acceptors, Log D), the number of HBDs is the most restrictive when it comes to intestinal membrane transport/absorption [18,75]. Two drugs breaking this rule (i.e., >5 HBDs and high fraction absorbed), tetracycline and rifampicin, were recently analyzed to evaluate their potential for crossing the intestinal membrane by passive lipoidal diffusion, regardless of their unfavorable properties [67]. A liposomal permeation assay showed that rifampicin and metoprolol permeated to a similar extent, and that tetracycline and labetalol permeated similarly, suggesting that these >5 HBD drugs can be absorbed by passive lipoidal diffusion to a substantial degree.

To explain why some drugs are absorbed by passive lipoidal diffusion, regardless of their unfavorable physicochemical properties, it is necessary to find more complex descriptions of the molecular interaction with the lipoidal membrane. Permanently charged molecules, for instance, vary in their degree of passive permeation according to their ability to spread the charge over several ring structures [66]. Several experimental studies (based on nuclear magnetic resonance and the crystalline form) have also shown that intramolecular hydrogen bonding can mask polar structures and thus increase membrane transport [76,77]. The principle is that the intramolecular hydrogen bonding reduces the thermodynamic penalty of dissolving in the membrane core [15].

This has also been shown in several molecular dynamics simulations of the transport of solutes across a lipid bilayer. A drug usually loses degrees of freedom when dissolving in the membrane core. The energy demand is reduced by intramolecular hydrogen bonding and with lipid head groups. By changing the type of intramolecular hydrogen bonding in β-blockers, the molecular conformation can be changed, depending on its position in the membrane bilayer. For instance, a more elongated shape is favored in the center of the lipid bilayer and a more folded structure is favored at the interface. The more elongated, flexible shape allowed in the center favors a flip flop to the other side, while also generally reducing the cost of dehydration, when dissolving in the bilayer by forming intramolecular hydrogen bonds [67,68]. Tetracycline is thus able to hide three of the six hydrogen donor groups by intramolecular hydrogen bonding, as shown experimentally by high-intensity synchrotron radiation [78].

The accuracy of QSAR predictions of intestinal absorption, based solely on the physicochemical descriptors of a molecule, is also significantly improved by including molecular dynamics simulations [79]. Molecular simulations have also been successfully used to predict the effects of cholesterol in the lipid membrane; cholesterol typically makes the bilayer more stiff and less permeable (also described as reduced membrane fluidity) [15]. Molecular simulation investigations have also been able to replicate experimental data on the relative permeation of a set of compounds (atenolol < pindolol < progesterone < testosterone), based on free energy transfer in different depths of the membrane bilayer [80].

The detailed discussion of the intestinal membrane transport of atenolol below is based on data from various sources, ranging from theoretical calculations to human pharmacokinetic data.

5. Atenolol

Transport mechanisms for a low molecular mass drug is often interpreted based on multiple techniques. Atenolol is a well-recognized BCS class III drug that has been proposed to be transported by transcellular, paracellular as well as with various CM processes (see below). Atenolol is therefore suitable for illustrating the complexity of classifying a drug's transport mechanisms, as data from various in silico, in vitro, in situ, and in vivo models are needed.

Following oral administration to humans, the plasma pharmacokinetics of atenolol are linear for doses of 25 to 200 mg for the area under the concentration-time curve (AUC), and for oral doses of 0.1 to 200 mg (1.4–2857 μg/kg) for the maximum concentration (Cmax) (Figure 5) [81–83]. There is a 1.5- and 1.6-fold higher AUC for doses of 0.03 and 0.1, respectively, and a 1.6-fold higher Cmax for the 0.03 mg oral dose, than for the average values in the clinical oral dose range [81,84]. These data from microdosing studies (0.03 and 0.1 mg) mean that there is some CM contribution to the intestinal permeation of atenolol at lower oral doses/luminal concentrations. Xenopus laevis oocyte transport studies suggest that OATP1A2 might be a plausible absorptive transporter for atenolol [85]. However, it should be mentioned that there was no statistical difference in AUC between 0.1 and 50 mg in one of the microdosing studies, which suggests that passive and non-saturable transmembrane transport might prevail in vivo for atenolol [81]. In addition, the difference in plasma exposure is unrelated to the elimination of atenolol, which is 100% renal (of parent drug) in both humans and rats, and is unaffected by oral doses in the range of 0.3–80 mg/kg [86–88]. Consequently, the dose of atenolol does not affect its renal clearance, which has been shown to be partly mediated by the efflux transporters OCT2 and MATE 1 and 2 [89]. This is also in accordance with their Km values (280, 32, and 76 μM, respectively), which are substantially higher than the maximum plasma concentration of 2 μM following an oral dose of 100 mg [88].

In humans, co-administration of oral atenolol with apple or orange juice in the fasted state decreases the plasma exposure of atenolol to 20–50% of that observed with water [90,91]. This interaction may be the result of inhibition of absorptive transporters, as observed for fexofenadine and celiprolol [92]. However, given the large volumes of apple juice (600–1200 mL) or orange juice (200 mL) used, and the notoriously high osmolarity of fruit juices, the reduced exposure is probably the result of an increased intestinal transit time. Similar results have been observed for oral atenolol when administered with a non-absorbable osmotic load (500–700 mOsm); the intestinal transit time was decreased from 180 to 60 min, and exposure was decreased from 1.7 to about 0.4 mg × h/L, compared to water [93].

Efflux ratios (B–A:A–B) of 2.3 and 3.5 were observed for atenolol in cell monolayer studies (Caco-2 and IPEC-J2); these were reduced to 1.7 and 1.1 with coadministration of the Pgp inhibitors verapamil and zosuquidar, respectively [94,95]. This suggests that atenolol might be a Pgp substrate. However, other Caco-2 studies (atenolol concentrations between 30 μM and 3.8 mM) have shown that the efflux ratio of atenolol is 1, is concentration independent, and differs between laboratories (ranging from 0.18 to 3.76) and between batches in the same laboratory [44,96,97]. The P_{app} of atenolol was also unaffected by verapamil in the mouse SPIP model, and after knockout of the Pgp gene [98,99]. Similarly, the absorption rate of atenolol was increased in the rat in an in situ jejunal loop study with co-administration of another Pgp inhibitor, cyclosporine [100]. In addition, atenolol has linear pharmacokinetics (AUC, Cmax) in rats following oral administration of doses between 0.55 μg and 5.5 mg (0.167–1670 μg/kg), and oral co-administration of the Pgp inhibitor itraconazole to humans did not affect its pharmacokinetics (Figure 5) [101,102].

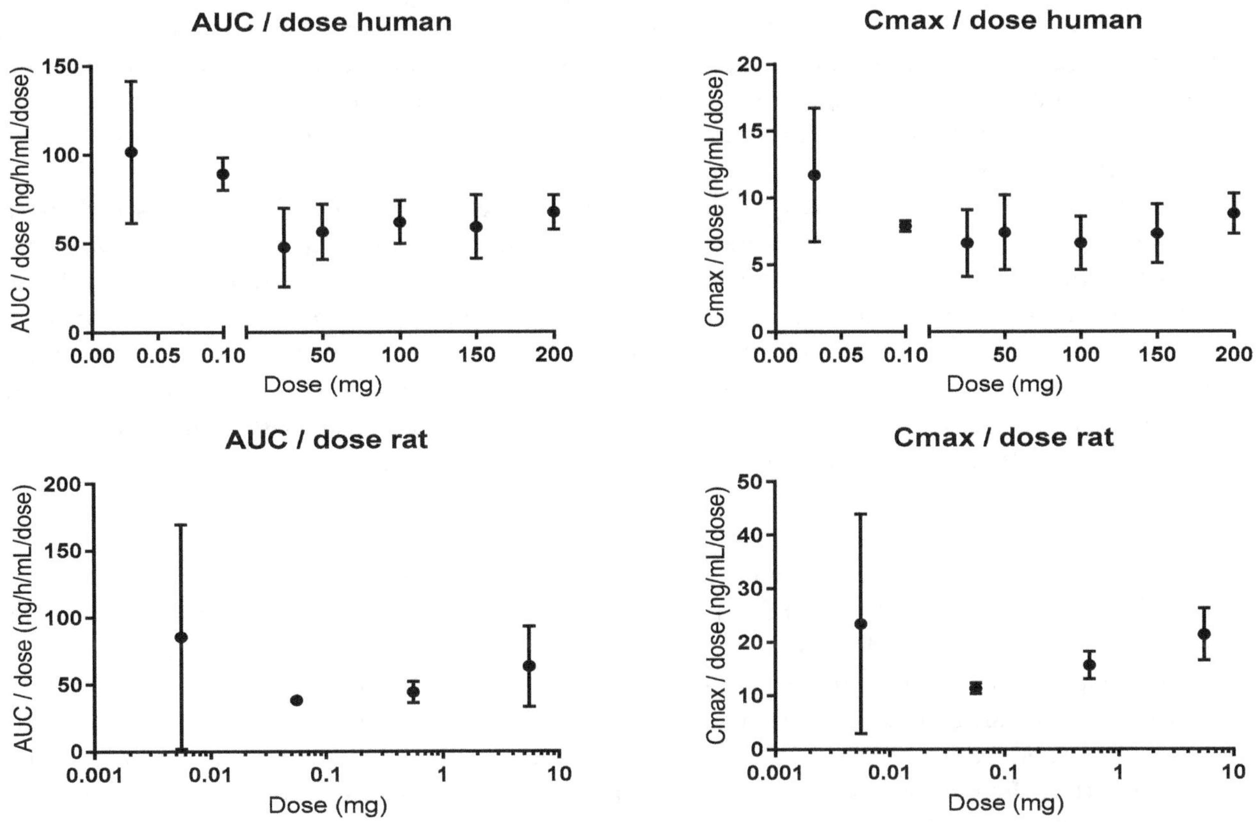

Figure 5. Dose proportionality in the area under the concentration-time curve (**AUC**) and maximum concentrations; (**Cmax**) of atenolol in humans (0.1–200 mg) and rats (0.55 μg–5.5 mg) [81–83,102]. Figures are made based on historical data.

In humans, the regional intestinal P_{eff} for atenolol was substantial (Figure 6A) [3]. However, this difference almost disappeared when the P_{eff} value was corrected for the regional intestinal difference in surface area (Figure 6B) [103]. These results indicate that passive membrane permeation is the predominant transport mechanism of atenolol.

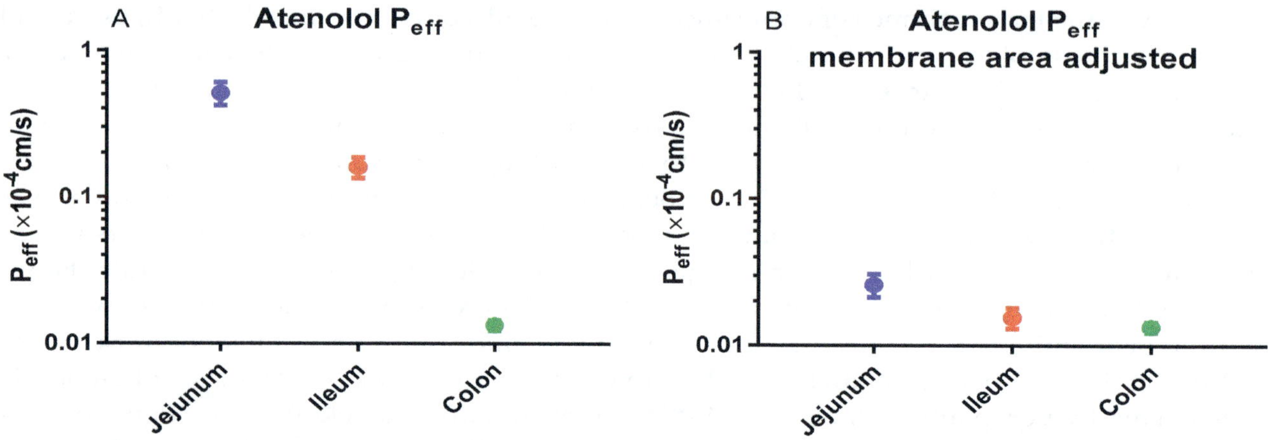

Figure 6. (**A**) Regional intestinal effective permeability (P_{eff}) of atenolol in humans [3]. (**B**) Surface area (villi and folds)-adjusted regional intestinal P_{eff} values for atenolol in humans: jejunum 19-fold, ileum 10-fold, colon 1-fold [103]. Figures are remade based on historical data.

Atenolol has generally been regarded as a passive permeability marker in blood-brain barrier (BBB) transport studies, based on the linear plasma clearance of the drug into the brain over time [104,105]. However, its use as a marker for passive permeability in the brain and intestines has been questioned recently [106]. based on the free fraction of atenolol in the brain extracellular fluid (3.5% of that in blood plasma at steady state), suggesting CM efflux of atenolol from the BBB by an unknown transporter protein. The paper did not address why the data from a rat study evaluating BBB transport should be valid for the intestine, however.

In summary, there are conflicting data regarding the contribution of CM transporters to the intestinal absorption of atenolol. Cell-based assays have indicated an affinity for efflux proteins, but one of two oral microdosing studies indicated an affinity for influx proteins. However, taking into account all the available data, including extensive oral plasma pharmacokinetic data from a wide dose range (0.1–100 mg), it seems likely that the influence of intestinal transporters on the intestinal absorption of atenolol is, at most, modest. Atenolol can be considered to be transported almost exclusively by the passive route (lipoidal and/or paracellular), especially at oral human doses > 1 mg (>14 μg/kg), representing an intestinal concentration of about 20 μM (1 mg in 250 mL).

6. Conclusions

Investigation of intestinal drug permeation processes is crucial for the development of oral pharmaceutical products. The prevailing hypothesis for the permeation of drugs through the intestine involves several parallel CM and passive permeation mechanisms (such as passive lipoidal diffusion, CM uptake transport, CM efflux, paracellular diffusion, mucus resistance, endocytosis and transcytosis). The determination of an intestinal P_{eff} for a drug is based on the technique, model and conditions applied and is influenced by the multiple interactions between the drug molecule and the biological membrane. Further development of the oral biopharmaceutics system requires the development of novel in vitro models and the use of human and animal in vivo techniques. For instance intestinal organoid technologies that bridge the gap between conventional two-dimensional cell line culture and in vivo models are expected to improve our mechanistic understanding. These innovative and more complex in vitro models need extensive comparison to high-quality in vivo data. Novel clinical techniques are expected to provide an improved understanding and high-quality data of biopharmaceutical relevant GI processes.

Abbreviations

API	Active pharmaceutical ingredient
AUC	Area under the concentration-time curve
BBB	Blood-brain barrier
BCS	Biopharmaceutics classification system
CM	Carrier-mediated
C_{max}	Maximum concentration
F	Bioavailability
F_{abs}	Fraction absorbed
FDA	US Food and Drug Administration
GI	Gastrointestinal
HBD	Hydrogen bond donor
MR	Modified-release
OrBiTo	Innovative Tools for Oral Biopharmaceutics
P_{eff}	Effective permeability
PBPK	Physiologically based pharmacokinetic
QSAR	Quantitative structure-activity relationship
SPIP	Single-pass intestinal perfusion

References

1. Hellriegel, E.T.; Bjornsson, T.D. Interpatient variability in bioavailability is related to the extent of absorption: Implications for bioavailability and bioequivalence studies. *Clin. Pharm. Ther.* **1996**, *60*, 601–607. [CrossRef]
2. Sjögren, E.; Abrahamsson, B.; Augustijns, P.; Becker, D.; Bolger, M.B.; Brewster, M.; Brouwers, J.; Flanagan, T.; Harwood, M.; Heinen, C.; et al. In vivo methods for drug absorption–comparative physiologies, model selection, correlations with in vitro methods (IVIVC), and applications for formulation/API/excipient characterization including food effects. *Eur. J. Pharm. Sci.* **2014**, *57*, 99–151.
3. Dahlgren, D.; Roos, C.; Lundqvist, A.; Abrahamsson, B.; Tannergren, C.; Hellström, P.M.; Sjögren, E.; Lennernäs, H. Regional intestinal permeability of three model drugs in human. *Mol. Pharm.* **2016**, *13*, 3013–3021. [CrossRef] [PubMed]
4. Sellers, R.S.; Morton, D. The Colon From Banal to Brilliant. *Toxicol. Pathol.* **2013**, *42*, 67–81. [CrossRef] [PubMed]
5. Tannergren, C.; Bergendal, A.; Lennernäs, H.; Abrahamsson, B. Toward an increased understanding of the barriers to colonic drug absorption in humans: Implications for early controlled release candidate assessment. *Mol. Pharm.* **2009**, *6*, 60–73. [CrossRef] [PubMed]
6. Amidon, G.L.; Lennernas, H.; Shah, V.P.; Crison, J.R. A theoretical basis for a biopharmaceutic drug classification: The correlation of in vitro drug product dissolution and in vivo bioavailability. *Pharm. Res.* **1995**, *12*, 413–420. [CrossRef] [PubMed]
7. Roos, C.; Dahlgren, D.; Tannergren, C.; Abrahamsson, B.; Sjögren, E.; Lennernas, H. Regional intestinal permeability in rats: A comparison of methods. *Mol. Pharm.* **2017**, *14*, 4252–4261. [CrossRef] [PubMed]
8. Heimbach, T.; Suarez-Sharp, S.; Kakhi, M.; Holmstock, N.; Olivares-Morales, A.; Pepin, X.; Sjögren, E.; Tsakalozou, E.; Seo, P.; Li, M. *Dissolution and Translational Modeling Strategies Toward Establishing an In Vitro-In Vivo Link—A Workshop Summary Report. ed.*; Springer: Berlin/Heidelberg, Germany, 2019.
9. Lennernas, H.; Lindahl, A.; Van Peer, A.; Ollier, C.; Flanagan, T.; Lionberger, R.; Nordmark, A.; Yamashita, S.; Yu, L.; Amidon, G. In vivo predictive dissolution (IPD) and biopharmaceutical modeling and simulation: Future use of modern approaches and methodologies in a regulatory context. *Mol. Pharm.* **2017**, *14*, 1307–1314. [CrossRef]

10. Lennernas, H. Intestinal permeability and its relevance for absorption and elimination. *Xenobiotica* **2007**, *37*, 1015–1051. [CrossRef]
11. Roffey, S.J.; Obach, R.S.; Gedge, J.I.; Smith, D.A. What is the objective of the mass balance study? A retrospective analysis of data in animal and human excretion studies employing radiolabeled drugs. *Drug Metab. Rev.* **2007**, *39*, 17–43. [CrossRef]
12. Food, Drug and Administration. *Guidance for Industry: Waiver of In Vivo Bioavailability and Bioequivalence Studies for Immediate-Release Solid Oral Dosage Forms Based on a Biopharmaceutics Classification System*; Food Drug Administrain: Rockville, MD, USA, 2000.
13. Gozalbes, R.; Jacewicz, M.; Annand, R.; Tsaioun, K.; Pineda-Lucena, A. QSAR-based permeability model for drug-like compounds. *Bioorg. Med. Chem.* **2011**, *19*, 2615–2624. [CrossRef]
14. Scior, T.; Medina-Franco, J.; Do, Q.T.; Martínez-Mayorga, K.; Yunes Rojas, J.; Bernard, P. How to recognize and workaround pitfalls in QSAR studies: A critical review. *Curr. Med. Chem.* **2009**, *16*, 4297–4313. [CrossRef]
15. Awoonor-Williams, E.; Rowley, C.N. Molecular simulation of nonfacilitated membrane permeation. *Biochim. Biophys. Acta (BBA) Biomembr.* **2016**, *1858*, 1672–1687. [CrossRef]
16. Lee, C.T.; Comer, J.; Herndon, C.; Leung, N.; Pavlova, A.; Swift, R.V.; Tung, C.; Rowley, C.N.; Amaro, R.E.; Chipot, C. Simulation-based approaches for determining membrane permeability of small compounds. *J. Chem. Inf. Model.* **2016**, *56*, 721–733. [CrossRef]
17. Mathiowetz, A.M. *Design Principles for Intestinal Permeability of Cyclic Peptides*; Cyclic Peptide Design, Ed.; Springer: Berlin/Heidelberg, Germany, 2019; pp. 1–15.
18. Lipinski, C.A.; Lombardo, F.; Dominy, B.W.; Feeney, P.J. Experimental and computational approaches to estimate solubility and permeability in drug discovery and development settings. *Adv. Drug Deliv. Rev.* **1997**, *23*, 3–25. [CrossRef]
19. Kostewicz, E.S.; Aarons, L.; Bergstrand, M.; Bolger, M.B.; Galetin, A.; Hatley, O.; Jamei, M.; Lloyd, R.; Pepin, X.; Rostami-Hodjegan, A.; et al. PBPK models for the prediction of in vivo performance of oral dosage forms. *Eur. J. Pharm. Sci.* **2013**, *57*, 300–321. [CrossRef]
20. Sugano, K. Introduction to computational oral absorption simulation. *Expert Opin. Drug Metab. Toxicol.* **2009**, *5*, 259–293. [CrossRef]
21. Sjögren, E.; Thörn, H.; Tannergren, C. In silico modeling of gastrointestinal drug absorption: Predictive performance of three physiologically based absorption models. *Mol. Pharm.* **2016**, *13*, 1763–1778. [CrossRef]
22. Jones, H.; Chen, Y.; Gibson, C.; Heimbach, T.; Parrott, N.; Peters, S.; Snoeys, J.; Upreti, V.; Zheng, M.; Hall, S. Physiologically based pharmacokinetic modeling in drug discovery and development: A pharmaceutical industry perspective. *Clin. Pharm. Ther.* **2015**, *97*, 247–262. [CrossRef]
23. Flanagan, T.; Van Peer, A.; Lindahl, A. Use of physiologically relevant biopharmaceutics tools within the pharmaceutical industry and in regulatory sciences: Where are we now and what are the gaps? *Eur. J. Pharm. Sci.* **2016**, *91*, 84–90. [CrossRef]
24. Margolskee, A.; Darwich, A.S.; Pepin, X.; Aarons, L.; Galetin, A.; Rostami-Hodjegan, A.; Carlert, S.; Hammarberg, M.; Hilgendorf, C.; Johansson, P. IMI–oral biopharmaceutics tools project–evaluation of bottom-up PBPK prediction success part 2: An introduction to the simulation exercise and overview of results. *Eur. J. Pharm. Sci.* **2017**, *96*, 610–625. [CrossRef]
25. Margolskee, A.; Darwich, A.S.; Pepin, X.; Pathak, S.M.; Bolger, M.B.; Aarons, L.; Rostami-Hodjegan, A.; Angstenberger, J.; Graf, F.; Laplanche, L. IMI–oral biopharmaceutics tools project–evaluation of bottom-up PBPK prediction success part 1: Characterisation of the OrBiTo database of compounds. *Eur. J. Pharm. Sci.* **2017**, *96*, 598–609. [CrossRef]
26. Darwich, A.S.; Margolskee, A.; Pepin, X.; Aarons, L.; Galetin, A.; Rostami-Hodjegan, A.; Carlert, S.; Hammarberg, M.; Hilgendorf, C.; Johansson, P. IMI–Oral biopharmaceutics tools project–Evaluation of bottom-up PBPK prediction success part 3: Identifying gaps in system parameters by analysing In Silico performance across different compound classes. *Eur. J. Pharm. Sci.* **2017**, *96*, 626–642. [CrossRef]
27. Wagner, C.; Zhao, P.; Pan, Y.; Hsu, V.; Grillo, J.; Huang, S.; Sinha, V. Application of physiologically based pharmacokinetic (PBPK) modeling to support dose selection: Report of an FDA public workshop on PBPK. *CPT Pharmacomet. Syst. Pharmacol.* **2015**, *4*, 226–230. [CrossRef]
28. Grønlund, D.; Poulsen, J.; Sandberg, T.; Olesen, A.; Madzak, A.; Krogh, K.; Frøkjaer, J.; Drewes, A. Established and emerging methods for assessment of small and large intestinal motility. *Neurogastroenterol. Motil.* **2017**, *29*, e13008. [CrossRef]

29. Amoako-Tuffour, Y.; Jones, M.L.; Shalabi, N.; Labbé, A.; Vengallatore, S.; Prakash, S. Ingestible gastrointestinal sampling devices: State-of-the-art and future directions. *Crit. Rev. ™ Biomed. Eng.* **2014**, *42*, 1–15. [CrossRef]
30. Lozoya-Agullo, I.; Gonzalez-Alvarez, I.; Zur, M.; Fine-Shamir, N.; Cohen, Y.; Markovic, M.; Garrigues, T.M.; Dahan, A.; Gonzalez-Alvarez, M.; Merino-Sanjuán, M. Closed-Loop Doluisio (Colon, Small Intestine) and Single-Pass Intestinal Perfusion (Colon, Jejunum) in Rat—Biophysical Model and Predictions Based on Caco-2. *Pharm. Res.* **2018**, *35*, 2. [CrossRef]
31. Dahlgren, D.; Roos, C.; Lundqvist, A.; Langguth, P.; Tannergren, C.; Sjöblom, M.; Sjögren, E.; Lennernas, H. Preclinical effect of absorption modifying excipients on rat intestinal transport of five model compounds and the intestinal barrier marker 51Cr-EDTA. *Mol. Pharm.* **2017**, *14*, 4243–4251. [CrossRef]
32. Sedin, J.; Sjöblom, M.; Nylander, O. The selective cyclooxygenase-2 inhibitor parecoxib markedly improves the ability of the duodenum to regulate luminal hypertonicity in anaesthetized rats. *Acta Physiol.* **2012**, *205*, 433–451. [CrossRef]
33. Dahlgren, D.; Roos, C.; Lundqvist, A.; Tannergren, C.; Sjöblom, M.; Sjögren, E.; Lennernas, H. Effect of absorption-modifying excipients, hypotonicity, and enteric neural activity in an in vivo model for small intestinal transport. *Int. J. Pharm.* **2018**, *549*, 239–248. [CrossRef]
34. Nylander, O. The impact of cyclooxygenase inhibition on duodenal motility and mucosal alkaline secretion in anaesthetized rats. *Acta Physiol.* **2011**, *201*, 179–192. [CrossRef]
35. Dahlgren, D.; Roos, C.; Peters, K.; Lundqvist, A.; Tannergren, C.; Sjögren, E.; Sjöblom, M.; Lennernäs, H. Evaluation of drug permeability calculation based on luminal disappearance and plasma appearance in the rat single-pass intestinal perfusion model. *Eur. J. Pharm. Biopharm.* **2019**, *142*, 31–37. [CrossRef]
36. Sjögren, E.; Dahlgren, D.; Roos, C.; Lennernas, H. Human in vivo regional intestinal permeability: Quantitation using site-specific drug absorption data. *Mol. Pharm.* **2015**, *12*, 2026–2039. [CrossRef]
37. Dahlgren, D.; Roos, C.; Johansson, P.; Tannergren, C.; Lundqvist, A.; Langguth, P.; Sjöblom, M.; Sjögren, E.; Lennernas, H. The effects of three absorption-modifying critical excipients on the in vivo intestinal absorption of six model compounds in rats and dogs. *Int. J. Pharm.* **2018**, *547*, 158–168. [CrossRef]
38. Dahlgren, D.; Roos, C.; Johansson, P.; Lundqvist, A.; Tannergren, C.; Abrahamsson, B.; Sjögren, E.; Lennernäs, H. Regional intestinal permeability in dogs: Biopharmaceutical aspects for development of oral modified-release dosage forms. *Mol. Pharm.* **2016**, *13*, 3022–3033. [CrossRef]
39. Baker, J.R.; Dickens, J.R.; Koenigsknecht, M.; Frances, A.; Lee, A.A.; Shedden, K.A.; Brasseur, J.G.; Amidon, G.L.; Sun, D.; Hasler, W.L. Propagation Characteristics of Fasting Duodeno-Jejunal Contractions in Healthy Controls Measured by Clustered Closely-spaced Manometric Sensors. *J. Neurogastroenterol. Motil.* **2019**, *25*, 100. [CrossRef]
40. Akamatsu, M.; Fujikawa, M.; Nakao, K.; Shimizu, R. In silico prediction of human oral absorption based on QSAR analyses of PAMPA permeability. *Chem. Biodivers.* **2009**, *6*, 1845–1866. [CrossRef]
41. Sjöberg, Å.; Lutz, M.; Tannergren, C.; Wingolf, C.; Borde, A.; Ungell, A.L. Comprehensive study on regional human intestinal permeability and prediction of fraction absorbed of drugs using the Ussing chamber technique. *Eur. J. Pharm. Sci.* **2013**, *48*, 166–180. [CrossRef]
42. Artursson, P. Epithelial transport of drugs in cell culture. I: A model for studying the passive diffusion of drugs over intestinal absorbtive (Caco-2) cells. *J. Pharm. Sci.* **1990**, *79*, 476–482. [CrossRef]
43. Nielsen, C.U.; Andersen, R.; Brodin, B.; Frokjaer, S.; Taub, M.E.; Steffansen, B. Dipeptide model prodrugs for the intestinal oligopeptide transporter. Affinity for and transport via hPepT1 in the human intestinal Caco-2 cell line. *J. Control. Release* **2001**, *76*, 129–138. [CrossRef]
44. Neuhoff, S.; Ungell, A.L.; Zamora, I.; Artursson, P. pH-dependent bidirectional transport of weakly basic drugs across Caco-2 monolayers: Implications for drug–drug interactions. *Pharm. Res.* **2003**, *20*, 1141–1148. [CrossRef]
45. Larregieu, C.A.; Benet, L.Z. Drug Discovery and Regulatory Considerations for Improving In Silico and In Vitro Predictions that Use Caco-2 as a Surrogate for Human Intestinal Permeability Measurements. *AAPS J.* **2013**, *15*, 483–497. [CrossRef]
46. Mochel, J.P.; Jergens, A.E.; Kingsbury, D.; Kim, H.J.; Martín, M.G.; Allenspach, K. Intestinal stem cells to advance drug development, precision, and regenerative medicine: A paradigm shift in translational research. *AAPS J.* **2018**, *20*, 17. [CrossRef]

47. Chandra, L.; Borcherding, D.C.; Kingsbury, D.; Atherly, T.; Ambrosini, Y.M.; Bourgois-Mochel, A.; Yuan, W.; Kimber, M.; Qi, Y.; Wang, Q. Derivation of adult canine intestinal organoids for translational research in gastroenterology. *BMC Biol.* **2019**, *17*, 33. [CrossRef]
48. Fujii, M.; Matano, M.; Toshimitsu, K.; Takano, A.; Mikami, Y.; Nishikori, S.; Sugimoto, S.; Sato, T. Human intestinal organoids maintain self-renewal capacity and cellular diversity in niche-inspired culture condition. *Cell Stem Cell.* **2018**, *23*, 787–793. [CrossRef]
49. Sato, T.; Clevers, H. Growing self-organizing mini-guts from a single intestinal stem cell: Mechanism and applications. *Science* **2013**, *340*, 1190–1194. [CrossRef]
50. Kell, D.B.; Dobson, P.D.; Bilsland, E.; Oliver, S.G. The promiscuous binding of pharmaceutical drugs and their transporter-mediated uptake into cells: What we (need to) know and how we can do so. *Drug Discov. Today* **2013**, *18*, 218–239. [CrossRef]
51. Kell, D.B.; Dobson, P.D.; Oliver, S.G. Pharmaceutical drug transport: The issues and the implications that it is essentially carrier-mediated only. *Drug Discov. Today.* **2011**, *16*, 704–714. [CrossRef]
52. Sugano, K.; Kansy, M.; Artursson, P.; Avdeef, A.; Bendels, S.; Di, L.; Ecker, G.F.; Faller, B.; Fischer, H.; Gerebtzoff, G.; et al. Coexistence of passive and carrier-mediated processes in drug transport. *Nat. Rev. Drug Discov.* **2010**, *9*, 597–614. [CrossRef]
53. Smith, D.; Artursson, P.; Avdeef, A.; Di, L.; Ecker, G.F.; Faller, B.; Houston, J.B.; Kansy, M.; Kerns, E.H.; Krämer, S.D. Passive lipoidal diffusion and carrier-mediated cell uptake are both important mechanisms of membrane permeation in drug disposition. *Mol. Pharm.* **2014**, *11*, 1727–1738. [CrossRef]
54. Thomae, A.V.; Wunderli-Allenspach, H.; Krämer, S.D. Permeation of aromatic carboxylic acids across lipid bilayers: The pH-partition hypothesis revisited. *Biophys. J.* **2005**, *89*, 1802–1811. [CrossRef]
55. Palm, K.; Luthman, K.; Ros, J.; Gråsjö, J.; Artursson, P. Effect of molecular charge on intestinal epithelial drug transport: pH-dependent transport of cationic drugs. *J. Pharm. Exp. Ther.* **1999**, *291*, 435–443.
56. Zheng, Y.; Benet, L.Z.; Okochi, H.; Chen, X. pH dependent but not P-gp dependent bidirectional transport study of S-propranolol: The importance of passive diffusion. *Pharm. Res.* **2015**, *32*, 2516–2526. [CrossRef]
57. Karasov, W.H. Integrative physiology of transcellular and paracellular intestinal absorption. *J. Exp. Biol.* **2017**, *220*, 2495–2501. [CrossRef]
58. Fagerholm, U.; Nilsson, D.; Knutson, L.; Lennernäs, H. Jejunal permeability in humans in vivo and rats in situ: Investigation of molecular size selectivity and solvent drag. *Acta Physiol. Scand.* **1999**, *165*, 315–324. [CrossRef]
59. Lingaraju, A.; Long, T.M.; Wang, Y.; Austin II, J.R.; Turner, J.R. Conceptual barriers to understanding physical barriers. *Semin. Cell Dev. Biol.* **2015**, *42*, 13–21. [CrossRef]
60. Van Itallie, C.M.; Fanning, A.S.; Anderson, J.M. Reversal of charge selectivity in cation or anion-selective epithelial lines by expression of different claudins. *Am. J. Physiol. Ren. Physiol.* **2003**, *285*, F1078–F1084. [CrossRef]
61. Price, E.R.; Brun, A.; Gontero-Fourcade, M.; Fernández-Marinone, G.; Cruz-Neto, A.P.; Karasov, W.H.; Caviedes-Vidal, E. Intestinal water absorption varies with expected dietary water load among bats but does not drive paracellular nutrient absorption. *Physiol. Biochem. Zool.* **2015**, *88*, 680–684. [CrossRef]
62. Günzel, D.; Yu, A.S. Claudins and the modulation of tight junction permeability. *Physiol. Rev.* **2013**, *93*, 525–569. [CrossRef]
63. Avdeef, A.; Tam, K.Y. How Well Can the Caco-2/Madin– Darby Canine Kidney Models Predict Effective Human Jejunal Permeability? *J. Med. Chem.* **2010**, *53*, 3566–3584. [CrossRef]
64. Wang, Y.T.; Mohammed, S.D.; Farmer, A.D.; Wang, D.; Zarate, N.; Hobson, A.R.; Hellström, P.M.; Semler, J.R.; Kuo, B.; Rao, S.S. Regional gastrointestinal transit and pH studied in 215 healthy volunteers using the wireless motility capsule: Influence of age, gender, study country and testing protocol. *Aliment. Pharm. Ther.* **2015**, *42*, 761–772. [CrossRef]
65. Sugano, K.; Nabuchi, Y.; Machida, M.; Asoh, Y. Permeation characteristics of a hydrophilic basic compound across a bio-mimetic artificial membrane. *Int. J. Pharm.* **2004**, *275*, 271–278. [CrossRef]
66. Fischer, H.; Kansy, M.; Avdeef, A.; Senner, F. Permeation of permanently positive charged molecules through artificial membranes—Influence of physico-chemical properties. *Eur. J. Pharm. Sci.* **2007**, *31*, 32–42. [CrossRef]
67. Krämer, S.D.; Aschmann, H.E.; Hatibovic, M.; Hermann, K.F.; Neuhaus, C.S.; Brunner, C.; Belli, S. When barriers ignore the "rule-of-five". *Adv. Drug Deliv. Rev.* **2016**, *101*, 62–74. [CrossRef]

68. Bemporad, D.; Luttmann, C.; Essex, J. Behaviour of small solutes and large drugs in a lipid bilayer from computer simulations. *Biochim. Biophys. Acta (BBA) Biomembr.* **2005**, *1718*, 1–21. [CrossRef]
69. Vorobyov, I.; Olson, T.E.; Kim, J.H.; Koeppe Ii, R.E.; Andersen, O.S.; Allen, T.W. Ion-induced defect permeation of lipid membranes. *Biophys. J.* **2014**, *106*, 586–597. [CrossRef]
70. Van Hell, A.J.; Melo, M.N.; Van Blitterswijk, W.J.; Gueth, D.M.; Braumuller, T.M.; Pedrosa, L.R.; Song, J.Y.; Marrink, S.J.; Koning, G.A.; Jonkers, J. Defined lipid analogues induce transient channels to facilitate drug-membrane traversal and circumvent cancer therapy resistance. *Sci. Rep.* **2013**, *3*, 1949. [CrossRef]
71. Xiang, T.X.; Anderson, B. Influence of a transmembrane protein on the permeability of small molecules across lipid membranes. *J. Membr. Biol.* **2000**, *173*, 187–201. [CrossRef]
72. Miller, J.M.; Dahan, A.; Gupta, D.; Varghese, S.; Amidon, G.L. Enabling the intestinal absorption of highly polar antiviral agents: Ion-pair facilitated membrane permeation of zanamivir heptyl ester and guanidino oseltamivir. *Mol. Pharm.* **2010**, *7*, 1223–1234. [CrossRef]
73. Neubert, R. Ion pair transport across membranes. *Pharm. Res.* **1989**, *6*, 743–747. [CrossRef]
74. Khavrutskii, I.V.; Gorfe, A.A.; Lu, B.; McCammon, J.A. Free energy for the permeation of Na+ and Cl− ions and their ion-pair through a zwitterionic dimyristoyl phosphatidylcholine lipid bilayer by umbrella integration with harmonic fourier beads. *J. Am. Chem. Soc.* **2009**, *131*, 1706–1716. [CrossRef]
75. Bickerton, G.R.; Paolini, G.V.; Besnard, J.; Muresan, S.; Hopkins, A.L. Quantifying the chemical beauty of drugs. *Nat. Chem.* **2012**, *4*, 90. [CrossRef]
76. Alex, A.; Millan, D.S.; Perez, M.; Wakenhut, F.; Whitlock, G.A. Intramolecular hydrogen bonding to improve membrane permeability and absorption in beyond rule of five chemical space. *Med. Chem. Comm.* **2011**, *2*, 669–674. [CrossRef]
77. Kuhn, B.; Mohr, P.; Stahl, M. Intramolecular hydrogen bonding in medicinal chemistry. *J. Med. Chem.* **2010**, *53*, 2601–2611. [CrossRef]
78. Clegg, W.; Teat, S.J. Tetracycline hydrochloride: A synchrotron microcrystal study. *Acta Crystallogr. Sect. C Cryst. Struct. Commun.* **2000**, *56*, 1343–1345. [CrossRef]
79. Bennion, B.J.; Be, N.A.; McNerney, M.W.; Lao, V.; Carlson, E.M.; Valdez, C.A.; Malfatti, M.A.; Enright, H.A.; Nguyen, T.H.; Lightstone, F.C. Predicting a drug's membrane permeability: A computational model validated with in vitro permeability assay data. *J. Phys. Chem. B.* **2017**, *121*, 5228–5237. [CrossRef]
80. Orsi, M.; Essex, J.W. Permeability of drugs and hormones through a lipid bilayer: Insights from dual-resolution molecular dynamics. *Soft Matter* **2010**, *6*, 3797–3808. [CrossRef]
81. Mahajan, R.; Parvez, A.; Gupta, K. Microdosing vs. Therapeutic dosing for evaluation of pharmacokinetic data: A comparative study. *J. Young Pharm.* **2009**, *1*, 290. [CrossRef]
82. Wakelkamp, M.; Alván, G.; Paintaud, G.; Hedman, A. Dose proportional absorption of 25–150 mg atenolol. *Eur. J. Clin. Pharmacol.* **1993**, *44*, 305–306. [CrossRef]
83. Fitzgerald, J.; Ruffin, R.; Smedstad, K.; Roberts, R.; McAinsh, J. Studies on the pharmacokinetics and pharmacodynamics of atenolol in man. *Eur. J. Clin. Pharm.* **1978**, *13*, 81–89. [CrossRef]
84. Ieiri, I.; Maeda, K.; Sasaki, T.; Kimura, M.; Hirota, T.; Chiyoda, T.; Miyagawa, M.; Irie, S.; Iwasaki, K.; Sugiyama, Y. Microdosing clinical study: Pharmacokinetic, pharmacogenomic (SLCO2B1), and interaction (grapefruit juice) profiles of celiprolol following the oral microdose and therapeutic dose. *J. Clin. Pharm.* **2012**, *52*, 1078–1089. [CrossRef]
85. Kato, Y.; Miyazaki, T.; Kano, T.; Sugiura, T.; Kubo, Y.; Tsuji, A. Involvement of influx and efflux transport systems in gastrointestinal absorption of celiprolol. *J. Pharm. Sci.* **2009**, *98*, 2529–2539. [CrossRef]
86. Reeves, P.R.; Barnfield, D.J.; Longshaw, S.; McIntosh, D.A.; Winrow, M.J. Disposition and metabolism of atenolol in animals. *Xenobiotica* **1978**, *8*, 305–311. [CrossRef]
87. Reeves, P.R.; McAinsh, J.; McIntosh, D.A.; Winrow, M.J. Metabolism of atenolol in man. *Xenobiotica* **1978**, *8*, 313–320. [CrossRef]
88. Mason, W.; Winer, N.; Kochak, G.; Cohen, I.; Bell, R. Kinetics and absolute bioavailability of atenolol. *Clin. Pharm. Ther.* **1979**, *25*, 408–415. [CrossRef]
89. Yin, J.; Duan, H.; Shirasaka, Y.; Prasad, B.; Wang, J. Atenolol Renal Secretion Is Mediated by Human Organic Cation Transporter 2 and Multidrug and Toxin Extrusion Proteins. *Drug Metab. Dispos.* **2015**, *43*, 1872–1881. [CrossRef]
90. Jeon, H.; Jang, I.J.; Lee, S.; Ohashi, K.; Kotegawa, T.; Ieiri, I.; Cho, J.Y.; Yoon, S.H.; Shin, S.G.; Yu, K.S.; et al. Apple juice greatly reduces systemic exposure to atenolol. *Br. J. Clin. Pharm.* **2013**, *75*, 172–179. [CrossRef]

91. Lilja, J.; Raaska, K.; Neuvonen, P. Effects of orange juice on the pharmacokinetics of atenolol. *Eur. J. Clin. Pharm.* **2005**, *61*, 337–340. [CrossRef]
92. Bailey, D.G. Fruit juice inhibition of uptake transport: A new type of food–drug interaction. *Br. J. Clin. Pharm.* **2010**, *70*, 645–655. [CrossRef]
93. Riley, S.; Kim, M.; Sutcliffe, F.; Kapas, M.; Rowland, M.; Turnberg, L. Effects of a non-absorbable osmotic load on drug absorption in healthy volunteers. *Br. J. Clin. Pharm.* **1992**, *34*, 40–46. [CrossRef]
94. Augustijns, P.; Mols, R. HPLC with programmed wavelength fluorescence detection for the simultaneous determination of marker compounds of integrity and P-gp functionality in the Caco-2 intestinal absorption model. *J. Pharm. Biomed. Anal.* **2004**, *34*, 971–978. [CrossRef]
95. Saaby, L.; Helms, H.C.C.; Brodin, B. IPEC-J2 MDR1, a novel high-resistance cell line with functional expression of human P-glycoprotein (ABCB1) for drug screening studies. *Mol. Pharm.* **2016**, *13*, 640–652. [CrossRef]
96. Hayeshi, R.; Hilgendorf, C.; Artursson, P.; Augustijns, P.; Brodin, B.; Dehertogh, P.; Fisher, K.; Fossati, L.; Hovenkamp, E.; Korjamo, T. Comparison of drug transporter gene expression and functionality in Caco-2 cells from 10 different laboratories. *Eur J. Pharm. Sci.* **2008**, *35*, 383–396. [CrossRef]
97. Tronde, A.; Nordén, B.; Jeppsson, A.B.; Brunmark, P.; Nilsson, E.; Lennernäs, H.; Bengtsson, U.H. Drug absorption from the isolated perfused rat lung–correlations with drug physicochemical properties and epithelial permeability. *J. Drug Target.* **2003**, *11*, 61–74. [CrossRef]
98. Mols, R.; Brouwers, J.; Schinkel, A.H.; Annaert, P.; Augustijns, P. Intestinal perfusion with mesenteric blood sampling in wild-type and knockout mice evaluation of a novel tool in biopharmaceutical drug profiling. *Drug Metab. Dispos.* **2009**, *37*, 1334–1337. [CrossRef]
99. Brouwers, J.; Mols, R.; Annaert, P.; Augustijns, P. Validation of a differential in situ perfusion method with mesenteric blood sampling in rats for intestinal drug interaction profiling. *Biopharm. Drug Dispos.* **2010**, *31*, 278–285. [CrossRef]
100. Terao, T.; Hisanaga, E.; Sai, Y.; Tamai, I.; Tsuji, A. Active secretion of drugs from the small intestinal epithelium in rats by P-glycoprotein functioning as an absorption barrier. *J. Pharm. Pharm.* **1996**, *48*, 1083–1089. [CrossRef]
101. Lilja, J.J.; Backman, J.T.; Neuvonen, P.J. Effect of itraconazole on the pharmacokinetics of atenolol. *Basic Clin. Pharm. Toxicol.* **2005**, *97*, 395–398. [CrossRef]
102. Ni, J.; Ouyang, H.; Aiello, M.; Seto, C.; Borbridge, L.; Sakuma, T.; Ellis, R.; Welty, D.; Acheampong, A. Microdosing assessment to evaluate pharmacokinetics and drug metabolism in rats using liquid chromatography-tandem mass spectrometry. *Pharm. Res.* **2008**, *25*, 1572–1582. [CrossRef]
103. Helander, H.F.; Fändriks, L. Surface area of the digestive tract-revisited. *Scand. J. Gastroenterol.* **2014**, *49*, 681–689. [CrossRef]
104. Van Bree, J.B.; Baljet, A.V.; van Geyt, A.; de Boer, A.G.; Danhof, M.; Breimer, D.D. The unit impulse response procedure for the pharmacokinetic evaluation of drug entry into the central nervous system. *J. Pharm. Biopharm.* **1989**, *17*, 441–462. [CrossRef]
105. Nakagawa, S.; Deli, M.A.; Kawaguchi, H.; Shimizudani, T.; Shimono, T.; Kittel, A.; Tanaka, K.; Niwa, M. A new blood–brain barrier model using primary rat brain endothelial cells, pericytes and astrocytes. *Neurochem. Int.* **2009**, *54*, 253–263. [CrossRef]
106. Chen, X.; Slättengren, T.; Lange, E.C.; Smith, D.E.; Hammarlund-Udenaes, M. Revisiting atenolol as a low passive permeability marker. *Fluids Barriers CNS* **2017**, *14*, 30. [CrossRef]

5

In Silico Prediction of Plasma Concentrations of Fluconazole Capsules with Different Dissolution Profiles and Bioequivalence Study Using Population Simulation

Marcelo Dutra Duque [1,2,*], **Daniela Amaral Silva** [1,3], **Michele Georges Issa** [1], **Valentina Porta** [1], **Raimar Löbenberg** [3] **and Humberto Gomes Ferraz** [1]

1 Department of Pharmacy, Faculty of Pharmaceutical Sciences, Universidade de São Paulo—USP, Av. Prof. Lineu Prestes, 580, São Paulo—SP 05508-000, Brazil; amaralsi@ualberta.ca (D.A.S.); michelegeorges@usp.br (M.G.I.); vporta@usp.br (V.P.); sferraz@usp.br (H.G.F.)

2 Department of Pharmaceutical Sciences, Institute of Environmental, Chemical and Pharmaceutical Sciences, Universidade Federal de São Paulo—UNIFESP, Rua São Nicolau, 210, Centro, Diadema—SP 09913-030, Brazil

3 Faculty of Pharmacy & Pharmaceutical Sciences, Katz Group-Rexall Centre for Pharmacy & Health Research, University of Alberta, 11361 – 87 Avenue, Edmonton, AB T6G 2E1, Canada; raimar@ualberta.ca

* Correspondence: marcelo.duque@unifesp.br

Abstract: A biowaiver is accepted by the Brazilian Health Surveillance Agency (ANVISA) for immediate-release solid oral products containing Biopharmaceutics Classification System (BCS) class I drugs showing rapid drug dissolution. This study aimed to simulate plasma concentrations of fluconazole capsules with different dissolution profiles and run population simulation to evaluate their bioequivalence. The dissolution profiles of two batches of the reference product Zoltec® 150 mg capsules, A1 and A2, and two batches of other products (B1 and B2; C1 and C2), as well as plasma concentration–time data of the reference product from the literature, were used for the simulations. Although products C1 and C2 had drug dissolutions < 85% in 30 min at 0.1 M HCl, simulation results demonstrated that these products would show the same in vivo performance as products A1, A2, B1, and B2. Population simulation results of the ln-transformed 90% confidence interval for the ratio of C_{max} and AUC_{0-t} values for all products were within the 80–125% interval, showing to be bioequivalent. Thus, even though the in vitro dissolution behavior of products C1 and C2 was not equivalent to a rapid dissolution profile, the computer simulations proved to be an important tool to show the possibility of bioequivalence for these products.

Keywords: fluconazole; biowaiver; dissolution; Biopharmaceutics Classification System (BCS); bioequivalence; GastroPlus™

1. Introduction

Bioavailability (BA) is the rate and extent of absorption of an active pharmaceutical ingredient from a dosage form when it becomes available at the site of action. Drug products that are pharmaceutical equivalents are considered bioequivalent and, therefore, interchangeable when BA is not statistically different between the two products after administration at the same dose and under similar experimental conditions in a bioequivalence (BE) study. For purposes of establishing BE, a test product must be compared to a reference product [1–3].

For highly soluble and highly permeable drugs, categorized as class I according to the Biopharmaceutics Classification System (BCS), the waiver of BE studies can be considered in immediate-release (IR) products [4]. In this case, the rate and extent of absorption are not dependent on drug dissolution but rather solely on gastric emptying [5]. In IR products containing BCS class I drugs with rapid (≥85% in 30 min) or very rapid (≥85% in 15 min) in vivo dissolution in relation to gastric emptying, BA is independent of drug dissolution or gastrointestinal transit time [4].

The Brazilian Health Surveillance Agency (ANVISA) guidance for biowaiver [6] allows the waiver of bioequivalence studies for BCS class I drugs that are described in a Normative Instruction [7], which was updated later [8]. For this purpose, the applicant should provide data demonstrating rapid drug dissolution from the IR dosage form, i.e., at least 85% of the drug dissolved within 30 min under all conditions tested for both test and reference products [6]. The dissolution test conditions accepted by ANVISA are suggested in the Pharmaceutical Equivalence and Comparative Studies of Dissolution Profiles guidance [9]: apparatus 1 at 100 rpm or apparatus 2 at 50 rpm; dissolution media pH 1.2 HCl or simulated gastric fluid without enzyme, pH 4.5 and pH 6.8 (or simulated intestinal fluid); 900 mL and temperature 37 ± 1 °C.

Fluconazole is a triazole antifungal agent indicated for superficial and systemic infections, and is available for oral administration in capsules containing 50–150 mg of the drug; it is generally well absorbed, showing a BA of about 90% [10]. Due to its clinical and biopharmaceutical characteristics, fluconazole is a candidate for BCS class I biowaiver [11,12]. This drug is described in the Brazilian Health Surveillance Agency's Normative Instruction list of drug candidates for the waiver of bioequivalence studies according to BCS [8].

Currently, the prediction of intestinal absorption of drugs based on computer simulations using advanced compartmental absorption and transit (ACAT) and physiologically-based pharmacokinetic (PBPK) models is a reality [13–21]. Computer software can be used to predict oral absorption of drugs from IR products containing different dissolution profiles, helping formulation scientists to decide on the best dissolution test conditions or formulation, gaining time, and reducing costs in drug development [17]. Computer simulations have been demonstrated to also be important for biowaiver extension for BCS class II [14,22,23] and class III drugs [24].

The dissolution criterion for the biowaiver (rapid or very rapid dissolution) of IR products containing 32 BCS class I drugs was evaluated by [25], which showed that very rapid dissolution is not necessary to guarantee BE according to BCS. However, considering the importance of appropriate dissolution tests and the possibility of requesting a waiver of BE studies when in vitro dissolution data are available for BCS class I drugs [3,6], the objective of this article was to use computer simulations to predict the plasma concentrations of fluconazole capsules with different dissolution profiles using the software GastroPlus™, comparing products with rapid or very rapid drug dissolution to products that do not meet this criterion, and evaluating whether they could be bioequivalent using simulated population studies.

2. Methods

2.1. Plasma Concentration Simulations

The software GastroPlus™ version 9.0 (Simulations Plus Inc., Lancaster, CA, USA) was used to predict the oral absorption of fluconazole 150 mg capsules from different manufacturers compared to the reference product in Brazil, Zoltec® 150 mg capsules (Laboratórios Pfizer Ltda, Guarulhos, Brazil).

For such, a fluconazole database was created in GastroPlus™. Input data consisted of values taken from the literature, including but not limited to drug solubility, pKa, and the logarithm of the partition coefficient (Log P), as well as other parameters obtained using the ADMET Predictor™ (Absorption, Distribution, Metabolism, Elimination and Toxicity Predictor) (Simulations Plus, Lancaster, CA, USA) module in GastroPlus™ (Table 1).

Table 1. Input data used in GastroPlus™ to simulate plasma concentrations.

Parameter	Value	Reference/Data Source
Solubility (mg/mL)	8.03 at pH 0.8; 6.91 at pH 4.5; 7.82 at pH 6.8; 6.90 at pH 7.4	[11,12]
pKa	2.56; 2.94; 11.01	[26,27]
Log P	0.82	ADMET Predictor™
Dose (mg)	150	[28,29]
Effective permeability, Peff (cm/s × 10^{-4})	4.06	ADMET Predictor™
Blood/plasma ratio	1.1	ADMET Predictor™
Unbound plasma (%)	27.41	ADMET Predictor™
Physiology	Human, fasting conditions	[28]
Body weight (kg)	61	[28]

Plasma concentrations of the reference product (Zoltec® 150 mg capsules) previously reported by [28] were extracted from the original figure using Web Plot Digitizer [30] and used in the PKPlus™ module in GastroPlus™ to build a compartmental pharmacokinetic (PK) model. PKPlus™ is an optional module in GastroPlus™ that uses intravenous or oral plasma concentration–time data to calculate the most appropriate modeling (one-, two-, or three-compartmental models) and generate PK parameters for simulations [31].

In the GastroPlus™ fluconazole database, records were created for two batches of three different products, namely A1, A2, B1, B2, C1, and C2, as previously described by [29]; A1 and A2 were batches #1 and #2, respectively, of the reference product Zoltec® 150 mg capsules, whereas B1, B2, C1, and C2 were batches #1 and #2 of two different products found in the Brazilian market. The dissolution tests were performed using the United States Pharmacopeia (USP) apparatus 1 (basket) with 900 mL of 0.1 M HCl at 37 ± 0.5 °C and 100 rpm for 30 min and yielded results (n = 6 for each product) [29] that were used in the software to simulate the plasma concentration for each product (A1, A2, B1, B2, C1, and C2).

The simulations were run in GastroPlus™ in order to obtain the predicted values of the plasma concentration. Concentration curves were compared to that of the reference product (Ref) with respect to regression parameters generated by the software: coefficient of determination (R^2), sum of square error (SSE), root mean square error (RMSE), and mean absolute error (MAE).

The pharmacokinetic parameters %F (% bioavailable), which is the percent of drug that reached the systemic circulation, T_{max}, C_{max}, and AUC (Area Under the Curve) were generated by GastroPlus™.

2.2. Population Simulations

Population Simulator is one of the simulation modes present in GastroPlus™. This mode allows the user to run simulated clinical trials for virtual subjects, combining physiology and pharmacokinetic variability within populations and considering formulation variables used as input data in the software. In this mode, Monte Carlo simulations are used to randomly generate each subject to have a unique set of parameters (gastrointestinal transit time and pH; pharmacokinetic parameters; plasma protein binding; small intestine, stomach, caecum and colon dimensions; and hepatic blood flow rate). Variations in each parameter are randomly generated for each simulated virtual subject [31].

In this way, population simulations were run in GastroPlus™ for each product (A1, A2, B1, B2, C1, and C2) considering in the Population Simulator mode the number of output data points to be saved for each virtual subject as 25. The number of virtual subjects chosen for the simulations was 28. This was the same number of volunteers enrolled in the bioequivalence study described by reference

#28. Bioequivalence between each product and the reference Zoltec® 150 mg capsules [28] from population simulation results were presented as 90% confidence interval (CI) for the ratio of C_{max} and AUC_{0-t} using ln-transformed data. GastroPlus™ automatically set in green the values of 90% CI for C_{max} and AUC_{0-t} that are within the 80–125% interval, according to regulatory agencies [32,33]. The end time used for the simulations was 96 h and the average AUC_{0-t}/AUC_{0-inf} ratio was calculated.

3. Results and Discussion

After adding plasma concentrations of the reference product, Zoltec® 150 mg capsules, in the software GastroPlus™ and selecting compartmental PK modeling, the PKPlus™ module calculated the most appropriate compartmental model (one, two, or three compartments) considering the administration of fluconazole 150 mg as IR capsules to subjects with an average weight of 61 kg under fasting conditions. Compartmental models were compared by evaluating R^2 and the Akaike Information Criterion (AIC). As shown in Table 2, the two-compartmental model presented the best fit due to the highest R^2 and lowest AIC value. Table 3 presents the PK parameters predicted using the selected model.

Table 2. Elimination half-life (T1/2), coefficient of determination (R^2), and Akaike Information Criterion (AIC) for compartmental models calculated by PKPlus™ module.

Compartmental Models	T1/2 (h)	R^2	AIC
One-compartmental	29.55	0.9936	−80.27
Two-compartmental	30.25	0.9977	−87.53
Three-compartmental	1523.50	0.9976	−83.84

Table 3. Pharmacokinetic (PK) parameters from the two-compartmental model calculated by the PKPlus™ module.

Parameter	Value
Clearance, CL (L/h)	0.99565
Central compartment volume, Vc (L)	30.66
Elimination half-life, T1/2 (h)	30.25
Distribution rate constant from C1 to C2, K12 (h^{-1})	0.16515
Distribution rate constant from C2 to C1, K21 (h^{-1})	0.41884
Distribution volume of second compartment, V2 (L/kg)	0.19817

Mean (± standard deviation, SD) clearance (CL) and central compartment volume (Vc) values for fluconazole in healthy subjects are reported in the literature as 1.272 ± 0.219 L/h and 46.3 ± 7.9 L (38.4 to 54.2 L), respectively [34], whereas T1/2 of fluconazole is about 30 h [10]. Thus, the CL value calculated using PKPlus™ is in accordance with the literature, and the calculated Vc is near to the lowest (38.4 L) value reported by [34].

Figure 1 shows the percent of fluconazole dissolved over time during dissolution tests of products A1, A2, B1, B2, C1, and C2 [29].

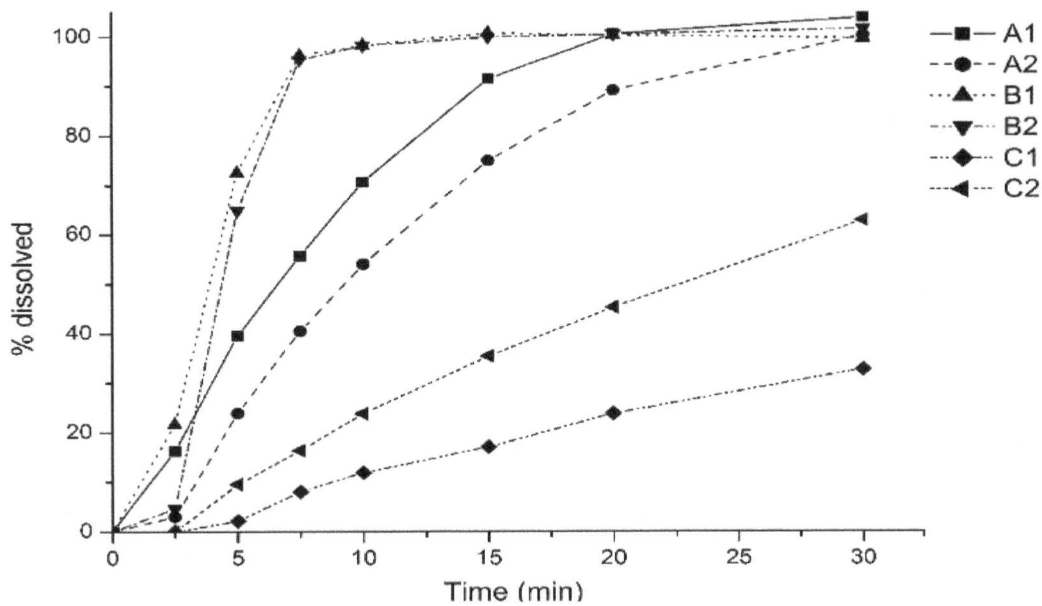

Figure 1. Dissolution profiles of products A1, A2, B1, B2, C1, and C2, obtained in USP Apparatus 1 (basket) with 900 mL of 0.1 M HCl at 37 ± 0.5 °C and 100 rpm for 30 min (adapted from [29], with permission from *Brazilian Journal of Pharmaceutical Sciences*, 2019).

Products A1, A2, B1, B2, C1, and C2 had 91.4%, 74.9%, 100.7%, 99.9%, 17.1%, and 35.4% of drug dissolved in 15 min, respectively. Although product A2 have shown less than 85% of the drug dissolved in 15 min, only products C1 and C2 had values that did not reach 85% of drug dissolved at the end of the test (Figure 1). Considering these findings, products C1 and C2 are not expected to be bioequivalent to the reference product.

Fluconazole is a high solubility and high permeability (BCS class I) drug, which is not expected to present problems in dissolution tests. However, Charoo et al. [35] described the influence of the polymorphism of fluconazole on dissolution. This drug exhibits the polymorphic forms I, II, III, and monohydrate. The solubility values of forms I and monohydrate were reported as 4.96 and 4.21 mg/mL, respectively, and form II as 6.59 mg/mL in water at 25 °C [36,37]. Low intrinsic dissolution rate was also reported for the form I [38,39]; the tendency of form II to convert into forms I and monohydrate in the presence of high humidity values have also been reported [40]. It is possible that products C1 and C2 contain polymorphic form I or monohydrate due to the lower in vitro dissolution rate in comparison to the other products, as shown in Figure 1.

GastroPlus™ was used to simulate plasma concentration–time curves for all the products, including C1 and C2, and the resulting profiles were then compared to the reference product (Ref) curve plotted with experimental values (Figure 2) in order to evaluate in vivo performance.

According to the predicted plasma concentration–time curves (Figure 2), all products would show in vivo performance equivalent to that of the reference product.

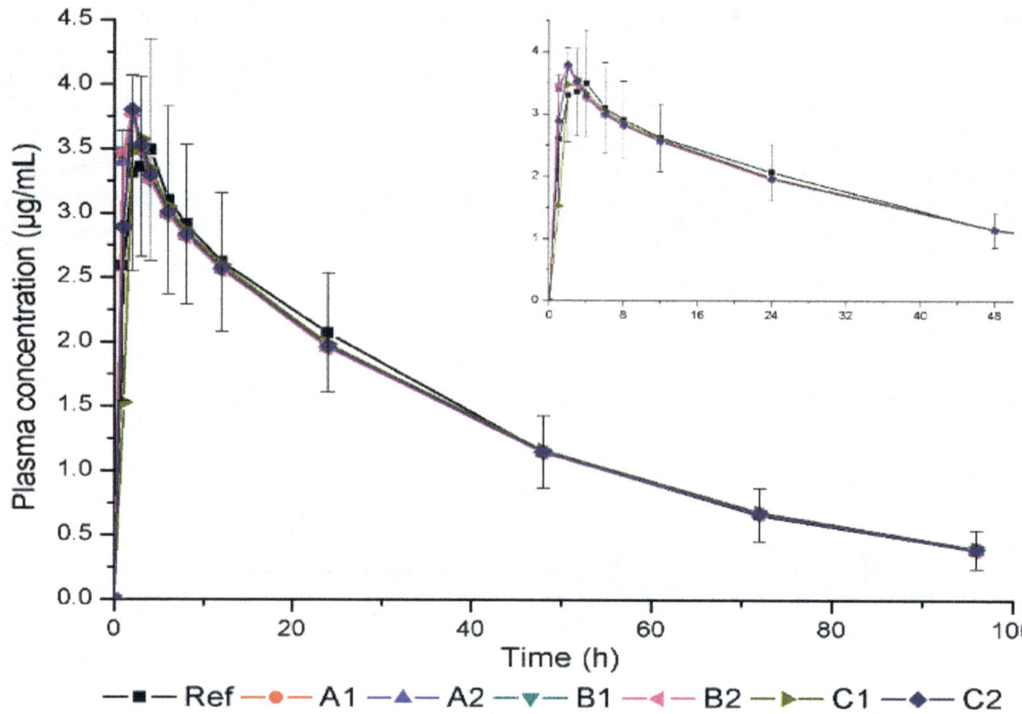

Figure 2. Plasma concentration-time curve of reference product (Ref) based on experimental values and of products A1, A2, B1, B2, C1, and C2 created using simulated values given by GastroPlus™; error bars represent the standard deviation for the reference plot. A zoom in of the time period 0–48 h is highlighted for better visualization.

Statistical parameters (R^2, SSE, RMSE e MAE) generated by the software for each predicted profile in comparison to the plasma concentration–time curve of the reference product [28] are shown in Table 4.

Table 4. Statistical parameters generated by GastroPlus™ for each predicted plasma concentration-time curve.

Product	R^2	SSE	RMSE	MAE
A1	0.987	1.482×10^{-1}	1.161×10^{-1}	7.561×10^{-2}
A2	0.936	9.806×10^{-1}	2.986×10^{-1}	1.833×10^{-1}
B1	0.929	1.097	3.158×10^{-1}	1.898×10^{-1}
B2	0.929	1.094	3.154×10^{-1}	1.897×10^{-1}
C1	0.832	2.382	4.653×10^{-1}	2.402×10^{-1}
C2	0.969	4.301×10^{-1}	1.977×10^{-1}	1.366×10^{-1}

R^2, coefficient of determination; SSE, sum of square error; RMSE, root mean square error; MAE, mean absolute error.

For all predicted profiles, low values were found for the prediction error parameters SSE, RMSE, and MAE (Table 4), indicating the viability of using GastroPlus™ to predict plasma concentrations of fluconazole from input data. High correlation (R^2) was demonstrated between the predicted plasma concentration–time curves of all products and the experimentally-determined reference curve.

The percent of drug dissolved less than 85% at 30 min for products C1 and C2 did not affect the predicted in vivo performance, as observed in the predicted plasma concentration–time curves (Figure 2) and statistical parameters (Table 4).

GastroPlus™ also calculates the amount of drug dissolved in vivo (AmtDiss), absorbed to the portal vein (AmtPV), total amount absorbed (AmtAbs), and the amount in the systemic circulation (AmtSC). These data are shown in Figure 3.

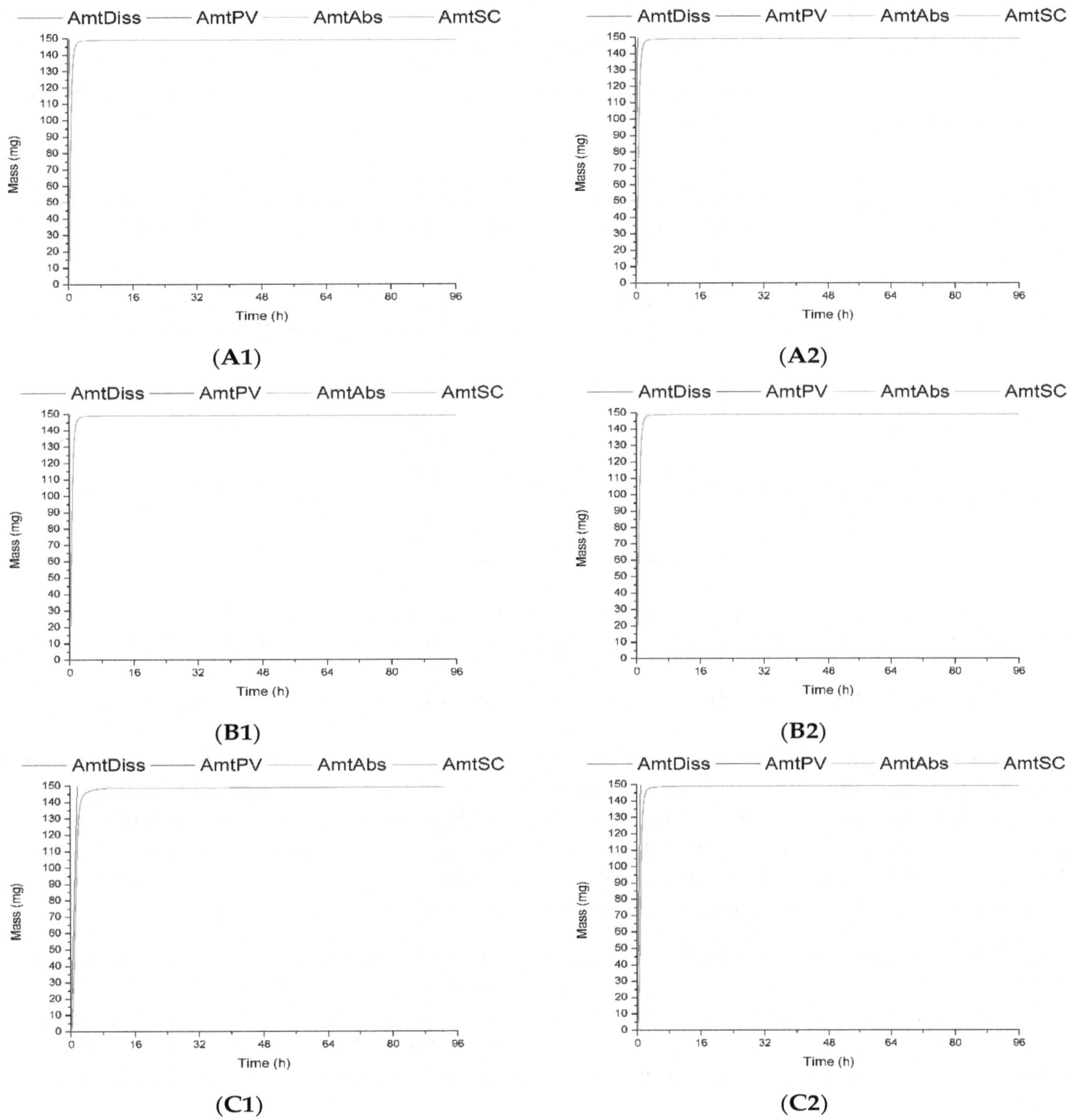

Figure 3. Amount of fluconazole dissolved in vivo (AmtDiss), amount absorbed to the portal vein (AmtPV), total amount absorbed (AmtAbs), and the amount in the systemic circulation (AmtSC) for products (**A1–C2**) calculated by GastroPlus™. Simulation time displayed is 8 h instead of the total simulation time (96 h) to provide better visualization.

It can be observed in Figure 3 that products A1, A2, B1, and B2 showed similar predicted in vivo dissolution behavior with a fast amount absorbed by enterocytes, then into the portal vein, and in the systemic circulation. The slow in vitro dissolution of products C1 and C2 (Figure 1) could be attributed to the presence of the low soluble polymorphic forms I and monohydrate. Despite a small displacement of the curves (Figure 3) corresponding to the predicted in vivo dissolution (AmDiss) of products C1 and C2 was observed, it did not affect the predicted fluconazole amount absorbed (AmtAbs) and the predicted amount in the systemic circulation (AmtSC). It is expected that for fluconazole, as for BCS class I drugs, dissolution is not the limiting step for absorption.

The C_{max} and AUC predicted values for products A1, A2, B1, B2, C1, and C2 and the experimental ones for the reference product (Ref) are shown in Table 5.

Table 5. Pharmacokinetic parameters of the reference product (Ref) based on the experimental curve and of products A1, A2, B1, B2, C1, and C2 obtained using simulated curves given by GastroPlus™.

Products	F%	T_{max} (h)	C_{max} (μg/mL)		AUC_{0-t} (μg h/mL)	
			Obs	Pred	Obs	Pred
Ref	90.0	4.00	3.49	–	135.77	–
A1	99.6	2.30	–	3.26	–	133.24
A2	99.6	1.66	–	3.82	–	132.48
B1	99.6	1.60	–	3.82	–	132.51
B2	99.6	1.60	–	3.82	–	132.51
C1	99.4	3.20	–	3.16	–	132.66
C2	99.6	1.80	–	3.81	–	132.37

%F, oral bioavailability: % of the drug that reached the systemic circulation; T_{max}, time of C_{max}; C_{max}, maximum plasma concentration; AUC, area under the plasma concentration-time curve; Obs, observed value.

As stated in the Methods section, in vivo data of the reference product (Ref) was extracted from a figure containing the plasma concentration–time curve of Zoltec® 150 mg capsules described by the reference #28, using WebPlotDigitizer [30]. These in vivo values were used as input data of Ref in GastroPlus™ and the pharmacokinetic parameters (F%, T_{max}, C_{max}, and AUC_{0-t}) presented as Obs (Table 5) were calculated by the software. These PK parameters are in accordance with those reported by reference #28 (T_{max} = 2.96 h (1.96 h–3.96 h), C_{max} = 3.64 μg/mL (2.85 μg/mL–4.43 μg/mL), and AUC_{0-t} = 135.72 μg h/mL (106.20 μg h/mL–165.24 μg h/mL)). Even with the small difference found in the value of T_{max}, the calculations made using GastroPlus™ were reasonable.

ANVISA recommendations for the waiver of BE studies according to BCS for class I drugs state that IR solid oral products must have rapid drug dissolution (≥85% in 30 min) in 0.1 M HCl, pH 4.5 and pH 6.8 [6]. In this study, even though the dissolution tests were carried out only in hydrochloric acid as the dissolution medium [29], products C1 and C2 that did not meet the requirements of the dissolution rate still showed in vivo performance equivalent to the reference product. Al-Tabakha et al. [41] evaluated different products containing amoxicillin trihydrate and potassium clavulanate. These authors observed that products considered as bioequivalents presented in vitro dissolution differences, showing that in some cases in vitro dissolution can be more discriminating than in vivo bioequivalence testing.

Population simulation results for products A1 and A2, B1 and B2, and C1 and C2 are presented in Table 6.

Table 6. Population simulation results: average pharmacokinetic (PK) parameters F%, C_{max}, T_{max}, $AUC_{0\text{–}inf}$, $AUC_{0\text{–}t}$, 90% CI ln-transformed for their ratio for A1, A2, B1, B2, C1, C2, and the reference product (Ref), and average $AUC_{0\text{–}t}/AUC_{0\text{–}inf}$ ratio.

PK Parameter	Ref	A1	A2	B1	B2	C1	C2
F%	90	99.62 (99.58–99.66)	99.53 (99.44–99.63)	99.55 (99.48–99.63)	99.58 (99.54–99.62)	99.25 (99.11–99.38)	99.64 (99.60–99.68)
C_{max} (μg/mL)	3.49	3.22 (3.06–3.40)	3.79 (3.61–3.98)	3.88 (3.71–4.07)	3.80 (3.65–3.96)	3.16 (3.02–3.31)	3.73 (3.58–3.89)
T_{max} (h)	4	2.24 (2.14–2.35)	1.66 (1.59–1.74)	1.60 (1.53–1.68)	1.60 (1.55–1.65)	3.36 (3.20–3.53)	1.77 (1.73–1.82)
$AUC_{0\text{–}inf}$ (μg h/mL)	153.56	135.06 (126.60–144.10)	146.81 (135.90–158.60)	156.58 (146.50–167.30)	157.02 (148.30–166.30)	141.3 (129.3–154.4)	150.58 (142.10–159.60)
$AUC_{0\text{–}t}$ (μg h/mL)	135.77	121.59 (115.70–127.80)	128.43 (121.50–135.70)	135.81 (129.30–142.60)	135.81 (129.30–142.70)	125.48 (117.20–134.40)	130.6 (124.90–136.60)
Average $AUC_{0\text{–}t}/AUC_{0\text{–}inf}$	0.88	0.90	0.87	0.87	0.86	0.88	0.87

The 90% CI ln-transformed of the ratio of C_{max} and AUC_{0-t} for the products and reference are within the 80–125% interval (Table 6), in accordance with the regulatory guidance of the FDA [32] and ANVISA [33] for bioequivalence evaluation of test and reference products. The average AUC_{0-t}/AUC_{0-inf} ratios for the reference and all products were between 0.86 and 0.90, showing that the end time (96 h) used in the simulations was appropriate (>80%) to provide a reliable estimate of the extent of absorption [32,42].

4. Conclusions

Plasma concentration profile predictions and population simulation using virtual subjects obtained for fluconazole capsules with dissolution profiles that meet (A1, A2, B1, and B2) and do not meet (C1 and C2) the regulatory criterion of rapid or very rapid dissolution showed their bioequivalence. Computer simulations can be used as a tool for screening formulations that could be bioequivalent, contributing to gaining time and reducing costs for pharmaceutical companies.

Author Contributions: Conceptualization, M.D.D., D.A.S. and M.G.I.; methodology, M.D.D., D.A.S. and M.G.I.; software, M.D.D. and D.A.S.; investigation, M.D.D., D.A.S. and M.G.I.; resources, M.G.I., R.L. and H.G.F.; writing—original draft preparation, M.D.D. and M.G.I.; writing—review and editing, M.D.D., M.G.I., R.L., V.P. and H.G.F.; supervision, R.L., V.P. and H.G.F.; funding acquisition, M.G.I., R.L. and H.G.F.

Acknowledgments: Portions of these results were generated by GastroPlus software provided by Simulations Plus, Inc., Lancaster, CA, USA.

References

1. Silva, M.F.; Schramm, S.G.; Kano, E.K.; Koono, E.D.M.; Porta, V.; Serra, C.H.R. Bioequivalence evaluation of single doses of two tramadol formulations: A randomized, open-label, two-period crossover study in healthy Brazilian volunteers. *Clin. Ther.* **2010**, *32*, 758–765. [CrossRef]
2. Kano, E.K.; Koono, E.E.M.; Schramm, S.G.; Serra, C.H.R.; Junior, E.A.; Pereira, R.; Freitas, M.S.T.; Iecco, M.C.; Porta, V. Average bioequivalence of single 500 mg doses of two oral formulations of levofloxacin: A randomized, open-label, two-period crossover study in healthy adult Brazilian volunteers. *Braz. J. Pharm. Sci.* **2015**, *51*, 203–211. [CrossRef]
3. FDA. Food and Drug Administration. Guidance for Industry: Bioavailability and Bioequivalence Studies Submitted in NDAs or INDs—General Considerations. Draft Guidance. U.S. Department of Health and Human Services, Center for Drug Evaluation and Research (CDER). 2014. Available online: https://www.fda.gov/downloads/Drugs/GuidanceComplianceRegulatoryInformation/Guidances/UCM389370.pdf (accessed on 7 June 2018).
4. FDA. Food and Drug Administration. Guidance for Industry: Waiver on In Vivo Bioavailability and Bioequivalence Studies for Immediate-Release Solid Oral Dosage Forms Based on a Biopharmaceutics Classification System. U.S. Department of Health and Human Services, Center for Drug Evaluation and Research (CDER). 2017. Available online: https://www.fda.gov/downloads/Drugs/GuidanceComplianceRegulatoryInformation/Guidances/UCM070246.pdf (accessed on 7 June 2018).
5. Modi, N.B. In vitro-in vivo correlation. In *Pharmaceutical Product Development: In Vitro-In Vivo Correlation*, 1st ed.; Chilukuri, D.M., Sunkara, G., Young, D., Eds.; Informa Healthcare: New York, NY, USA, 2007; Volume 1, pp. 107–112.
6. BRASIL. Brazilian Health Surveillance Agency (ANVISA). Resolução da Diretoria Colegiada RDC nº 37 de 03 de agosto de 2011. Dispõe sobre o guia para isenção e substituição de estudos de biodisponibilidade relativa/bioequivalência e dá outras providências. CFAR/GTFAR/CGMED/ANVISA. 2011. Available online: http://portal.anvisa.gov.br/documents/33880/2568070/rdc0037_03_08_2011.pdf/13c41657-e93b-4d09-99eb-377f760f3aa0 (accessed on 7 June 2018).
7. BRASIL. Brazilian Health Surveillance Agency (ANVISA). Instrução Normativa IN nº 04 de 03 de agosto de 2011. Dispõe sobre a lista de fármacos candidatos à biosenção baseada no sistema de classificação biofarmacêutica (SCB) e dá outras providências. CFAR/GTFAR/CGMED/ANVISA. 2011. Available online: http://bvsms.saude.gov.br/bvs/saudelegis/anvisa/2011/int0004_03_08_2011.html (accessed on 7 June 2018).

8. BRASIL. Brazilian Health Surveillance Agency (ANVISA). Instrução Normativa IN nº 07 de 21 de agosto de 2014. Determina a publicação da lista de fármacos candidatos à biosenção baseada no sistema de classificação biofarmacêutica (SCB) e dá outras providências. CFAR/GTFAR/CGMED/ANVISA. 2014. Available online: http://portal.anvisa.gov.br/documents/33836/349509/IN%2B07%2B2014.pdf/0996340b-24e5-4855-8bfd-0756765e422e?version=1.0 (accessed on 7 June 2018).
9. BRASIL. Brazilian Health Surveillance Agency (ANVISA). Resolução da Diretoria Colegiada RDC nº 31 de 11 de agosto de 2010. Dispõe sobre a realização dos estudos de equivalência farmacêutica e de perfil de dissolução comparativo. CFAR/GTFAR/CGMED/ANVISA. 2010. Available online: http://portal.anvisa.gov.br/documents/33880/2568070/res0031_11_08_2010.pdf/5e157d15-d3d5-4bb9-98db-5667e4d9e0c8 (accessed on 7 June 2018).
10. Sweetman, S.C. *Martindale: The Complete Drug Reference*, 36th ed.; Pharmaceutical Press: London, UK, 2009; pp. 532–534.
11. Charoo, N.; Cristofoletti, R.; Graham, A.; Lartey, P.; Abrahamsson, B.; Groot, D.W.; Kopp, S.; Langguth, P.; Polli, J.; Shah, V.P.; et al. Biowaiver monograph for immediate-release solid oral dosage forms: Fluconazole. *J. Pharm. Sci.* **2014**, *103*, 3843–3858. [CrossRef] [PubMed]
12. Charoo, N.A.; Cristofoletti, R.; Dressman, J.B. Risk assessment for extending the Biopharmaceutics Classification System-based biowaiver of immediate release dosage forms of fluconazole in adults to the paediatric population. *J. Pharm. Pharmacol.* **2015**, *67*, 1156–1169. [CrossRef] [PubMed]
13. Okumo, A.; Dimaso, M.; Löbenberg, R. Dynamic dissolution testing to establish in vitro/in vivo correlations for montelukast sodium, a poorly soluble drug. *Pharmaceut. Res.* **2008**, *12*, 2778–2785. [CrossRef] [PubMed]
14. Okumo, A.; Dimaso, M.; Löbenberg, R. Computer simulations using GastroPlus™ to justify a biowaiver for etoricoxib solid oral drug products. *Eur. J. Pharm. Biopharm.* **2009**, *72*, 91–98. [CrossRef] [PubMed]
15. Wei, H.; Dalton, C.; Dimaso, M.; Kanfer, I.; Löbenberg, R. Physicochemical characterization of file glyburide powders: A BCS based approach to predict oral absorption. *Eur. J. Pharm. Biopharm.* **2008**, *69*, 1046–1056. [CrossRef] [PubMed]
16. Honório, T.S.; Pinto, E.C.; Rocha, H.V.A.; Esteves, V.S.D.; Santos, T.C.; Castro, H.C.R.; Rodrigues, C.R.; Sousa, V.P.; Cabral, L. In vitro-in vivo correlation of efavirenz tablets using GastroPlus®. *AAPS PharmSciTech* **2013**, *14*, 1244–1254. [CrossRef]
17. Kostewicz, E.S.; Aarons, L.; Bergstrand, M.; Bolger, M.B.; Galetin, A.; Hatley, O.; Jamei, M.; Lloyd, R.; Pepin, X.; Rostami-Hodjegan, A.; et al. PBPK models for the prediction of in vivo performance of oral dosage forms. *Eur. J. Pharm. Sci.* **2014**, *57*, 300–321. [CrossRef] [PubMed]
18. Almukainzi, M.; Jamali, F.; Aghazadeh-Habashi, A.; Löbenberg, R. Disease specific modeling: Simulation of the pharmacokinetics of meloxicam and ibuprofen in disease state vs. healthy conditions. *Eur. J. Pharm. Biopharm.* **2016**, *100*, 77–84. [CrossRef]
19. Kesisoglou, F.; Ghung, J.; Van Asperen, J.; Heimbach, T. Physiologically based absorption modeling to impact biopharmaceutics and formulation strategies in drug development- industry case studies. *J. Pharm. Sci.* **2016**, *105*, 2723–2734. [CrossRef]
20. Almukainzi, M.; Gabr, R.; Abdelhamid, G.; Löbenberg, R. Mechanistic understanding of the effect of renal impairment on metformin oral absorption using computer simulations. *J. Pharm. Investig.* **2017**, *47*, 151–161. [CrossRef]
21. Silva, D.A.; Duque, M.D.; Davies, N.M.; Löbenberg, R.; Ferraz, H.G. Application of in silico tools in clinical practice using ketoconazole as model drug. *J. Pharm. Pharm. Sci.* **2018**, *21*, 242s–253s. [CrossRef]
22. Tubic-Grozdanis, M.; Bolger, M.G.; Langguth, P. Application of gastrointestinal simulation for extensions for biowaivers of highly permeable compounds. *AAPS J.* **2008**, *10*, 213–226. [CrossRef] [PubMed]
23. Kovačević, I.; Parojčić, J.; Homšek, I.; Tubić-Grozdanis, M.; Langguth, P. Justification of biowaiver for carbamazepine, a low soluble high permeable compound, in solid dosage forms based on IVIVC and gastrointestinal simulation. *Mol. Pharm.* **2009**, *6*, 40–47. [CrossRef]
24. Tsume, Y.; Amidon, G.L. The biowaiver extension for BCS class III drugs: The effect of dissolution rate on the bioequivalence of BCS class III immediate-release drugs predicted by computer simulation. *Mol. Pharm.* **2010**, *7*, 1235–1243. [CrossRef] [PubMed]
25. Kortejärvi, H.; Shawahna, R.; Koski, A.; Malkki, J.; Ojala, K.; Yliperttula, M. Very rapid dissolution is not needed to guarantee bioequivalence for biopharmaceutics classification system (BCS) I drugs. *J. Pharm. Sci.* **2010**, *99*, 621–625. [CrossRef] [PubMed]

26. Chen, Z.-F.; Ying, G.-G.; Jiang, Y.-X.; Yang, B.; Lai, H.-J.; Liu, Y.-S.; Pan, C.-G.; Peng, F.-Q. Photodegradation of the azole fungicide fluconazole in aqueous solution under UV-254: Kinetics, mechanistic investigations and toxicity evaluation. *Water Res.* **2014**, *52*, 83–91. [CrossRef] [PubMed]
27. Corrêa, J.C.R.; Vianna-Soares, C.D.; Salgado, H.R.N. Development and validation of dissolution test for fluconazole capsules by HPLC and derivative UV spectrophotometry. *Chromatogr. Res. Int.* **2012**, *610427*, 1–8. [CrossRef]
28. Porta, V.; Chang, K.H.; Storpirtis, S. Evaluation of the bioequivalence of capsules containing 150 mg of fluconazole. *Int. J. Pharm.* **2005**, *288*, 81–86. [CrossRef] [PubMed]
29. Porta, V.; Yamamichi, E.; Storpirtis, S. Avaliação biofarmacêutica in vitro de cápsulas de fluconazol. *Braz. J. Pharm. Sci.* **2002**, *38*, 333–343. [CrossRef]
30. Rohatgi, A. WebPlotDigitizer: Web Based Tool to Extract Data from Plot, Images, and Maps. Version 4.1. January 2018. Available online: https://automeris.io/WebPlotDigitizer/citation.html (accessed on 17 March 2019).
31. Simulations Plus. *GastroPlus™ Version 9.0 Manual*; Simulations Plus: Lancaster, CA, USA, 2015.
32. FDA. Food and Drug Administration. Guidance for Industry: Statistical Approaches to Establishing Bioequivalence. U.S. Department of Health and Human Services, Center for Drug Evaluation and Research (CDER). 2001. Available online: https://www.fda.gov/downloads/Drugs/GuidanceComplianceRegulatoryInformation/Guidances/UCM070244.pdf (accessed on 7 June 2018).
33. BRASIL. AGÊNCIA NACIONAL DE VIGILÂNCIA SANITÁRIA (ANVISA). Resolução RE nº 1.170 de 19 de abril de 2006. Guia para provas de biodisponibilidade relativa/bioequivalência de medicamentos. CFAR/GTFAR/CGMED/ANVISA. 2006. Available online: http://portal.anvisa.gov.br/documents/10181/2718376/%281%29RE_1170_2006_COMP.pdf/52326927-c379-45b4-9a7e-9c5ecabaa16b (accessed on 7 June 2018).
34. Debruyne, D. Clinical pharmacokinetics of fluconazole in superficial and systemic mycoses. *Clin. Pharmacokinet.* **1997**, *33*, 52–77. [CrossRef]
35. Charoo, N.A.; Cristofoletti, R.; Kim, S.K. Integrating biopharmaceutics risk assessment and in vivo absorption model in formulation development of BCS class I drug using the QbD approach. *Drug Dev. Ind. Pharm.* **2017**, *43*, 668–677. [CrossRef]
36. Alkhamis, K.A.; Obaidat, A.A.; Nuseirat, A.F. Solid-state characterization of fluconazole. *Pharm. Dev. Technol.* **2002**, *7*, 491–503. [CrossRef]
37. Park, H.J.; Kim, M.S.; Kim, J.S.; Cho, W.; Park, J.; Cha, K.H.; Kang, Y.S.; Hwang, S.J. Solid-state carbon NMR characterization and investigation of intrinsic dissolution behavior of fluconazole polymorphs, anhydrate forms I and II. *Chem. Pharm. Bull.* **2010**, *58*, 1243–1247. [CrossRef] [PubMed]
38. Modha, N.B.; Chotai, N.P.; Patel, V.A.; Patel, B.G. Preparation, characterization and evaluation of fluconazole polymorphs. *Int. J. Res. Pharm. Biomed. Sci.* **2010**, *1*, 124–127.
39. Desai, S.R.; Dharwadkar, S.R. Study of process induced polymorphic transformations in fluconazole drug. *Acta Pol. Pharm. Drug Res.* **2009**, *66*, 115–122.
40. Obaidat, R.M.; Alkhamis, K.A.; Salem, M.S. Determination of factors affecting kinetics of solid-state transformation of fluconazole polymorph II to polymorph I using diffuse reflectance Fourier transform spectroscopy. *Drug Dev. Ind. Pharm.* **2010**, *36*, 570–580. [CrossRef] [PubMed]
41. Al-Tabakha, M.M.; Fahelelbom, K.M.S.; Obaid, D.E.E.; Sayed, S. Quality attributes and in vitro bioequivalence of different brands of amoxicillin trihydrate tablets. *Pharmaceutics* **2017**, *9*, 18. [CrossRef]
42. EMEA. European Medicines Agency. Committee for Medical Products for Human Use (CHMP). Guideline on the Investigation of Bioequivalence. 2010. Available online: https://www.ema.europa.eu/en/documents/scientific-guideline/guideline-investigation-bioequivalence-rev1_en.pdf (accessed on 22 March 2019).

6

Development of a New Ex Vivo Lipolysis-Absorption Model for Nanoemulsions

Lu Xiao [1,†], Ying Liu [2,†] and Tao Yi [3,*]

1 Department of Basic Medicine, Zunyi Medical University, Zhuhai Campus, Zhuhai 519041, China; xl1527@163.com
2 Pharmacy Department, Wuhan Medical Treatment Center, Wuhan 430023, China; winter_ling@163.com
3 School of Health Sciences, Macao Polytechnic Institute, Macau 999078, China
* Correspondence: yitao@ipm.edu.mo
† These authors contributed equally to this work.

Abstract: The use of lipid-based formulations (LBFs) in improving the absorption of poorly water-soluble drugs has now well established. Because the in vivo evaluation of LBFs is labor-intensive, in vitro or ex vivo approaches could provide advantages. In this study, a new ex vivo lipolysis-absorption model (*ev*LAM) composed of an intestinal digestion system and an intestinal tissue system was developed to evaluate and predict the in vivo absorption performances of LBFs. Model factors, including the pH of the system and concentrations of D-glucose and pancreatic lipase, were investigated and optimized by a Box-Behnken design. To evaluate this new model, a lipid formulation of indomethacin, which was chosen based on preliminary studies of pseudo-ternary phase diagrams, emulsion droplets, and solubility, was further investigated by an in vivo pharmacokinetic study of rats, the everted gut sac model, and the *ev*LAM, respectively. The absorption percentages obtained from the *ev*LAM were much more similar to the data of rats in vivo than those from the everted gut sac model, showing a preferable in vitro-in vivo correlation ($r = 0.9772$). Compared with the conventional in vitro and in vivo methods, the *ev*LAM, which allowed precise insights into the in vivo absorption characteristics without much time or a complicated process, could be a better tool for assessing LBFs of poorly water-soluble drugs.

Keywords: lipid-based formulations; lipolysis; absorption; poorly water-soluble drugs; model

1. Introduction

For the oral delivery of poorly water-soluble drugs, lipid-based formulations (LBFs) have gained increasing attention due to enhanced oral bioavailability [1,2]. The main mechanism for the enhanced bioavailability of LBFs [3–8] was probably the pre-dissolved state of drugs in LBFs, which could reduce the energy associated with the solid-to-liquid phase transition process and cause the enhanced drug solubilization by colloidal structures. The formations of colloidal structures were the results of interactions among LBFs, their digestion products, and endogenous surfactants such as bile salts and phospholipids [9–13]. The powerful digestive system in the intestine could play an important role in the fate of LBFs [14,15].

It is very important to provide a fast and accurate method to evaluate the in vitro and in vivo characteristics of LBFs. Because the in vivo pharmacokinetics study is expensive and labor-intensive, the evaluation of LBFs by in vitro or ex vivo assays could present important advantages. Conventional in vitro methods for screening formulation and evaluating characteristics of LBFs are based on the pseudo-ternary phase diagram, the comparison of droplet size and solubility, and the in vitro lipolysis [16,17]. Phase diagram, emulsion droplet size, and in vitro solubility assays are important for the preliminary choice of a lipid-based formulation, especially for microemulsions and self-microemulsifying drug delivery systems. However, the in vitro findings in these assays only correlate poorly with the in vivo absorption characteristics.

The in vitro lipolysis model for assessing the fate of drugs of LBFs, whether they were soluble or precipitated in the intestinal digestive system, has been well-recognized [18–24]. The standard in vitro lipolysis assay was performed using a pH-stat to maintain the pH of the system, adding porcine pancreatin to serve as a lipase-colipase model for human pancreatic juice, and using bile salt-lecithin mixed micelles to provide a solubilization environment. The data generated from the pH-stat could be used to quantify the rate and extent of lipolysis through recording the amounts of free fatty acids released from LBFs. After the reaction had been terminated, the products of lipolysis could be examined to determine the fate of the drug after lipolysis [5,19]. The in vitro lipolysis model is useful for the optimization of LBFs and has been used for lipid nanoparticles [25]. Since the pancreatic extract contained both the pancreatic lipase and carboxyl ester hydrolase, the in vitro lipolysis model was improved by using porcine pancreatic extract, as it was therefore permitted to mimic the duodenal digestive lipolysis in a biorelevant manner. However, the in vitro lipolysis model may not be predictive for actual in vivo absorptions due to the lack of effective simulation of the internal physiological environment. However, the in vitro lipolysis model may not be predictive for actual in vivo absorptions due to the lack of effective simulation of the internal physiological environment [24].

The everted gut sac model (EGSM), commonly using intact intestinal mucosal epithelium of rats to mimic the in vivo conditions, has been widely used to pharmacokinetic studies such as drug absorption, drug metabolism in intestinal segments, efflux transport, multidrug resistance, and drug interactions [26]. The viability of intestinal segments under in vitro conditions was impacted by experimental factors such as pH, aeration, temperature, and the concentration of the substance. The EGSM provides a relatively large surface area available for absorption and a mucus layer. Consequently, results from EGSM have been in agreement with in vivo findings for many drugs [26]. However, the EGSM could not accurately evaluate LBFs due to the lack of the simulation of the lipolytic condition. Therefore, it was hypothesized that the combination of the EGSM and the in vitro lipolysis model could form a new ex vivo model which should be much closer to the in vivo conditions and, resultantly, could evaluate LBFs more accurately.

The first aim of this study was to establish a new ex vivo lipolysis-absorption model (*ev*LAM) for evaluating and predicting the in vivo performance of LBFs. In this study, the *ev*LAM composed of an intestinal digestion system (a pH-stat to maintain the pH of the system, adding porcine pancreatin to serve as a lipase-colipase model for human pancreatic juice, and using bile salt-lecithin mixed micelles to provide a solubilization environment) and an intestinal tissue system (intestinal segments under physiological medium to obtain absorption data). The new *ev*LAM was much closer to the in vivo conditions and resultantly could evaluate LBFs more accurately. Model factors, including the pH of the system and concentrations of Ca^{2+}, D-glucose, K^+, and pancreatic lipase, were investigated and optimized by a three-level Box-Behnken design. The pH of the system, concentrations of D-glucose, and pancreatic lipase were chosen as the independent variables; the intestinal tissue activity and the fatty acid concentration were the dependent variables [19,27,28].

Furthermore, the in vitro absorptions obtained from the new *ev*LAM and the conventional EGSM were compared with the pharmacokinetics data of rats. The in vitro-in vivo correlations of absorption curves obtained from the two models were further compared to indicate the advantages of the new model in evaluating and predicting the in vivo performance of LBFs.

2. Experimental Section

2.1. Materials

Sodium taurodeoxycholate (97%), porcine pancreatin (8 × USP specifications activity), and Trizma maleate (99.5%) were purchased from Sigma Chemical Co. (St. Louis, MO, USA). Medium chain mono- and di-glyceride (Capmul MCM) were kindly donated by Abitec Co. (Janesville, WI, USA). Lecithin (approximately 80% pure phosphatidylcholine) was a gift from Q.P. Co. (Fuchu-Shi, Tokyo, Japan). Indomethacin (99.5%) was purchased from Zizhu Pharmaceutical Co. (Beijing, China). The Naproxen sodium reference substance (99.9%) and indomethacin reference substance (99.9%) were purchased from the China Institute for the Control of Drugs and Biological Products (Beijing, China). A lactate dehydrogenase Assay Kit was purchased from the Nanjing Jiancheng Bioengineering Institute (Nanjing, China). Other chemicals were of HPLC or analytical grade.

2.2. Preparation of the Intestinal Tissue Medium in the Fasted State

1.25 mM of lecithin was dissolved in chloroform in a round bottom flask, and then chloroform was evaporated off under vacuum, resulting in a thin film of lecithin around the bottom of the flask. After the addition of 5 mM of sodium taurodeoxycholate, 50 mM of Trizma maleate, and 150 mM of NaCl and Ca^{2+} solution (at 1, 3, 5 or 10 mM), the mixed solution was adjusted with NaOH or HCl to a pH of 7.500 ± 0.001 and then stirred and equilibrated for 12 h; after which, it finally formed a clear and slightly yellow solution. At last, D-glucose solution (at 0, 5, 10 or 15 mM) and K^+ solution (at 0, 3.5, 5.5 or 6.5 mM) were added in before use.

2.3. Preparation of Intestinal Segments

All surgical and experimental procedures were approved by the Animal Research Ethics Committee of Zunyi Medical University (No.: ZMCER2018A051). Male Wistar rats (Chongqing, China) 11–12 weeks old, 250 ± 20 g in weight, and fasted for 24 h prior to the experiment were anaesthetized intraperitoneally with 3.5% chloral hydrate (1 mL·100 g^{-1}). The small intestine was removed out and washed three times with saline (0.9% NaCl solution) at 37 °C. The intestine was immediately placed in an oxygenated (O_2: CO_2 = 95:5% v/v) intestinal tissue medium (pH 7.5, 37 °C). The intestinal segment (5–7 cm in length) was everted on a tube (2.5 cm in diameter), and then one end was sealed with a clamp.

2.4. Establishment of the evLAM

A new *ev*LAM, composed of an intestinal tissue system (intestinal segment, medium, temperature controlled stirrer, vents, and O_2/CO_2) and an intestinal digestion system (pH-stat meter controller, NaOH autoburette, pH electrodes, and computer) was set up based on characteristics of intestinal digestion of LBFs. As shown in Figure 1, the intestinal segment was filled with fresh and oxygenated intestinal tissue medium using a 1 mL glass syringe and then incubated in a centrifuge tube containing oxygenated intestinal tissue medium with the lipid-based formulation to be assayed at 37 °C. Lipase and pancreatin were used to mimic the intestinal digestive lipolysis in a biorelevant manner. Then, the pancreatic lipase extract, which was prepared by adding 1 g of porcine pancreatic lipase powder into 5 mL of digestion buffer (Trizma maleate, NaCl, Ca^{2+}, pH 7.5) and stirred for 15 min followed by centrifugation at 1,600× g and 5 °C for 15 min, was added to initiate lipolysis. In the process of the lipolysis, the pH of the system was sustained by a pH-stat automatic titration unit with 0.2 M NaOH. At designated intervals of 2 h experiment, samples of 200 μL were collected from the gut sac and conserved at −20 °C until analysis. Each experiment was performed by three parallel treatments, and the average value was used. At the same time, the fresh intestinal tissue medium with the same volume was added.

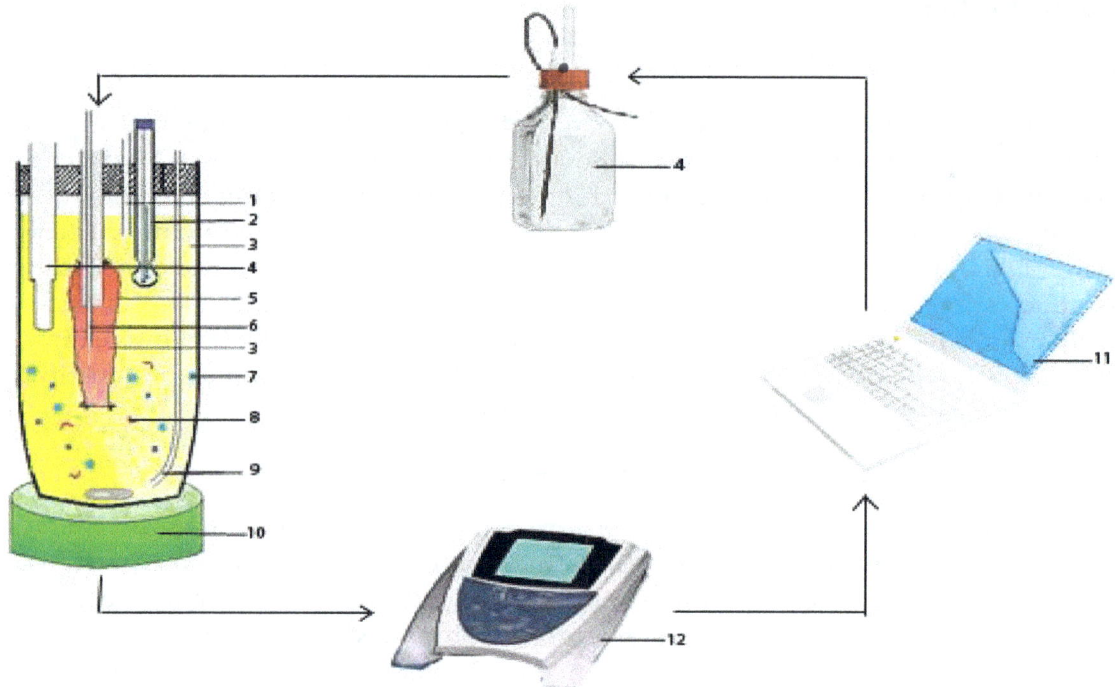

Figure 1. The new lipolysis-absorption model for lipid-based formulations: (**1**) Vent; (**2**) pH electrode; (**3**) intestinal tissue medium; (**4**) NaOH autoburette; (**5**) intestinal segment; (**6**) sampler; (**7**) a lipid-based formulation; (**8**) pancreatic lipase/colipase; (**9**) O_2/CO_2; (**10**) temperature controlled stirrer; (**11**) computer; and (**12**) pH-stat meter controller.

2.5. *Optimization of the evLAM*

2.5.1. Measurement of the Attenuation Rate of Intestinal Tissue Activity

The concentrations of lactate dehydrogenase in the sample at every time point was measured by the lactate dehydrogenase assay kit. The determination was performed three times, and the average value was used. The attenuation rate (AR) of intestinal tissue activity was calculated as follows.

$$AR = (CLDH_{end} - CLDH_0)/\text{time interval} \quad (1)$$

where $CLDH_{end}$ was the concentration of lactate dehydrogenase at the end, and $CLDH_0$ was the concentration of lactate dehydrogenase at the beginning. The release of lactate dehydrogenase increased with the increasing damage of intestinal tissue. The faster intestinal tissue activity decreased, the faster the attenuation rate was.

2.5.2. Analysis of the Amount of Fatty Acids

The release of free fatty acids from the lipolysis of LBFs was monitored using a titration method [29]. The amount of fatty acids in each sample was determined by the end-point titration with 0.2 M of NaOH. The determination was performed by three parallel treatments, and the average value was used.

2.5.3. Three-Level Box-Behnken Design

A three-level Box-Behnken design comprised of 15 experimental runs was constructed by Design-Expert (Version 8.0.0, Stat-Ease Inc., Minneapolis, MN, USA) [30]. Independent variables and dependent variables are listed in Table 1 along with their low, medium, and high levels and target value, which were selected based on results from preliminary experiment.

Table 1. Variables and their levels in the Box-Behnken design.

Factor	Levels used, Actual (Coded)		
	Low (−1)	Medium (0)	High (+1)
Independent variables			
X_1 = the pH of the system	6.5	7.5	8.5
X_2 = D-glucose concentration (mM)	5	10	15
X_3 = pancreatic lipase concentration (unit·mL^{-1})	2500	4250	6000
Dependent variables		Target value	
Y_1 = Attenuation rate of intestinal tissue activity (U·L^{-1}·min^{-1})		Minimize	
Y_2 = Amount of Fatty Acids (mmol)		4.468~4.703	

2.6. *Evaluation of the evLAM*

2.6.1. Choosing a Lipid-Based Formulation of Indomethacin

A lipid formulation of indomethacin was chosen as follows: Solubility and pseudo-ternary phase diagrams were first studied to obtain four formulations, Formulation I to IV (shown in Supplementary Figures S1 and S2). Then, in vitro characteristics of these four formulations, such as the droplet size, self-emulsifying efficiency, and solubility, were determined (shown in Supplementary Table S1). Based on the results, the optimal formulation of indomethacin, Formulation II composed of Labrafac@Lipohile WL1349, Cremophor RH40, and Transcutol P (20:60:20, *w/w*), was chosen for further studies. The solubility of indomethacin in Formulation II was 32.19 mg/g, and the drug content of indomethacin in Formulation II was 16.0 mg/g. After lipolysis, the proportion of drug dispersed in aqueous phase and precipitation phase was 86.95 $\pm$ 0.75% and 12.50 $\pm$ 0.26%, respectively.

2.6.2. HPLC Analysis of Indomethacin

The concentration of indomethacin was determined by an HPLC analysis system (Agilent 1200, Agilent Technologies, Santa Clara, CA, USA) with an Agilent ODS-C18 column (250 $\times$ 4.6 mm, 5 μm). The column temperature was 25 °C, and the injection volume was 10 μL. The mobile phase was a mixture of acetonitrile and 0.1 M sodium acetate at a ratio of 40:60 (*v/v*), with pH of 5.0 adjusted by acetic acid. The detection was carried out at a wavelength of 320 nm, with a flow rate of 1.0 mL/min. The percent relative standard deviation (RSD%) of method precision was lower than 2%. The observed-to-expected ratios for spiking recovery ranged from 100.8% to 101.1%, showing the acceptable accuracy of the method. The sensitivity of the method represented by limit of quantitation was 0.1 μg/mL.

2.6.3. Comparison of the In Vitro Absorption between evLAM and EGSM

The *ev*LAM optimized above was used to investigate the in vitro intestinal absorption of indomethacin of Formulation II. Briefly, a known quantity of Formulation II (250 mg formulation per 10 mL intestinal tissue medium) was crudely emulsified in the intestinal tissue medium in a centrifuge tube. Lipolysis was initiated by the addition of pancreatic lipase extract into the gut sac. Samples were collected at designated intervals, and drug concentrations were measured by HPLC as described above. The in vitro cumulative absorption percentage (P_a) was calculated as follows:

$$P_a = \frac{(V_{\text{mea}} \times C_{\text{n}} \times \frac{V_{\text{bal}}}{V_{\text{sam}}} + V_{\text{mea}} \times \sum_{t=1}^{n-1} C_{\text{i}})/V}{C} \times 100\% \tag{2}$$

where C_{n} was the drug concentration of each sample; V_{bal} was the volume of the intestinal tissue medium before balance; V_{sam} was the volume of samples collected at each time point; V_{mea} was the volume of samples measured at each time point; V was the total volume of the intestinal tissue medium in the gut sac; and C was the initial drug concentration.

The conventional EGSM was also used to study the in vitro intestinal absorption of indomethacin of Formulation II. After anesthesia of rats, an intestinal segment (about 6 cm) was removed rapidly. The segment was washed with saline at 4 °C and everted over a glass rod gently. One end of the everted segment was tied with suture, and then the intestinal segment was filled with Krebs solution at 37 °C by needle tubing. The other end of the filled intestinal segment was hanged up with a tie. Finally, the intestinal segment was put into a beaker containing 20 mL medium with Formulation II at 37 °C. Samples of 0.1 mL were collected at designated intervals, and the drug concentrations were measured by HPLC as described above. The blank medium of 0.1 mL was replenished at each time point. The value of P_a was also calculated as described above.

2.6.4. In Vivo Absorption Study of Indomethacin LBF

A pharmacokinetic study was designed to investigate the in vivo absorption of the indomethacin LBF, Formulation II. Five Male Wistar rats (250 ± 10 g), which had been acclimatized for at least 1–2 weeks before the experiment, were fasted for 24 h prior to drug administration but allowed free access to water. Formulation II was administered intragastrically to each rat at a dose of 4.5 $mg \cdot kg^{-1}$ of indomethacin. About 200 μL of blood sample was collected from the rat tail vein into heparinized tubes at designated time intervals [31]. Plasma was separated by centrifugation and stored at −20 °C until analysis.

The concentration of indomethacin in plasma was determined by HPLC [32] as follows: 10 μL of internal standard solution (200 $mg \cdot L^{-1}$ naproxen sodium solution) was added into 150 μL of plasma and mixed for 5 min. Then, 15 μL of a phosphate buffer (pH 7.0) and 20 mg of NaCl were added. The sample was extracted with 375 μL acetidin by vortex-mixing for 10 min and centrifuging at 10,000× g. The supernatant was transferred to a clean tube and evaporated by nitrogen purging. The residue was reconstituted in 50 μL methanol. After vortex-mixing for 10 min, 20 μL of the sample was used for HPLC as described above. The 3p97 computer program and a Wagner-Nelson method were employed to analyze the plasma concentration-time data. The in vivo absorption percentage (f_a) was calculate as follows.

$$f_a = \frac{C_t + K_e \int_0^{\tau} C_t dt}{K_e \int_0^{\infty} C_t dt} \times 100\% \quad (3)$$

where C_n was the drug concentration at each time point, and K_e was the elimination rate constant.

2.7. Statistical Analysis

All data were expressed as mean ± SD. Statistical analysis and data fitting were performed using SPSS 16.0 (SPSS Inc., Chicago, IL, USA). One-way analysis of variance (ANOVA) was performed to test differences for statistical significance. Difference between mean values was considered statistically significant at $p < 0.05$ and very statistically significant at $p < 0.001$.

3. Results and Discussion

3.1. Effects of Components of the evLAM on Activity of Intestinal Tissue

As a new model for assessing the in vitro absorption of LBFs, it was important to simulate the actual dynamics of intestinal fluids. Because the viability of intestinal tissue under in vitro conditions was impacted by many factors, it was also important to select components of this new *ev*LAM based on the minimal tissue damage. Components of the *ev*LAM and their concentration ranges were all chosen as a compromise between in vivo values as the literatures reported [27,28,33–37] and pre-experiments in our laboratory. Trizma maleate was chosen at the concentration of 50 mM, which was similar to that used in other studies [19,38–42]. Sodium taurodeoxycholate and phosphatidylcholine were both added because that the administered exogenous lipids and their digestion products could intercalate into endogenous sodium taurodeoxycholate and phosphatidylcholine structures, changing the nature of solubilizing species, promoting micelle swelling and further increasing solubilization capacity [10,15,33]. Concentrations of sodium taurodeoxycholate and phosphatidylcholine in intestinal fluid after oral administration of LBFs have not been reported, so 5 mM of sodium taurodeoxycholate and 1.25 mM phosphatidylcholine were chosen in the *ev*LAM based on their typical concentrations in the fasted state as the literatures reported [10,15,33].

Influences of Ca^{2+}, D-glucose, K^+, pH, and pancreatic lipase on the activity of intestinal segments in the *ev*LAM were investigated. Value ranges of these model factors were set up based on the literatures. The same amount of Formulation II was used in the *ev*LAM with different levels of model factors. Attenuation rates of the activity of intestinal segments under different conditions were measured and are shown in Figure 2.

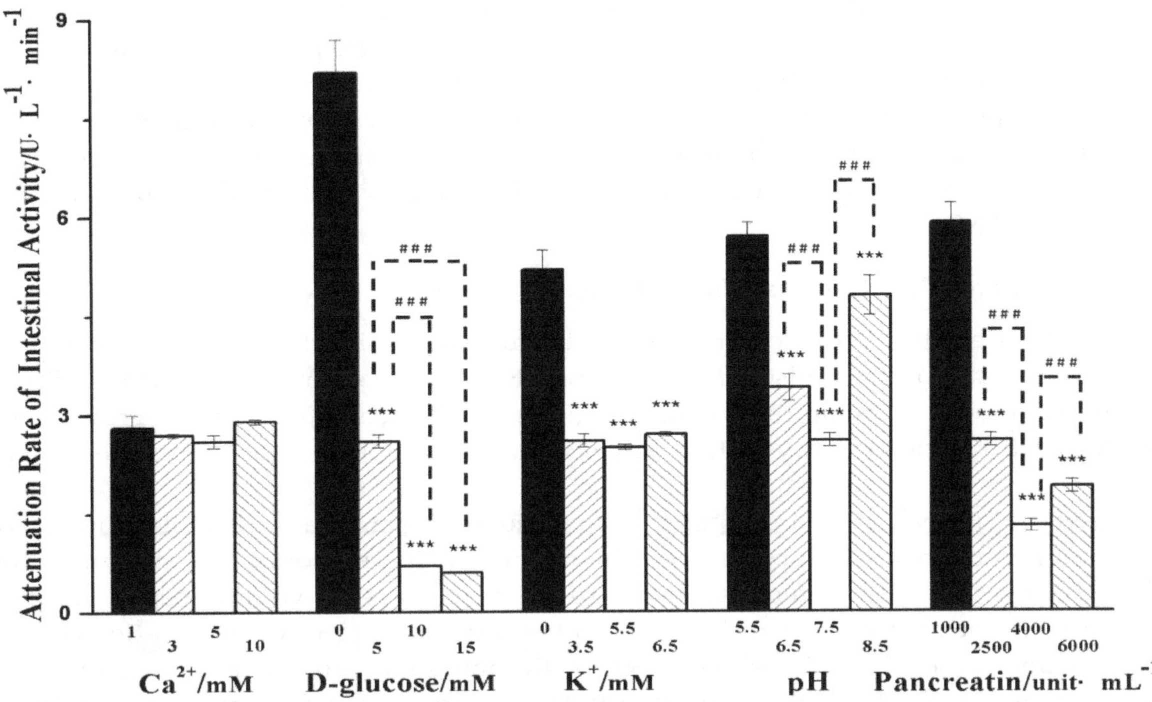

Figure 2. Influences of Ca^{2+}, D-glucose, K^+, pH, and pancreatic lipase on the attenuation rate of the intestinal tissue activity of the ex vivo lipolysis-absorption model. (Mean ± S.D., $n = 5$). *** very statistically significant ($p < 0.001$) compared with D-glucose of 0 mM, K^+ of 0 mM, pancreatic lipase of 1000 uint·mL^{-1} and pH of 5.5, respectively. ### very statistically significant ($p < 0.001$) difference in pairwise comparison.

Though there was no mention of a calcium binding site in the 3-D structure of pancreatic lipase/co-lipase complex [34,35], Ca^{2+} was necessary for the activity of pancreatic lipase. The formation of Ca^{2+}-soaps could draw the equilibrium towards the ionized fatty acids and maintain lipolysis in the presence of bile [36]. The mean concentration of Ca^{2+} in the fasted state was 0.5–3 mM in the duodenum, and Ca^{2+} of 1–10 mM was investigated in the previous studies [27,28,37]. As shown in Figure 2, no significant differences in the attenuation rate of intestinal tissue activity were seen in a range of Ca^{2+} concentrations, which suggested that Ca^{2+} did not directly influence the activity of intestinal tissue.

The attenuation rate of intestinal tissue activity decreased with the increasing concentration of D-glucose in the range of 0–15 mM, suggesting that the higher concentration of D-glucose could maintain the activity of intestinal tissue for a much longer time. It was probably due to that D-glucose was the energy source for cell metabolism.

The attenuation rate of intestinal tissue activity was significantly decreased after adding K^+. This could be due to the fact that the Na^+ pump was usually activated upon K^+, benefitting the secondary active transport of D-glucose [43] and providing more energy to intestinal tissue cells. However, when the amount of K^+ was sufficient in the concentration range of 3.5–6.5 mM, there were no significant changes in attenuation rate of intestinal tissue activity.

The pH value of the in vitro lipolysis model showed a high variability ranging from 5.8 to 8.5 [27,28]. As shown in Figure 2, the decreased attenuation rate of intestinal tissue activity appeared significantly at the pH range of 5.5 to 7.5, but the increased attenuation rate of intestinal activity was observed at pH 8.5. It was suggested that it was important for the activity of intestinal tissue to select a moderate pH.

The pancreatic lipase had an activity of 500–600 unit·mL^{-1} in the fasted state and 800–1800 unit·mL^{-1} in the fed state, respectively [14,34,35]. In some previous studies, the pancreatic lipase reached up to 10,000 unit·mL^{-1} [19]. As shown in Figure 2, the attenuation rate of intestinal tissue activity was significantly decreased when the pancreatic lipase concentration increased from 1000 to 4000 unit·mL^{-1}, but the attenuation rate increased when the pancreatic lipase reached up to 6000 unit·mL^{-1}. It was suggested that excessive pancreatic lipase might damage intestinal tissue.

From the results above, it could be seen that the pH of the system, concentrations of D-glucose, and pancreatic lipase had much more influence on the activity of intestinal tissue than the other model factors. Therefore, these three factors were chosen as independent variables of Box-Behnken design for optimizing the *ev*LAM.

3.2. Optimization of the evLAM by Box-Behnken Design

All the responses observed for 15 experimental runs were simultaneously fitted to first order, second order, and quadratic models by Design Expert 8.0. It was observed that the best-fitted model was the quadratic model. Comparative values are given in Table 2 along with the regression equations generated for each response. Only statistically significant ($p < 0.05$) coefficients were included in the equations.

A positive value indicated an effect that favored the optimization, while a negative value represented an inverse relationship between the factor and the response. As shown in Table 2, it was evident that the pH of the system (X_1) had positive effects on the two responses—the attenuation rate of intestinal tissue activity (Y_1) and the amount of fatty acids (Y_2). Concentrations of D-glucose (X_2) and pancreatic lipase (X_3) had positive effects on the amount of fatty acids but had negative effects on the attenuation rate of intestinal tissue activity. More than one factor term or the coefficients with higher order terms in the regression equation represented, respectively, interaction terms or quadratic relationships, which suggests that the relationships between factors and responses were not always linear. As shown in Table 2, the interaction effect of concentrations of D-glucose and pancreatic lipase was only positive for the attenuation rate of intestinal tissue activity, but interaction effects between pH and D-glucose concentration, pH, and pancreatic lipase concentration were unfavorable for the amount of fatty acids. Higher and positive quadratic effects of pH and D-glucose concentration were observed for both the attenuation rate of intestinal tissue activity and the amount of fatty acids. Quadratic effects of pancreatic lipase concentration were positive or negative for the attenuation rate of intestinal tissue activity and the amount of fatty acids, respectively.

Table 2. Regression analysis for responses for fitting to quadratic model.

	R^2	Adjusted R^2	Predicted R^2	SD	% CV
Y_1	0.9999	0.9996	0.9982	0.026	1.31
Y_2	0.9966	0.9921	0.9656	0.16	3.32
Regression equations of the fitted quadratic model					
$Y_1 = 0.40 + 0.69X_1 - 0.99X_2 - 0.40X_3 - 0.08X_1X_2 - 0.049X_1X_3 + 0.064X_2X_3 + 1.33X_1{}^2 + 0.74X_2{}^2 + 0.82X_3{}^2$					
$Y_2 = 4.55 + 2.13X_1 + 0.27X_2 + 0.75X_3 - 0.089X_1X_2 - 0.20X_1X_3 + 0.72X_1{}^2 + 0.10X_2{}^2 - 0.41X_3{}^2$					

Three-dimensional response surface plots, which could represent interactions of all factors on the responses more clearly, are shown in Figures 3 and 4. When the third factor was kept at a constant level, these plots were very useful in study of the effects of another two factors on the response at the same time.

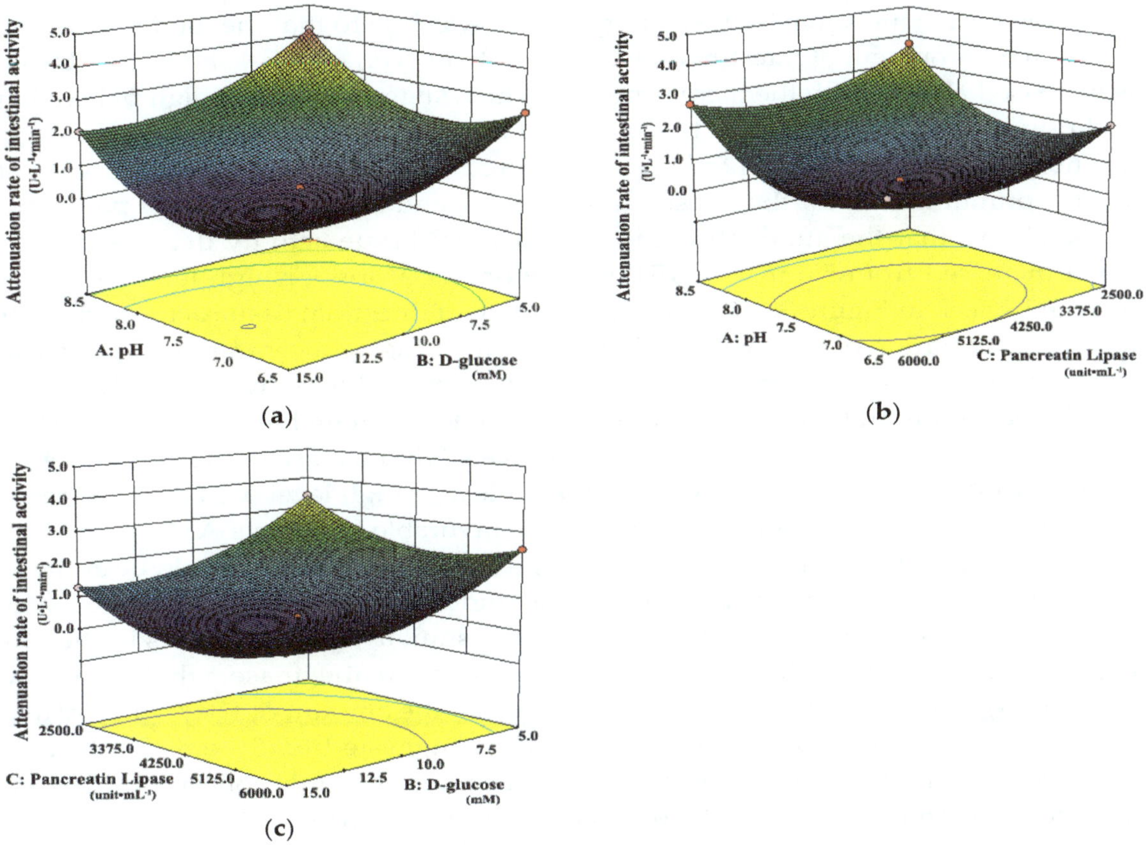

Figure 3. Response surface plots showing interaction effects of pH, D-glucose, and pancreatic lipase on the attenuation rate of intestinal tissue activity when (**a**) pancreatic lipase, (**b**) D-glucose, and (**c**) pH held constant, respectively.

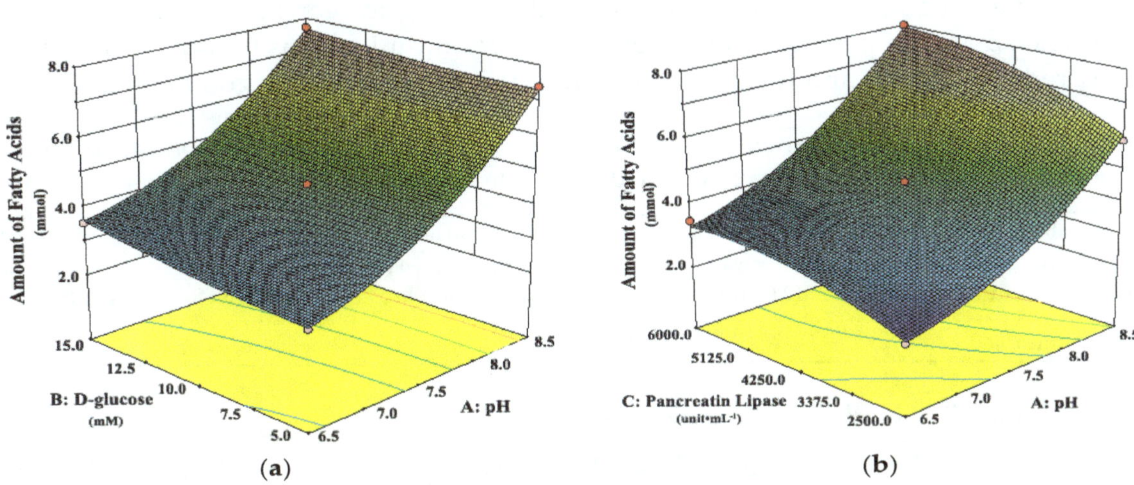

Figure 4. Response surface plots showing interaction effects of pH, D-glucose, and pancreatic lipase on the amount of fatty acids from digestion when (**a**) pancreatic lipase or (**b**) D-glucose held constant, respectively.

As shown in Figure 3a, when the pH of the system was 6.5 or 8.5, the attenuation rates of intestinal tissue activity were higher than those at other moderate levels of pH, regardless of the D-glucose concentration. A similar observation can be seen in Figure 3b. The attenuation rate of intestinal tissue activity increased when the pH of the system changed from the middle to the both ends of the range of 6.5 to 8.5, whether at low or high concentration of pancreatic lipase. It suggested that the moderate pH was favorable for the intestinal tissue activity, which was due to that the moderate pH simulated the physiological environment of intestinal tract in vivo. However, Figure 4 shows that the amount of fatty acids increased always with the increasing pH, which suggests that the high pH could promote the in vitro lipolysis. It might be due to that pancreatic lipase showed the highest catalytic activity in vitro around pH of 8 [35,40–42]. In the literature [28,35,40–42], the pH was usually set about 7.4, which was the optimum value for the intestinal cell culture and the best activity of pancreas lipase.

Figure 3a shows that the attenuation rate of intestinal tissue activity decreased as D-glucose concentration increased from 5.0 mM to 15.0 mM, whether at low or high level of pH. A similar observation can be seen in Figure 3c. The attenuation rate of intestinal tissue activity decreased with the increasing concentration of D-glucose, whether at low or high concentration of pancreatic lipase. The possible explanation was that more energy source from D-glucose was provided for intestinal tissue cells at higher concentrations of D-glucose, which could maintain the activity of intestinal tissues well in vitro. Moreover, Figure 4a shows that there was a slight increase in the amount of fatty acids with the increase of D-glucose concentration, whether at low or high level of pH. All the results above suggested that the high concentration of D-glucose was favorable for the *ev*LAM.

As shown in Figure 3b, the attenuation rate of intestinal tissue activity would be at the least level when the concentration of pancreatic lipase was in the middle of the range of 2500 to 6000 unit·mL^{-1}, whatever the pH of the system was. Figure 3c shows the similar variation trends in the attenuation rate of intestinal tissue activity with the concentration of pancreatic lipase, whether at low or high concentration of D-glucose. However, Figure 4b shows that the amount of fatty acids increased with the increasing concentration of pancreatic lipase, which suggested that the high concentration of pancreatic lipase could promote the in vitro lipolysis. Thus, the optimal concentration of pancreatic lipase should be a compromise between the optimal conditions in vitro for the intestinal tissue activity and the lipolysis.

The optimum *ev*LAM was selected based on the criteria for attaining the optimum value of the model by applying constraints on the attenuation rate of intestinal tissue activity (minimum) and the amount of fatty acids ($4.468 \leq Y_2 \leq 4.703$). Based on 'trading of' various response variables and comprehensive evaluation of feasibility search and exhaustive grid search, the *ev*LAM with pH of 7.37, D-glucose of 12.06 mM, and pancreatic lipase of 4.94×10^3 unit·mL^{-1} was found to fulfill the optimum model. The predicted values and the observed values were in reasonably good agreement (Table 3).

Table 3. Optimized values obtained by the constraints applied on the attenuation rate of intestinal tissue activity (Y_1) and the amount of fatty acids (Y_2) (Mean ± S.D., n = 5).

Variable	Nominal Values	Response	Predicted Values	Observed Values
X_1 (the pH of the system)	7.37	Y_1 (U·L^{-1}·min^{-1})	0.041	0.047 ± 0.002
X_2 (D-glucose concentration)	12.06 (mM)	Y_2 (mmol)	4.629	4.355 ± 0.720
X_3 (pancreatic lipase concentration)	4.94×10^3 (unit·mL^{-1})			

3.3. Evaluate of the evLAM by the Pharmacokinetics in Rats

The first aim of this study was to establish the ex vivo lipolysis-absorption model for evaluating and predicting the in vivo performance of LBFs. We conducted the in vivo pharmacokinetic studies to obtain the real absorption of formulations in vivo. Figure 5 shows that absorption percentages obtained from the new *ev*LAM (P_{a1}) were far higher than those from the conventional EGSM (P_{a2}) within 2 h. The EGSM provided a relatively large surface area available for absorption and a mucus layer [26] but lacked the simulation of lipolytic condition, resulting in the inadequate absorption in vitro of LBFs. On the contrary, the *ev*LAM provided the almost real environment for the digestion of LBFs. Therefore, the in vitro absorption of poorly water-soluble drugs in LBFs could be obtained more accurately by the *ev*LAM.

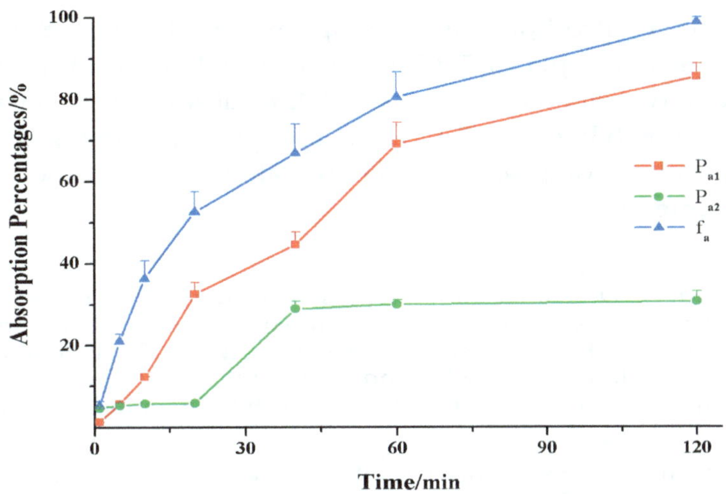

Figure 5. Absorption percentages of the lipid-based formulation of indomethacin from the new ex vivo lipolysis-absorption model (■, P_{a1}), the conventional everted gut sac model (•, P_{a2}) and pharmacokinetics test of rats (▲, f_a) within 2 h. ($n = 5$).

Figure 6 shows the in vitro-in vivo correlations (IVIVC) of absorption curve obtained from the new *ev*LAM and the conventional EGSM. The regression correlation coefficient (r) of IVIVC for the *ev*LAM ($r_1 = 0.9773$, $n = 7$) was far higher than the critical correlation coefficient ($r = 0.8740$, $P < 0.01$, $n = 7$), while r for the EGSM ($r_2 = 0.7852$, $n = 7$) was below the critical correlation coefficient. Therefore, there was a significant correlation between the absorption curve from the *ev*LAM and the in vivo absorption curve of rats. It was suggested that the *ev*LAM possessed good ability to predict the in vivo performance of lipid formulations. On the contrary, there was no significant correlation between the absorption curve from the EGSM and the in vivo absorption curve of rats. Indeed, these results demonstrated that the *ev*LAM, allowed precise insights into the in vivo absorption characteristics of LBFs, which suggests that it should be an attractive and great potential method for screening formulation and evaluating characteristics of LBFs.

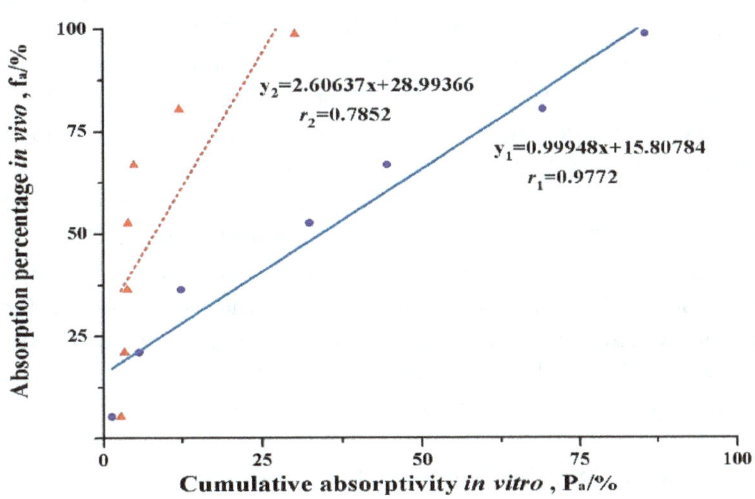

Figure 6. Plots of the in vivo-in vitro correlation of absorption curve for the lipid-based formulation of indomethacin obtained from the conventional everted gut sac model (▲) and the new ex vivo lipolysis-absorption model (•), respectively.

4. Conclusions

In this paper, a new *ev*LAM was developed to predict the intestinal absorptions of poorly water-soluble drugs in LBFs. This new model was composed of an intestinal digestion system and an intestinal tissue system. D-glucose, pancreatic lipase, and pH significantly affected the in vitro activity of intestinal tissue and the in vitro lipolysis. The optimal model parameters by the Box-Behnken design were set up as follows: a pH of 7.37, D-glucose of 12.06 mM, and a pancreatic lipase of 4.94×10^3 unit·mL^{-1}. For a typical lipid-based formulation, absorption percentages obtained from the optimal *ev*LAM showed a much better IVIVC with absorption percentages of rats in vivo. The new *ev*LAM could make up for the inadequacy of conventional methods and be a better tool for assessing LBFs of poorly water-soluble drugs.

Supplementary Materials:
Figure S1. Pseudo-ternary Phase Diagrams: "Me" represented microemulsion area; (A) the mixing ratio of Cremophor RH40 and Transcutol P was 3:1; (B) the mixing ratio of Cremophor RH40 and Transcutol P was 1:1; (C) the mixing ratio of Cremophor RH40 and Transcutol P was 1:3. Figure S2. The microscopic images of the four formulations. Formulations were showed as labeled and the ruler was in the bottom right corner of the diagram. Table S1. Self-emulsifying Time, droplet Size, appearance and solubility of indomethacin for the nanoemulsions (mean, $n = 5$).

Author Contributions: All authors contributed to this work. T.Y. designed and conducted the study. Y.L. performed the experiments. L.X analyzed the data and prepared the original draft. T.Y. revised the manuscript and also supervised this work.

References

1. Esfanjani, A.F.; Assadpour, E.; Jafari, S.M. Improving the bioavailability of phenolic compounds by loading them within lipid-based nanocarriers. *Trends Food Sci. Technol.* **2018**, *76*, 56–66. [CrossRef]
2. Jafari, S.M.; Mcclements, D.J. Nanotechnology Approaches for Increasing Nutrient Bioavailability. *Adv. Food Nutr. Res.* **2017**, *81*, 1–30.
3. Zeng, N.; Gao, X.; Hu, Q.; Song, Q.; Xia, H.; Liu, Z.; Gu, G.; Jiang, M.; Pang, Z.; Chen, H.; et al. Lipid-based liquid crystalline nanoparticles as oral drug delivery vehicles for poorly water-soluble drugs: Cellular interaction and in vivo absorption. *Int. J. Nanomed.* **2012**, *7*, 3703–3718.
4. Wasan, K.M. Formulation and physiological and biopharmaceutical issues in the development of oral lipid-based drug delivery systems. *Drug Dev. Ind. Pharm.* **2001**, *27*, 267–276. [CrossRef]
5. Pouton, C.W. Formulation of poorly water-soluble drugs for oral administration: Physicochemical and physiological issues and the lipid formulation classification system. *Eur. J. Pharm. Sci.* **2006**, *29*, 278–287. [CrossRef]
6. Pouton, C.W.; Porter, C.J. Formulation of lipid-based delivery systems for oral administration: Materials, methods and strategies. *Adv. Drug Deliv. Rev.* **2008**, *60*, 625–637. [CrossRef]
7. Porter, C.J.H.; Pouton, C.W.; Cuine, J.F.; Charman, W.N. Enhancing intestinal drug solubilisation using lipid-based delivery systems. *Adv. Drug Deliv. Rev.* **2008**, *60*, 673–691. [CrossRef]
8. Trevaskis, N.L.; Charman, W.N.; Porter, C.J. Lipid-based delivery systems and intestinal lymphatic drug transport: A mechanistic update. *Adv. Drug Deliv. Rev.* **2008**, *60*, 702–716. [CrossRef]
9. Hur, S.J.; Joo, S.T.; Lim, B.O.; Decker, E.A.; McClements, J.D. Impact of salt and lipid type on in vitro digestion of emulsified lipids. *Food Chem.* **2011**, *126*, 1559–1564. [CrossRef] [PubMed]
10. Kossena, G.A.; Boyd, B.J.; Porter, C.J.H.; Charman, W.N. Separation and characterization of the colloidal phases produced on digestion of common formulation lipids and assessment of their impact on the apparent solubility of selected poorly water-soluble drugs. *J. Pharm. Sci.* **2003**, *92*, 634–648. [CrossRef]
11. Kossena, G.A.; Charman, W.N.; Boyd, B.J.; Porter, C.I.H. Influence of the intermediate digestion phases of common formulation lipids on the absorption of a poorly water-soluble drug. *J. Pharm. Sci.* **2005**, *94*, 481–492. [CrossRef]
12. Kossena, G.A.; Charman, W.N.; Boyd, B.J.; Dunstan, D.E.; Porter, C.J. Probing drug solubilization patterns in the gastrointestinal tract after administration of lipid-based delivery systems: A phase diagram approach. *J. Pharm. Sci.* **2004**, *93*, 332–348. [CrossRef]
13. Wiedmann, T.S.; Kamel, L. Examination of the solubilization of drugs by bile salt micelles. *J. Pharm. Sci.* **2002**, *91*, 1743–1764. [CrossRef]

14. Armand, M.; Borel, P.; Pasquier, B.; Dubois, C.; Senft, M.; Andre, M.; Peyrot, J.; Salducci, J.; Lairon, D. Physicochemical characteristics of emulsions during fat digestion in human stomach and duodenum. *Am. J. Physiol.* **1996**, *271 (Pt 1)*, G172–G183. [CrossRef]
15. Hernell, O.; Staggers, J.E.; Carey, M.C. Physical-chemical behavior of dietary and biliary lipids during intestinal digestion and absorption. 2. Phase analysis and aggregation states of luminal lipids during duodenal fat digestion in healthy adult human beings. *Biochemistry* **1990**, *29*, 2041–2056. [CrossRef]
16. Kim, H.J.; Yoon, K.A.; Hahn, M.; Park, E.S.; Chi, S.C. Preparation and in vitro evaluation of self-microemulsifying drug delivery systems containing idebenone. *Drug Dev. Ind. Pharm.* **2000**, *26*, 523–529. [CrossRef]
17. Cirri, M.; Mura, P.; Mora, P.C. Liquid spray formulations of xibornol by using self-microemulsifying drug delivery systems. *Int. J. Pharm.* **2007**, *340*, 84–91. [CrossRef]
18. Dai, W.G. In vitro methods to assess drug precipitation. *Int. J. Pharm.* **2010**, *393*, 1–16. [CrossRef]
19. Sek, L.; Porter, C.J.H.; Charman, W.N. Characterisation and quantification of medium chain and long chain triglycerides and their in vitro digestion products, by HPTLC coupled with in situ densitometric analysis. *J. Pharm. Biomed.* **2001**, *25*, 651–661. [CrossRef]
20. Brogard, M.; Troedsson, E.; Thuresson, K.; Ljusberg-Wahren, H. A new standardized lipolysis approach for characterization of emulsions and dispersions. *J. Colloid Interface Sci.* **2007**, *308*, 500–507. [CrossRef]
21. Zangenberg, N.H.; Mullertz, A.; Kristensen, H.G.; Hovgaard, L. A dynamic in vitro lipolysis model. I. Controlling the rate of lipolysis by continuous addition of calcium. *Eur. J. Pharm. Sci.* **2001**, *14*, 115–122. [CrossRef]
22. Han, S.F.; Yao, T.T.; Zhang, X.X.; Gan, L.; Zhu, C.; Yu, H.Z.; Gan, Y. Lipid-based formulations to enhance oral bioavailability of the poorly water-soluble drug anethol trithione: Effects of lipid composition and formulation. *Int. J. Pharm.* **2009**, *379*, 18–24. [CrossRef] [PubMed]
23. Li, Y.; Hu, M.; McClements, D.J. Factors affecting lipase digestibility of emulsified lipids using an in vitro digestion model: Proposal for a standardised pH-stat method. *Food Chem.* **2011**, *126*, 498–505. [CrossRef]
24. Dahan, A.H.A. Use of a dynamic in vitro lipolysis model to rationalize oral formulation development for poor water soluble drugs: Correlation with in vivo data and the relationship to intra-enterocyte processes in rats. *Pharm. Res.* **2006**, *23*, 2165–2174. [CrossRef] [PubMed]
25. Jannin, V.; Dellera, E.; Chevrier, S.; Chavant, Y.; Voutsinas, C.; Bonferoni, C.; Demarne, F. In vitro lipolysis tests on lipid nanoparticles: Comparison between lipase/co-lipase and pancreatic extract. *Drug Dev. Ind. Pharm.* **2015**, *41*, 1582–1588. [CrossRef] [PubMed]
26. Alam, M.A.; Al-Jenoobi, F.I.; Al-Mohizea, A.M. Everted gut sac model as a tool in pharmaceutical research: Limitations and applications. *J. Pharm. Pharmacol.* **2012**, *64*, 326–336. [CrossRef] [PubMed]
27. Alvarez, F.J.; Stella, V.J. The role of calcium ions and bile salts on the pancreatic lipase-catalyzed hydrolysis of triglyceride emulsions stabilized with lecithin. *Pharm. Res.* **1989**, *6*, 449–457. [CrossRef]
28. Hu, M.; Li, Y.; Decker, E.A.; McClements, D.J. Role of calcium and calcium-binding agents on the lipase digestibility of emulsified lipids using an in vitro digestion model. *Food Hydrocoll.* **2010**, *24*, 719–725. [CrossRef]
29. Mun, S.; Decker, E.A.; Park, Y.; Weiss, J.; McClements, D.J. Influence of interfacial composition on in vitro digestibility of emulsified lipids: Potential mechanism for chitosan's ability to inhibit fat digestion. *Food Biophys.* **2006**, *1*, 21–29. [CrossRef]
30. Williams, H.D.; Sassene, P.; Kleberg, K.; Bakala-N'Goma, J.C.; Calderone, M.; Jannin, V.; Igonin, A.; Partheil, A.; Marchaud, D.; Jule, E.; et al. Toward the establishment of standardized in vitro tests for lipid-based formulations, part 1: Method parameterization and comparison of in vitro digestion profiles across a range of representative formulations. *J. Pharm. Sci.* **2012**, *101*, 3360–3380. [CrossRef]
31. Zhou, J.; Zhu, F.; Li, J.; Wang, J. Concealed body mesoporous silica nanoparticles for orally delivering indometacin with chiral recognition function. *Mater. Sci. Eng. C* **2018**, *90*, 314–324. [CrossRef] [PubMed]
32. Al Za'abi, M.A.; Dehghanzadeh, G.H.; Norris, R.L.; Charles, B.G. A rapid and sensitive microscale HPLC method for the determination of indomethacin in plasma of premature neonates with patent ductus arteriousus. *J. Chromatog. B Anal. Technol. Biomed. Life Sci.* **2006**, *830*, 364–367. [CrossRef] [PubMed]
33. Ali, H.N.M.; Zaghloul, A.A.; Nazzal, S. Comparison between lipolysis and compendial dissolution as alternative techniques for the in vitro characterization of alpha-tocopherol self-emulsified drug delivery systems (SEDDS). *Int. J. Pharm.* **2008**, *352*, 104–114. [CrossRef] [PubMed]

34. van Tilbeurgh, H.; Sarda, L.; Verger, R.; Cambillau, C. Structure of the pancreatic lipase-procolipase complex. *Nature* **1992**, *359*, 159–162. [CrossRef] [PubMed]
35. Di Maio, S.; Carrier, R.L. Gastrointestinal contents in fasted state and post-lipid ingestion: In vivo measurements and in vitro models for studying oral drug delivery. *J. Control. Release Off. J. Control. Release Soc.* **2011**, *151*, 110–122. [CrossRef] [PubMed]
36. Hofmann, A.F.; Mysels, K.J. Bile acid solubility and precipitation in vitro and in vivo: The role of conjugation, pH, and Ca2+ ions. *J. Lipid Res.* **1992**, *33*, 617–626. [PubMed]
37. Lindahl, A.; Ungell, A.L.; Knutson, L.; Lennernas, H. Characterization of fluids from the stomach and proximal jejunum in men and women. *Pharm. Res.* **1997**, *14*, 497–502. [CrossRef] [PubMed]
38. Sek, L.P.C.; Kaukonen, A.M.; Charman, W.N. Evaluation of the in-vitro digestion profiles of long and medium chain glycerides and the phase behaviour of their lipolytic products. *J. Pharm. Pharm.* **2002**, *54*, 29–41. [CrossRef]
39. Kaukonen, A.M.; Boyd, B.J.; Porter, C.J.; Charman, W.N. Drug solubilization behavior during in vitro digestion of simple triglyceride lipid solution formulations. *Pharm. Res.* **2004**, *21*, 245–253. [CrossRef]
40. Kaukonen, A.M.; Boyd, B.J.; Charman, W.N.; Porter, C.J. Drug solubilization behavior during in vitro digestion of suspension formulations of poorly water-soluble drugs in triglyceride lipids. *Pharm. Res.* **2004**, *21*, 254–260. [CrossRef]
41. Porter, C.J.H.; Kaukonen, A.M.; Boyd, B.J.; Edwards, G.A.; Charman, W.N. Susceptibility to lipase-mediated digestion reduces the oral bioavailability of danazol after administration as a medium-chain lipid-based microemulsion formulation. *Pharm. Res.* **2004**, *21*, 1405–1412. [CrossRef]
42. Porter, C.J.H.; Kaukonen, A.M.; Taillardat-Bertschinger, A.; Boyd, B.J.; O'Connor, J.M.; Edwards, G.A.; Charman, W.N. Use of in vitro lipid digestion data to explain the in vivo performance of triglyceride-based oral lipid formulations of poorly water-soluble drugs: Studies with halofantrine. *J. Pharm. Sci.* **2004**, *93*, 1110–1121. [CrossRef] [PubMed]
43. Burgstaller, W. Transport of small Ions and molecules through the plasma membrane of filamentous fungi. *Crit. Rev. Microbiol.* **1997**, *23*, 1–46. [CrossRef] [PubMed]

7

Drug Transport Across Porcine Intestine Using an Ussing Chamber System: Regional Differences and the Effect of P-Glycoprotein and CYP3A4 Activity on Drug Absorption

Yvonne E. Arnold [1], Julien Thorens [2,3], Stéphane Bernard [2] and Yogeshvar N. Kalia [1,*]

1 School of Pharmaceutical Sciences, University of Geneva & University of Lausanne, CMU-1 rue Michel Servet, 1211 Geneva 4, Switzerland; Yvonne.Arnold@unige.ch

2 Debiopharm International SA, Chemin Messidor 5-7, 1006 Lausanne, Switzerland; julienthorens@hotmail.com (J.T.); stephane.bernard@debiopharm.com (S.B.)

3 Present address: Pharmacie des fins, 3 rue de Frontenex, 74000 Annecy, France

* Correspondence: yogi.kalia@unige.ch

Abstract: Drug absorption across viable porcine intestines was investigated using an Ussing chamber system. The apparent permeability coefficients, $P_{app,pig}$, were compared to the permeability coefficients determined in humans in vivo, $P_{eff,human}$. Eleven drugs from the different Biopharmaceutical Classification System (BCS) categories absorbed by passive diffusion with published $P_{eff,human}$ values were used to test the system. The initial experiments measured $P_{app,pig}$ for each drug after application in a Krebs–Bicarbonate Ringer (KBR) buffer and in biorelevant media FaSSIF V2 and FeSSIF V2, mimicking fasted and fed states. Strong sigmoidal correlations were observed between $P_{eff,human}$ and $P_{app,pig}$. Differences in the segmental $P_{app,pig}$ of antipyrine, cimetidine and metoprolol confirmed the discrimination between drug uptake in the duodenum, jejunum and ileum (and colon); the results were in good agreement with human data in vivo. The presence of the P-gp inhibitor verapamil significantly increased $P_{app,pig}$ across the ileum of the P-gp substrates cimetidine and ranitidine ($p < 0.05$). Clotrimazole, a potent CYP3A4 inhibitor, significantly increased $P_{app,pig}$ of the CYP3A4 substrates midazolam, verapamil and tamoxifen and significantly decreased the formation of their main metabolites. In conclusion, the results showed that this is a robust technique to predict passive drug permeability under fasted and fed states, to identify regional differences in drug permeability and to demonstrate the activity of P-gp and CYP3A4.

Keywords: intestinal permeability; regional drug absorption; Ussing chamber; biorelevant media; P-gp; CYP3A4

---

1. Introduction

Methods to predict intestinal drug absorption in humans in vivo range from purely in silico computational techniques to preclinical animal studies in vivo. In vitro tests range from relatively simple solubilization or permeation studies to more advanced systems, mimicking several steps or even the complete passage through the gastrointestinal tract [1–7]. High-throughput methods (e.g., PAMPA or Caco-2 cell lines) are frequently used in early, preclinical stages. The monolayer cell culture system is limited by the absence of a full physiological membrane and the specific properties of the individual cell types present in the different segments of the intestine. These models are usually used to evaluate the permeability of the API alone since they are not sufficiently robust to support either biorelevant media or "real" formulations. Indeed, to better approach the physiological conditions, mucus-producing HT29-MTX cells and M cells inducing Raji B cells were introduced into the Caco-2 monolayer [8–13]. Although in vivo studies cannot necessarily provide insight into regional differences in drug absorption, this has been attempted to be addressed in rats by the single-pass intestinal perfusion technique or, with appropriate adjustments, the closed-loop Doluisio method [14].

In order to have comprehensive permeability data for the selection of lead drug candidates and to predict the absorption in humans in vivo, it is crucial to have a physiologically and anatomically similar model that can address the following points: (i) the identification of absorption sites (crucial for modified-release formulations and poorly soluble compounds), (ii) a full physiological membrane evaluation (including mucus layer), (iii) the influence of excipients on drug permeability, (iv) drug metabolism in epithelial cells, (v) the effect of active transporters and efflux systems, and (vi) the drug/drug interactions: These will determine the relevance of the model for humans, i.e., its predictive power.

One approach is to use an Ussing chamber system, which enables transport experiments to be performed using viable intestinal tissue ex vivo [15–21]; tissue integrity is monitored by the continuous measurement of transepithelial resistance. Human intestine is obviously the most suitable tissue for ex vivo evaluations, and there have been some studies over the last twenty years [22–27]. Much work was done by the Drug Metabolism and Pharmacokinetics group at AstraZeneca R&D, which published a landmark paper in 2013 that compiled 15 years of data on drug absorption focusing mainly on transport across the human jejunum and colon and the effect of pre-systemic metabolism and efflux transporters [28]. However, the availability of viable human intestine is extremely limited-samples are usually obtained from patients suffering from malignancies [23,26,28,29]. To circumvent this, rat intestines have been the traditional animal model of choice for ex vivo/in vivo permeation studies [24,30–32]. However, it has a number of limitations, including differences in intestinal morphology and other distinct physiological differences that can make extrapolation to humans difficult [33]. Although the major drug transporters in humans and rats are in good correlation, the enzyme expression between human and rat intestines is different: For example, rat intestine displays pre-systemic cytochrome P450 activity, but this does not correlate to the activity in the human intestine [34]. In addition to the scientific issues concerning relevance, ethical concerns can also be cited with the use of rats as they have to be sacrificed for such evaluations.

Like humans, pigs are large omnivorous mammals, and porcine intestine shows greater similarities to human intestine than the intestinal tissue from other animals [33–36]. For nutritional studies, the porcine model is known to be superior to other non-primate animal models: Despite some anatomic differences, the physiology of digestion and the associated metabolic processes are much alike between humans and pigs [37]. The gross anatomical features of the GI tract of pigs and humans are similar, although the divisions between the duodenum, jejunum and ileum are not as distinct in porcine small intestine [35]. Microscopically, the intestinal villus structure and component epithelial cell types are very alike, and the pH variations of the different regions of the gastrointestinal tract in pigs and human are, again, similar [33].

At a molecular level, the metabolic activities for Phase 1 and Phase 2 enzymes in humans and pigs are closely related [34]. Porcine intestine appears to possess a high cytochrome P450 CYP3A activity, and there is more homology between human and porcine CYP3A enzymes than with those in the rat [38,39]. In both humans and pigs, P-gp is coded by a single gene (ABCB1 (ATP-binding cassette B1) or MDR1 (multidrug resistance 1)) (cf. two P-gp homologues in rats). The alignment of the porcine and human P-gp sequences resulted in a homology of 90.8%, with a high homology in the predicted transmembrane domains known to be important for substrate binding [40]. Moreover, P-gp expression was shown to increase from the proximal to distal regions in the small intestine of Yucatan micropigs—as is the case in humans [41,42]. Multidrug-resistance-associated protein (MRP2), breast cancer-resistant protein (BCRP), peptide transporter-1 (PepT1) and organic anion-transporting polypeptide (OATP) are present in porcine intestine [34].

The objective of the present study was to demonstrate that the Ussing chamber system with porcine intestine could be a useful surrogate to predict intestinal absorption in humans. Reports describing the use of porcine intestine to model drug absorption using the Ussing chamber or related systems and with diffusion cells are scarce [43–55], e.g., indeed, Ussing chamber investigations have only been performed on the uptake of polyphenols present in apples [43] and in coffee [44]. To our knowledge, the only detailed investigation to date into the feasibility of using porcine intestine to predict human intestinal absorption employed a diffusion cell-based system with a view to enable the development of a "medium throughput" technique [45].

The systematic approach employed in the present study was similar to that used by Sjöberg et al. with an extension to include the use of physiologically relevant media [28]. The specific aims were (i) to investigate the absorption of a training set of 11 molecules across viable porcine intestine from a Krebs–Bicarbonate Ringer (KBR) buffer and, with a view approaching more physiologic conditions, from the biorelevant media Fasted State Simulated Intestinal Fluid Version 2 (FaSSIF V2) and Fed State Simulated Intestinal Fluid Version 2 (FeSSIF V2) and to correlate the experimental $P_{app,pig}$ with $P_{eff,human}$ values determined in humans in vivo; (ii) to demonstrate the ability of the model to detect the regional variation in drug absorption in the different segments of the small intestine (i.e., duodenum, jejunum and ileum)—furthermore, uptake in the colon was also evaluated—(iii) to determine $P_{app,pig}$ of the P-gp substrates, cimetidine and ranitidine, in the presence and absence of the P-gp inhibitor, verapamil, to demonstrate that the efflux transporter retained its activity in the porcine intestine ex vivo; and likewise, (iv) to determine $P_{app,pig}$ of the CYP3A4 substrates, midazolam, tamoxifen and verapamil, in the presence and absence of the potent CYP3A4 inhibitor, clotrimazole, to confirm that the enzyme retained activity. Furthermore, the respective metabolites, hydroxymidazolam, N-desmethyl-tamoxifen and norverapamil, were also quantified.

2. Materials and Methods

2.1. Chemicals

Antipyrine, cimetidine, clotrimazole, N-desmethyl-tamoxifen hydrochloride, furosemide, hydrochlorothiazide, ketoprofen, maleic acid, (+/−)-metoprolol-(+)-tartrate, (+/−)-norverapamil hydrochloride, piroxicam, tamoxifen, terbutaline hemisulfate and (+/−)-verapamil hydrochloride 99% were purchased from Sigma-Aldrich (St. Louis, MO, USA); (+/−)-propranolol hydrochloride and ranitidine hydrochloride were obtained from Alfa Aesar GmbH & Co KG (Karlsruhe, Germany), and carbamazepine was purchased from Acros Organics (New Jersey, USA). Midazolam and α-hydroxymidazolam were purchased from Lipomed AG (Arlesheim, Switzerland), and agar, calcium chloride dihydrate, glucose hydrate, magnesium chloride hexahydrate, potassium chloride, sodium chloride, sodium hydroxide, sodium phosphate monobasic and sodium hydrogencarbonate were obtained from Hänseler AG (Herisau, Switzerland). Sodium taurocholate was purchased from Prodotti Chimici e Alimentari S.p.A., (Basaluzzo, Italy) and lecithin (grade EPCS > 98% phospholipids) was obtained from Lipoid GmbH (Ludwigshafen, Germany).

2.2. Porcine Intestinal Tissue

Porcine intestinal tissue from 6-month-old female Swiss noble pigs (weight: 100–120 kg) was supplied by two local abattoirs (Abattoir de Meinier; Meinier, Switzerland and Abattoir de Loëx; Bernex, Switzerland) and was collected immediately after slaughter. In order to remove the luminal debris, the tissue was rinsed with ice-cold KBR (120 mM NaCl, 5.5 mM KCl, 2.5 mM $CaCl_2$, 1.2 mM $MgCl_2$, 1.2 mM NaH_2PO_4, 20 mM $NaHCO_3$ and 11 mM glucose; pH 7.4) [56]. During transport from the slaughterhouse to the laboratory, the tissue was stored in ice-cold KBR and constantly bubbled with a 95% O_2/5% CO_2 gas mixture (PanGas AG; Dagmersellen, Switzerland).

Once in the laboratory, the intestinal tissue was prepared using previously published protocols [46,57]. Briefly, the intestine was opened along the mesenteric border and rinsed with ice-cold KBR. The muscle layer was carefully removed using a scalpel and fine forceps. The remaining tunica mucosa and submucosa were cut into segments of approximately 1.5 cm^2. Areas including Peyer's patches were avoided. During the whole procedure, which took 5–10 min, the tissue was stored in ice-cold KBR and constantly bubbled with a gas mixture of 95% O_2/5% CO_2.

2.3. Ussing Chamber Setup and Procedures for Intestinal Absorption Experiments

A six Ussing chamber system coupled to a VCC MC6 MultiChannel Voltage–Current Clamp (Physiologic Instruments; San Diego, CA, USA) with a heating block and six input modules with integral dummy membranes was used for the permeation studies. A circulating water bath (ED-5, Julabo GmbH, Seelbach, Germany) was used to regulate the temperature. The Ussing chambers were set up using the method reported by Neirinckx et al. [46]. First, the Ag/AgCl electrodes were put in tips containing a congealed mixture of 3% agar in 3 M KCl. Then, the electrodes were inserted into the Ussing chambers, and the donor and acceptor compartments were filled with preheated KBR (38°C). The buffer solution was constantly bubbled with a 95% O_2/5% CO_2 gas mixture; in addition to oxygenating the tissue, this ensured mixing and circulation of the buffer in the two compartments. Any voltage difference between the electrodes and the transepithelial electrical resistance due to the buffer solution was eliminated. The chambers were emptied, the intestinal tissue was mounted on the sliders with an exposed surface area of 1.26 cm^2 and the sliders were inserted into the Ussing chambers. The intestine was mounted in the Ussing chamber 45 min after harvesting from the animal. KBR (7 mL) was added to the donor and acceptor compartments and left to equilibrate for 30 min, at which point both the donor and acceptor compartments were emptied and the acceptor phase was replaced with the same volume of fresh KBR (7 mL) so as to minimize the potential impact of endogenous material released during the 30 min equilibration period.

The composition of the solution in the donor compartment was dependent on the experiments: (i) in the first study into passive drug absorption, each API from the training set of 11 molecules (Table 1) was dissolved in KBR (7 mL) to prepare a 100 μM solution; (ii) in the second series of experiments, which investigated the effect of using fasted state biorelevant media on drug absorption, each API (100 μM) was dissolved in FaSSIF V2 (7 mL; 68.62 mM NaCl, 34.8 mM NaOH, 19.12 mM maleic acid, 3 mM Na taurocholate and 3 mM lecithin; pH 6.5) [58]; (iii) in the third series, which investigated the effect of fed state conditions on drug uptake, the API was dissolved in FeSSIF V2 (7 mL; 125.5 mM NaCl, 69.9 mM NaOH, 55.02 mM maleic acid, 10 mM Na taurocholate, 2 mM lecithin, 0.8 mM glycerol monooleate and 0.8 mM sodium oleate; pH 5.8) [58].

Table 1. The chemical structures and physicochemical properties of the drug molecules tested using the Ussing chamber system.

API	MW (g/mol)	log *P*	log *D* [59] Octanol/H_2O pH 7.4	pH 6.5	pH 5.5	Solubility (n = 3) (mg/mL) KBR	FaSSIF V2	FeSSIF V2	Study
BCS I									
Antipyrine (1) $C_{11}H_{12}N_2O$	188.23	0.38	0.6	0.6	0.6	103.00 ± 54.61	261.10 ± 132.29	564.44 ± 83.12	Passive [b] Regional [c]
Ketoprofen (2) $C_{16}H_{14}O_3$	254.28	3.12	0.1	0.8	1.8	2.82 ± 0.62	6.73 ± 2.70	6.37 ± 1.52	Passive
(+/−)-Metoprolol (3) $C_{15}H_{25}NO_3$	267.36	1.88	0.0	−0.5	−0.6	298.03 ± 13.86	43.85 ± 15.81	380.69 ± 33.79	Passive Regional
Midazolam $C_{18}H_{13}ClFN_3$	325.77	3.89	3.0 [a]	3.6 [a]	3.9 [a]	n.a.	n.a.	n.a.	CYP3A4 [d]
Propranolol (4) $C_{16}H_{21}NO_2$	259.34	3.48	1.4	0.9	0.7	158.69 ± 4.34	247.53 ± 7.47	222.57 ± 2.00	Passive
Verapamil $C_{27}H_{38}N_2O_4$	454.60	3.79	3.8 [a]	3.8 [a]	3.8 [a]	1.04 ± 0.09	5.60 ± 1.04	17.60 ± 0.98	CYP3A4
BCS II									
Carbamazepine (5) $C_{15}H_{12}N_2O$	236.27	2.1	2.45	2.45	2.45	0.20 ± 0.02	0.32 ± 0.01	0.73 ± 0.01	Passive
Naproxen (6) $C_{14}H_{14}O_3$	230	3.18	0.3	1.1	2.1	4.51 ± 0.04	14.59 ± 1.19	13.00 ± 2.37	Passive
Piroxicam (7) $C_{15}H_{13}N_3O_4S$	331.35	3.06	0.2 [a]	1.1 [a]	2.0 [a]	0.43 ± 0.02	0.29 ± 0.02	0.06 ± 0.00	Passive
Tamoxifen $C_{26}H_{29}NO$	371.51	5.93	5.6 [a]	5.9 [a]	5.9 [a]	23.32 ± 1.54	32.19 ± 0.42	27.87 ± 0.66	CYP3A4

Table 1. *Cont.*

API	MW (g/mol)	log *P*	log *D* [59] Octanol/H_2O			Solubility (n = 3) (mg/mL)			Study
			pH 7.4	pH 6.5	pH 5.5	KBR	FaSSIF V2	FeSSIF V2	
BSC III									
Atenolol (8) $C_{14}H_{22}N_2O_3$	365.40	0.75	−2.0	−2.0	−2.0	35.57 ± 7.29	33.73 ± 2.06	41.28 ± 1.16	Passive
Cimetidine $C_{14}H_{22}N_2O_3$	252.34	0.40	0.4 [a]	0.4 [a]	0.4 [a]	5.65 ± 0.13	5.88 ± 0.26	0.36 ± 0.26	Regional P-gp [e]
Ranitidine $C_{14}H_{22}N_2O_3$	314.40	0.27	0.2 [a]	0.3 [a]	0.3 [a]	19.64 ± 2.78	15.89 ± 1.47	807.51 ± 70.47	P-gp
Terbutaline (9) $C_{14}H_{22}N_2O_3$	225.28	0.9	−1.4	−1.3	−1.3	213.73 ± 15.18	372.59 ± 18.86	305.07 ± 124.48	Passive
BCS IV									
Furosemide (10) $C_{12}H_{11}ClN_2O_5S$	330.74	2.03	−0.9	−0.5	0.4	5.62 ± 0.10	24.90 ± 2.84	19.68 ± 2.59	Passive
Hydrochlorothiazide (11) $C_7H_8ClN_3O_4S_2$	297.74	−0.16	−0.2	−0.2	−0.2	0.81 ± 0.17	1.18 ± 0.14	1.04 ± 0.19	Passive

[a] The log *D* value was not taken from Reference [54] but was calculated using the following equation: $\log D = \log P + \log(\frac{1}{1+10^{pH-pKa}})$; [b] Passive: the drug used to study passive drug permeation from KBR and biorelevant media; [c] Regional: the drug used to study drug permeation in different intestinal segments; [d] CYP3A4: the drug used to study CYP3A4 activity; [e] P-gp: the drug used to study P-gp activity.

For the experiments investigating the effect of P-gp, verapamil hydrochloride (a known P-gp inhibitor) was added to the formulation in the donor compartment, again at 100 μM and similar to the concentration reported in the literature [60]. For the study investigating the activity of CYP3A4 present in the intestinal membrane, the experiments were performed in the presence/absence of clotrimazole—a potent CYP3A4 inhibitor (K_i = 18 nM)—again at 100 μM [61]. Given the experimental setup, all experiments were performed in sextuplicate.

The cumulative drug permeation across the intestinal epithelium was determined by taking aliquots (400 μL) from the acceptor compartment every 20 min (t = 20, 40, 60, 80, 100 and 120 min); the volume removed was replaced with a fresh buffer. During the experiment, the viability of the intestinal tissue was monitored by measuring the variation of the voltage during the intermittent application of a 50 μA current pulse (duration 200 ms) applied every minute. Using Ohm's law, the transepithelial electrical resistance was calculated and used as a measure for tissue viability. Preliminary studies were performed to define the threshold transepithelial electrical resistance value below which the tissue integrity was considered to be impaired or not viable. Based on these measurements, tissues with a transepithelial electrical resistance below 15 $\Omega.cm^2$ were considered not to be viable or intact and were not used for the calculation of the permeability coefficients.

Upon completion of the experiment (t = 120 min), in addition to the sample from the acceptor, a 400 μL aliquot was withdrawn from the donor compartment. The intestinal slices were cut into small pieces and extracted for 6 h using the mobile phase used for the UHPLC-MS/MS analytical method (see below). This enabled the amount of API retained in the intestinal tissue to be determined. Prior to analysis, all samples were centrifuged for 10 min at 14 000 rpm using an Eppendorf Centrifuge 5804 (Vaudaux-Eppendorf AG; Schönenbuch, Switzerland).

2.4. Analytical Methods

The samples were analyzed using UHPLC-MS/MS. The system consisted of a Waters ACQUITY UPLC® core system and a Waters XEVO® TQ-MS tandem quadrupole mass spectrometer (Milford, MA, USA). Chromatographic separation was achieved using an ACQUITY UPLC® BEH C18 column, 1.7 μm, 25 × 2.1 mm, attached to an ACQUITY UPLC® BEH C18 Van Guard™ Pre-column, 1.7 μm, 5 × 2.1 mm. Tandem mass spectrometry was performed in the multiple reaction monitoring (MRM), mode and the majority of the APIs (Supplementary Material, Table S1) were analyzed with positive ion electrospray ionization (ESI). Furosemide, hydrocholorothiazide, ketoprofen and piroxicam were analyzed with negative ESI (Table S1). The complete details of the isocratic UHPLC-MS/MS methods are reported in the Supplementary Material (Table S1 and Table S2). Data acquisition was done using the MassLynx™ software, version 4.1.

2.5. Data Analysis

2.5.1. Permeability Calculations

The apparent permeability coefficient for transport across the porcine intestinal tissue ($P_{app,pig}$) was calculated using the following equation:

$$P_{app,\ pig} = \frac{dc}{dt} \times \frac{V}{A \times C_0} \left(\frac{cm}{s}\right) \quad (1)$$

where *dc/dt* is the change in the acceptor concentration calculated from the slope of the concentration–time curve between 20 and 80 min, V is the buffer volume in the donor compartment, A is the exposed surface area (1.26 cm^2) and C_0 is the initial concentration of the API in the donor compartment [62].

2.5.2. Data Fitting

The experimental permeability values $P_{app,pig}$ were fitted to the in vivo permeability $P_{eff,human}$ values using a four parameter logistic equation (SigmaPlot software, version 12.5—Systat Software Inc.; San Jose, CA, USA) as used by Sjöberg et al., where y_0 is the minimum value of $P_{eff,human}$, X_{50} is the $P_{app,pig}$ when $P_{eff,human}$ is at half the maximum value, a is a scaling factor and b is the slope factor [28].

$$P_{eff,\ human} = y_0 + \frac{a}{1 + \left(\frac{P_{app,\ pig}}{X_{50}}\right)^b} \tag{2}$$

2.5.3. Evaluation of the Relative Contributions of Drug Deposition and Permeation During Intestinal Transport: The Transport Index (TI)

Conventional approaches to evaluate intestinal drug absorption use the permeability coefficient as the reference parameter. This does not take into account drug retention in the membrane. The quantification of drug deposition in addition to permeation is routinely carried out in investigations into the transport of drugs across other biological membranes [63–66]. In this context, Miyake et al. recently introduced the concept of the transport index (*TI*) to reflect the sum of the amounts accumulated in the intestine (Q_{DEP}) and permeated across the tissue (Q_{PERM}) as a percentage of the amount applied in the donor compartment [27,67]. This is analogous to a "delivery efficiency", which is again used in topical and transdermal delivery studies to indicate the fraction of drugs delivered from a formulation into or across the skin [68–70].

In the conditions used in the present study, Q_{DEP} and Q_{PERM} are calculated as follows:

$$Q_{DEP} = \frac{m_{int\ 2h}}{m_{donor\ 0h}} \times 100\ (\%) \tag{3}$$

$$Q_{PERM} = \frac{m_{acc\ 2h}}{m_{donor\ 0h}} \times 100\ (\%) \tag{4}$$

where $m_{int\ 2h}$ and $m_{acc\ 2h}$ represent the amounts deposited in and permeated across the intestine at 2 h and $m_{donor\ 0h}$ is the amount present in the donor compartment at t = 0.

2.6. *Statistical Analysis*

The data were expressed as the mean ± SD. The results were evaluated statistically using analysis of variance (one-way ANOVA) followed by Bonferroni's multiple comparisons test or Student's *t*-test. The level of significance was fixed at $\alpha = 0.05$.

3. Results and Discussion

3.1. *Intestinal Absorption of Drugs from KBR and FaSSIF V2 and FeSSIF V2*

The first part of the study involved the validation of the setup. This was done by determining the $P_{app,pig}$ of 11 drugs from the four BCS categories (seven high and four low permeability) formulated in KBR and in FaSSIF V2 and FeSSIF V2 followed by a comparison to the $P_{eff,human}$ reported in the literature (Tables 1 and 2). The mean initial transepithelial resistance of the jejunum, 41.77 ± 13.78 $\Omega.cm^2$ (n = 155), was similar to the resistance of the human intestine (duodenum/jejunum; 34 ± 12 $\Omega.cm^2$) [28], and its monitoring for the duration of the experiment reported on the tissue viability in the presence of KBR and, importantly, the effect of biorelevant media in the donor compartment. The ability to use biorelevant media that simulate more physiological conditions is a major advantage of this system since it enables a better approximation of the food effects on drug permeation [71]; this can be difficult with Caco-2 cells due to the cytotoxic effects [72] (necessitating the development of more complex systems [13,73–75]). As seen with other ex vivo models, the $P_{app,pig}$ values were, in general, smaller than the effective permeability $P_{eff,human}$ determined in humans in vivo with the Loc-I-Gut single-pass perfusion technique [76]. This can be explained by the differences between the physiological and experimental conditions. For example, $P_{app,pig}$ (and the apparent permeability coefficients with other species) calculated from Ussing chamber data ex vivo are derived from the drug concentration gradient observed in the acceptor compartment as the amount permeated across a small piece of intestine with a defined area gradually increasing with time. They do not take into account the amount of drug that is retained in the intestinal tissue, which can be significant for certain molecules (Table 1). In contrast, $P_{eff,human}$ calculated in vivo using the Loc-I-Gut technique is dependent upon the difference in concentration over a given length of tissue:

$$P_{eff,\ human} = \frac{Q_{in}}{A}\, ln\left(\frac{C_{out}}{C_{in}}\right) \tag{5}$$

where Q_{in} is the input rate, C_{in} and C_{out} are the drug concentrations at the start and end of the intestinal segment and A is the surface area for absorption. Thus, any process contributing to the loss of the drug from the intestinal fluid will contribute to an increase in $P_{eff,human}$. The surface area for absorption in the Loc-I-Gut model has typically been modelled as a smooth, flat cylinder, ignoring the presence of villi and microvilli, which significantly increase the effective surface area through which drug absorption can occur. A correction of the absorption area to take into account the presence of the additional surface provided by the villi/microvilli would result in a new estimate for the area, which, by definition, would be greater than that of the smooth cylinder and, hence, reduce the value of $P_{eff,human}$. The impact of this additional surface area was recently shown by Olivares-Morales et al., who demonstrated that the estimated $P_{eff,human}$ changed dramatically upon including a physiologically relevant estimate of the intestinal surface area available for drug absorption [77]. A correction of the surface area decreased $P_{eff,human}$ and brought the values closer to the permeability coefficients reported ex vivo. The comparison of these corrected $P_{eff,human}$ and the $P_{app,pig}$ obtained here using the Ussing chamber system shows excellent agreement (Table 2).

Table 2. The apparent permeability coefficients for passive absorption across porcine intestine, $P_{app,pig}$, from KBR and the biorelevant media FaSSIF V2 and FeSSIF V2 and the Q_{DEP} and Q_{PERM} values determined with viable porcine intestine ex vivo ($n \geq 3$): The effective permeability coefficients[a,b] for absorption in vivo in humans, $P_{eff,\,human}$, are given for comparison.

Drug	$P_{app,pig}$ Ex Vivo (10^{-6} cm/s)			$P_{eff,human}$ [a]	$P_{eff,human}$ [b]	KBR			FaSSIF V2			FeSSIF V2		
	KBR (n)	FaSSIF V2 (n)	FeSSIF V2 (n)	In Vivo (10^{-6} cm/s)	In Vivo (10^{-6} cm/s)	Q_{DEP} (%)	Q_{PERM} (%)	(n) [c]	Q_{DEP} (%)	Q_{PERM} (%)	(n) [c]	Q_{DEP} (%)	Q_{PERM} (%)	(n) [c]
BCS I														
(1) Antipyrine	8.06 ± 7.91 (10)	6.18 ± 2.18 (4)	7.47 ± 0.95 (3)	560 ± n.a. [31]	19–29 [77]	0.72 ± 0.20	2.18 ± 0.53	(6)	1.07 ± 0.22	0.33 ± 0.16	(4)	2.90 ± 0.26	1.03 ± 0.28	(3)
(2) Ketoprofen	26.31 ± 1.49 (3)	6.34 ± 2.63 (5)	6.42 ± 2.44 (4)	870 ± n.a. [31]	29–45 [77]	11.57 ± 2.65	6.25 ± 0.92	(6)	4.49 ± 1.61	0.90 ± 0.46	(5)	0.37 ± 0.08	0.97 ± 0.54	(4)
(3) Metoprolol	10.64 ± 2.92 (3)	7.62 ± 1.41 (3)	5.79 ± 1.38 (3)	850 ± n.a. [31]	5.2–7.9 [77]	0.28 ± 0.04	0.18 ± 0.05	(6)	0.12 ± 0.03	0.89 ± 0.19	(3)	0.22 ± 0.01	0.74 ± 0.08	(3)
(4) Propranolol	6.01 ± 3.41(5)	0.71 ± 0.24 (3)	0.93 ± 0.55 (3)	280 ± 130 [31]	9.3–14 [77]	0.35 ± 0.06	0.04 ± 0.05	(6)	4.17 ± 0.15	0.27 ± 0.03	(3)	1.61 ± 0.57	0.27 ± 0.30	(3)
BCS II														
(5) Carbamazepine	7.81 ± 5.69 (16)	5.97 ± 0.52 (4)	4.26 ± 0.96 (6)	430 ± n.a. [31]	-	1.44 ± 0.16	2.39 ± 0.42	(6)	n.a.	n.a.	-	3.45 ± 0.52	0.58 ± 0.22	(6)
(6) Naproxen	12.14 ± 4.83 (3)	9.33 ± 3.36 (3)	45.47 ± 7.97 (5)	850 ± n.a. [31]	27–42 [77]	n.a.	n.a.	-	n.a.	n.a.	-	4.74 ± 1.04	8.11 ± 1.22	(5)
(7) Piroxicam	8.93 ± 2.03 (3)	10.83 ± 3.70 (3)	5.14 ± 0.78 (4)	665 ± n.a. [31]	-	4.12 ± 0.15	2.52 ± 0.70	(3)	5.63 ± 0.26	2.32 ± 0.79	(3)	0.21 ± 0.04	1.13 ± 0.46	(5)
BCS III														
(8) Atenolol	3.05 ± 0.73 (6)	3.70 ± 1.28 (6)	4.53 ± 1.71 (5)	20 ± n.a. [31]	1.8–2.8 [77]	7.38 ± 3.11	0.67 ± 0.13	(6)	0.25 ± 0.06	0.48 ± 0.09	(6)	0.55 ± 0.11	0.61 ± 0.12	(5)
(9) Terbutaline	5.33 ± 1.95 (17)	4.47 ± 0.62 (5)	3.30 ± 0.68 (6)	30 ± 30 [78]	1.7–2.6 [77]	0.52 ± 0.11	0.66 ± 0.22	(6)	39.47 ± 2.51	0.54 ± 0.29	(5)	0.04 ± 0.00	0.39 ± 0.10	(6)
BCS IV														
(10) Furosemide	1.69 ± 0.89 (16)	3.34 ± 1.46 (4)	3.83 ± 0.77 (6)	5 ± n.a. [31]	1–1.6 [77]	n.a.	n.a.	-	2.22 ± 0.17	0.43 ± 0.09	(4)	1.52 ± 0.24	1.38 ± 0.24	(6)
(11) Hydrochlorothiazide	2.88 ± 2.84 (17)	0.2 ± 0.25 (3)	1.37 ± 0.53 (6)	4 ± n.a. [31]	-	n.a.	n.a.	-	0.22 ± 0.11	0.11 ± 0.05	(3)	0.74 ± 0.09	0.23 ± 0.08	(6)

[a] $P_{eff,human}$ determined using the Loc-I-Gut method was performed in living humans. A jejunal segment of 10 cm was isolated and perfused with a solution with a known drug concentration. The difference in drug concentrations across the isolated segment was used to estimate the drug absorption, and this amount together with the assumption of a cylindrical surface area for uptake enabled the estimation of $P_{eff,human}$; [b] $P_{eff,human}$ calculated using the Loc-I-Gut method was performed in living humans but with the inclusion of physiological estimates of the surface area for absorption [77]; [c] Number of replicates.

The $P_{eff,human}$ (uncorrected)/$P_{app,pig}$ ratios for high permeability drugs were approximately 20-fold greater than those for low permeability drugs. The permeation surface for high permeability drugs, normally absorbed via the transcellular pathway, is larger compared to that of low permeability drugs, which are absorbed by the paracellular pathway. Therefore, a reduction in or a lack of blood flow, motility or lymphatic drainage in ex vivo experiments influences high permeability drugs much more than low permeability drugs—hence, their higher $P_{eff,human}$ / $P_{app,pig}$ ratios.

In a next step, the published $P_{eff,human}$ values were plotted against the ln $P_{app, pig}$ values for the three experimental setups KBR/KBR, FaSSIF V2/KBR, and FeSSIF V2/KBR (Figure 1). In every case, strong sigmoidal correlations (R^2 = 0.97 for KBR/KBR, R^2 = 0.91 for FaSSIF V2/KBR and R^2 = 0.76 for FeSSIF V2/KBR) were obtained and it was possible to distinguish clearly between high and low permeability drugs. The data were fitted using a four parameter logistic equation (see Section 2.5.2) [28]; in general, $P_{app, pig}$ decreased going from KBR to FaSSIF V2 and FeSSIF V2, and the correlation curves were translated to the left. The quality of the fit decreased going from KBR/KBR to FeSSIF V2/KBR. A trend towards a decreased permeability with an increasing concentration of sodium taurocholate and lecithin in the biorelevant media was found. This was in good agreement with previous findings, where it was observed that, depending on the drug characteristics, permeability decreased with an increasing concentration of solubility enhancers since poorly water soluble drugs were increasingly solubilized in the micelles, and therefore, less free drug was available for permeation [79,80]. Thus, the composition of FeSSIF V2 makes it more likely to influence the solubility and absorption of certain drugs, and this additional complexity might affect the quality of the correlation.

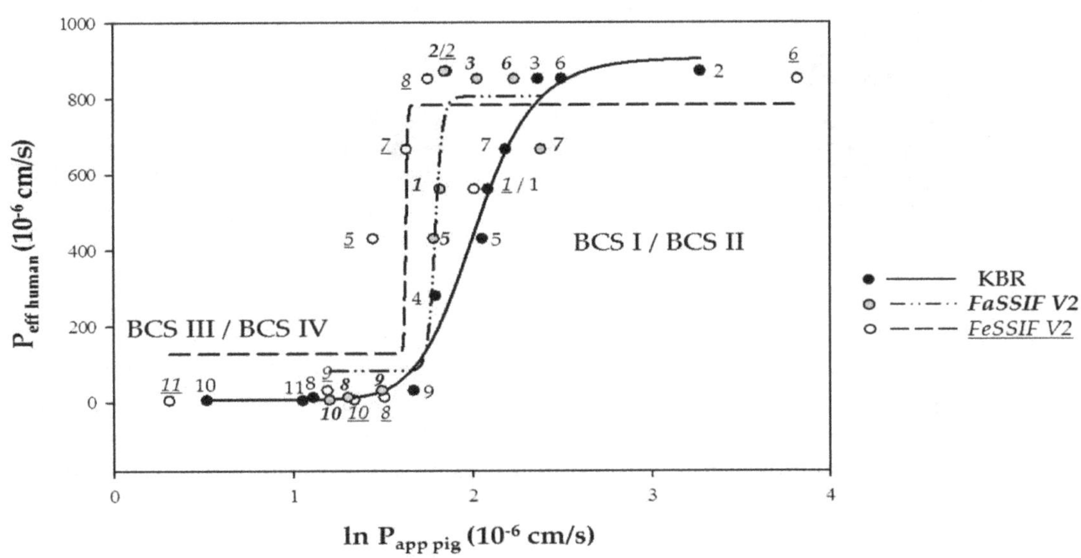

Figure 1. The correlation between the effective permeability coefficient in vivo, $P_{eff,human}$ (literature values derived assuming smooth cylindrical representation of the surface area for absorption) and the permeability coefficient calculated using porcine intestine ex vivo and the Ussing chamber technique ($P_{app,pig}$): The drug absorption was tested using KBR, and the biorelevant media, FaSSIF V2, and FeSSIF V2. BCS I/II (High permeability drugs): 1. Antipyrine, 2. Ketoprofen, 3. Metoprolol, 4. Propranolol, 5. Carbamazepine, 6. Naproxen and 7. Piroxicam; BCS III/IV (Low permeability drugs): 8. Atenolol, 9. Terbutaline, 10. Furosemide and 11. Hydrochlorothiazide (for n, see Table 2). A 100 µM solution of each drug was prepared in (i) KBR, (ii) FaSSIF V2 and (iii) FeSSIF V2. A four parameter logistic model was used to derive the fit between $P_{eff,human}$ and $P_{app,pig}$ (see Section 2.5.2) [28].

As the $P_{eff,human}$ values are obtained for more molecules, further experiments can be carried out with the porcine intestine to determine the corresponding $P_{app,pig}$ and so to expand the dataset.

3.2. *Segmental Intestinal Drug Permeation: Regional Variations in Drug Uptake*

Physiological factors such as variation of the surface, "tightness" of the tight junctions, variable expression of uptake and efflux transporters as well as enzymes can result in regional differences in drug absorption [81]. The identification of segmental drug permeation differences at an early stage can be advantageous since it can be used to optimize formulation development. Interestingly, the mean transepithelial resistances of the four intestinal segments at the start of the experiments were found to be in the same range: 57.33 ± 20.66 Ω.cm^2 (n = 14) for the duodenum, 41.77 ± 13.79 Ω.cm^2 (n = 155) for the jejunum, 40.85 ± 15.08 Ω.cm^2 (n = 31) for the ileum and 35.71 ± 16.56 Ω.cm^2 (n = 18) for the colon. The ability of the model to identify segmental differences in intestinal drug permeation was tested by determining $P_{app,pig}$ of antipyrine and metoprolol (two high permeability drugs; BCS I) and cimetidine (low permeability drug; BCS III) across the duodenum, jejunum, ileum and colon (Figure 2 and Table 3). Due to their lipophilicity, antipyrine and metoprolol are absorbed passively via the transcellular pathway [82]. Cimetidine, in contrast, is transported by the paracellular pathway, and it is also a P-gp substrate [83]. The results were compared with the permeability data determined in humans [84].

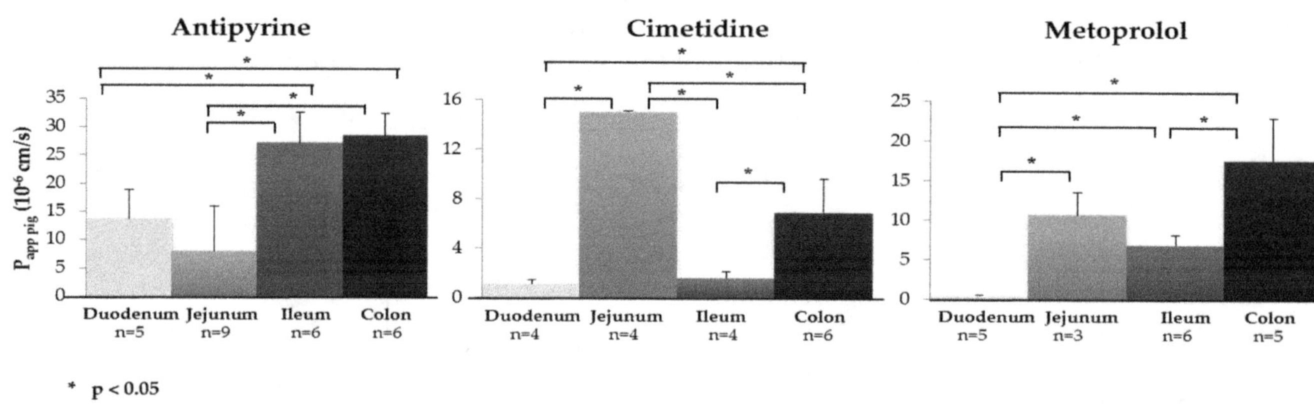

Figure 2. The porcine ex vivo model was able to identify regional variations in intestinal absorption ($P_{app,pig}$) for metoprolol, cimetidine and antipyrine in the duodenum, jejunum, ileum and colon. A 100 µM solution of each drug was prepared in KBR (Mean ± SD; n = number of replicates). A statistical analysis was performed using one-way ANOVA followed by a Bonferroni's multiple comparisons ad hoc test.

Table 3. The apparent drug permeability coefficients, $P_{app,pig}$ and Q_{DEP} and Q_{PERM}, for drugs in different segments of the small intestine (duodenum, jejunum and ileum) and the colon.

Drug	$P_{app,pig}$ Ex Vivo (10^{-6} cm/s)				Q_{DEP} (%) Q_{PERM} (%) (n) [a]							
	Duodenum (n)	Jejunum (n)	Ileum (n)	Colon (n)	Duodenum		Jejunum		Ileum		Colon	
Antipyrine	13.69 ± 5.24 (5)	8.06 ± 7.91 (9)	27.26 ± 5.47 (6)	28.56 ± 3.97 (6)	1.10 ± 0.47	1.57 ± 0.58 (5)	0.72 ± 0.20	2.18 ± 0.53 (5)	1.97 ± 0.34	1.39 ± 0.56 (6)	0.87 ± 0.16	3.79 ± 0.80 (5)
Cimetidine	1.12 ± 0.30 (4)	15.01 ± 0.07 (4)	1.66 ± 0.48 (4)	6.91 ± 2.74 (6)	0.67 ± 0.06	0.91 ± 0.27 (4)	3.28 ± 0.56	1.66 ± 0.64 (6)	0.07 ± 0.01	0.26± 0.08 (3)	0.05 ± 0.01	0.81 ± 0.25 (6)
Metoprolol	0.39 ± 0.16 (5)	10.64 ± 2.92 (3)	6.87 ± 1.23 (6)	17.55 ± 5.41 (6)	2.35 ± 0.25	0.14 ± 0.08 (5)	0.27 ± 0.04	0.18 ± 0.05 (4)	1.89 ± 0.67	0.83 ± 0.09 (5)	0.02 ± 0.00	1.65 ± 0.87 (6)

[a] Number of replicates.

In the case of antipyrine, $P_{app,pig}$ across the ileum was significantly greater than that for uptake across the duodenum and jejunum ($p < 0.05$), i.e., an improved permeation on passing from the proximal to the distal small intestine. It was noted that $P_{app,pig}$ for uptake in the colon was equivalent to that in the ileum. A similar behavior was observed with metoprolol, where a statistically significant increase in $P_{app,pig}$ from the proximal to the distal gastrointestinal tract was observed ($p < 0.05$). As mentioned above, in contrast to antipyrine and metoprolol, which are BCS I drugs, cimetidine is a BCS III drug, and it behaved differently: In this case, $P_{app,pig}$ was significantly higher in the jejunum as compared to all the other segments ($p < 0.05$).

To date, few in vivo data regarding a regional variation in drug permeability in humans are available. Of the drugs tested here, $P_{eff,human}$ has only been determined for cimetidine [85], and the same trend was observed: The $P_{eff,human}$ across jejunum was significantly higher than that across the other segments (although the absolute value of $P_{app,pig}$ was approx. 50-fold lower than (uncorrected) $P_{eff,human}$). It was found that $P_{eff,human}$ decreased three-fold going from the jejunum to the ileum (from 75×10^{-6} cm/s to 25×10^{-6} cm/s), in comparison, $P_{app,pig}$ decreased approx. eight-fold.

In terms of ex vivo data from human intestine in the Ussing chamber ($P_{app,human}$), (i) for antipyrine, the $P_{app,human}$ values increased approximately two-fold on going from the duodenum to the colon ($26.3 \pm 6.99 \times 10^{-6}$ cm/s to $54.6 \pm 13.0 \times 10^{-6}$ cm/s) [28] and were similar to $P_{app,pig}$ measured here ($13.7 \pm 5.2 \times 10^{-6}$ cm/s and $28.6 \pm 4.0 \times 10^{-6}$ cm/s, respectively); (ii) for cimetidine, $P_{app,human}$ was only determined for the jejunum ($3.74 \pm 0.47 \times 10^{-6}$ cm/s) and was approximately two-fold higher than $P_{app,pig}$ ($1.50 \pm 0.07 \times 10^{-6}$ cm/s); and (iii) for metoprolol, $P_{app,pig}$ was in the same range as $P_{app,human}$ in the jejunum ($10.64 \pm 2.92 \times 10^{-6}$ cm/s vs. $15.9 \pm 3.69 \times 10^{-6}$ cm/s, respectively) and in the colon ($17.55 \pm 5.41 \times 10^{-6}$ cm/s vs.$18.8 \pm 4.0 \times 10^{-6}$ cm/s, respectively) (Table 3) [28]. In general, there was a good agreement between $P_{app,human}$ and $P_{app,pig}$ (although $P_{app,human}$ was usually a little higher) confirming that healthy porcine intestinal tissue was able to identify regional differences in drug absorption consistent with those reported with human intestine [28].

3.3. Demonstrating Activity of the P-gp Efflux Transporter

The transport of two low permeability drugs, cimetidine and ranitidine (both BCS III), which are known substrates of P-gp [81,83,86], in the jejunum and ileum was investigated in the presence and absence of the P-gp inhibitor verapamil (Figure 3). BCS III substances were chosen since P-gp plays a minimal role in the drug permeation of high permeability drugs (BCS I and II) [87]. No statistically significant difference in $P_{app,pig}$ was observed for transport across the jejunum in the presence or absence of verapamil (Table 4). In contrast, the presence of verapamil significantly increased $P_{app,pig}$ in the ileum for both cimetidine and ranitidine. In human intestine, P-pg expression in the proximal intestine is lower than in the distal small intestine [41,84]. The more pronounced effect of verapamil on the absorption in the ileum suggested that the same P-gp distribution might be present in porcine intestine. However, since it is reported that verapamil is a modulator of the organic cation transporter, the effect—if any—of this activity needs to be investigated [88,89].

Table 4. The apparent drug permeability coefficients, $P_{app,pig}$ and Q_{DEP} and Q_{PERM}, in the jejunum and ileum for the drug substrates of the P-gp efflux transporter in the presence (+VER) and absence (−VER) of the P-gp inhibitor, verapamil.

Drug	$P_{app,pig}$ Ex Vivo (10^{-6} cm/s)				Q_{DEP} (%) Q_{PERM} (%) (*n*) [a]							
	Jejunum		Ileum		Jejunum (−VER)		Jejunum (+VER)		Ileum (−VER)		Ileum (+VER)	
	(−VER) (*n*)	(+VER) (*n*)	(−VER) (*n*)	(+VER) (*n*)								
Cimetidine	15.01 ± 0.07 (4)	10.07 ± 4.80 (6)	1.66 ± 0.48 (4)	4.28 ± 0.70 (4)	2.98 ± 0.29	1.38 ± 0.03 (4)	4.32 ± 0.97	1.49 ± 0.67(6)	0.07 ± 0.01	0.26 ± 0.08 (3)	0.08 ± 0.02	0.71 ± 0.14 (4)
Ranitidine	5.42 ± 0.61 (6)	4.92 ± 0.30 (5)	1.04 ± 0.83 (5)	4.78 ± 0.31 (6)	1.32 ± 0.31	0.67 ± 0.12 (6)	5.47 ± 0.75	0.23 ± 0.15 (5)	1.10 ± 0.59	0.55 ± 0.35 (4)	7.91 ± 0.74	0.25 ± 0.03 (6)

[a] Number of replicates.

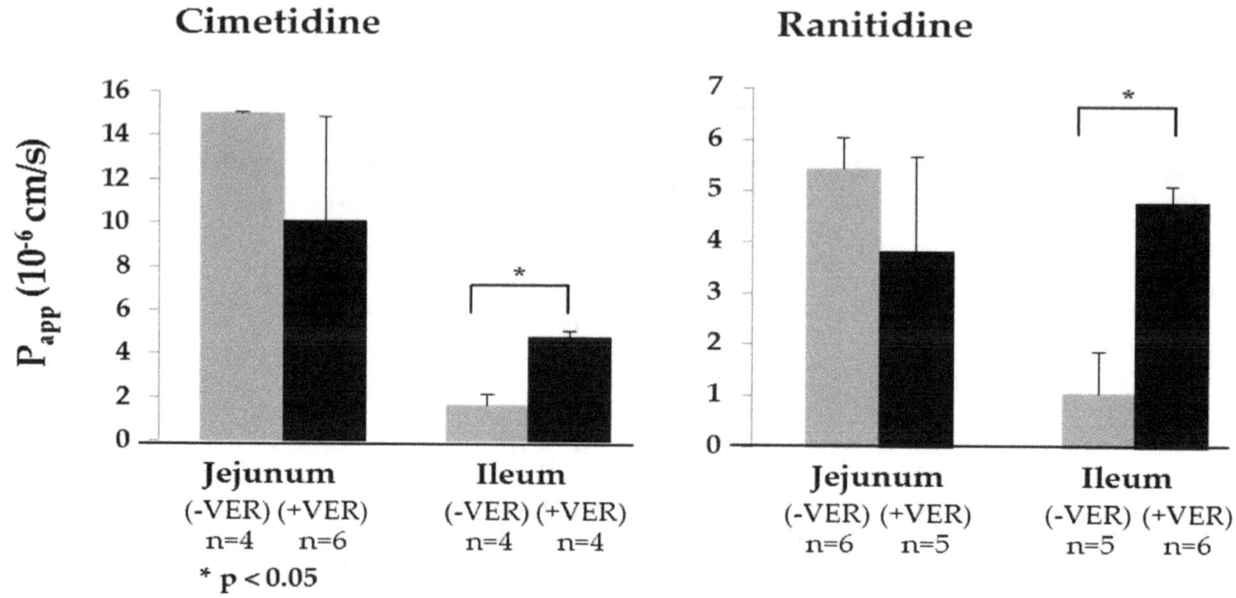

Figure 3. The activity of the P-gp efflux transporter was confirmed by measuring $P_{app,pig}$ of the P-gp substrates, cimetidine and ranitidine (both prepared at a concentration of 100 μM in KBR), in the jejunum and the ileum in the presence (+VER; 100 μM) or absence (−VER) of verapamil (a P-gp inhibitor). Statistically significant differences (Student's t-test) were observed for the ileum, which was consistent with the reports for humans in vivo. (Mean ± SD; n = number of replicates).

3.4. Demonstrating that CYP3A4 Retains Activity in the Porcine Intestine Ex Vivo

Another crucial process during drug permeation in vivo is the pre-systemic metabolism in the gut wall—principally due to CYP3A4 activity. To test whether CYP3A4 activity was retained in porcine intestine ex vivo, the intestinal permeation of three CYP3A4 substrates, midazolam, tamoxifen and verapamil, was investigated in the presence and absence of clotrimazole, a potent CYP3A4 inhibitor. The $P_{app,pig}$ of all three substances significantly increased in the presence of clotrimazole (Table 5); furthermore, the amount of each of the principal metabolites—α-hydroxymidazolam, N-desmethyl-tamoxifen, and norverapamil—in the intestinal tissue was significantly decreased (Figure 4).

Table 5. The apparent drug permeability coefficients, $P_{app,\,pig}$ and Q_{DEP} and Q_{PERM}, in the jejunum for drug substrates of CYP3A4 in the presence (+CLOTR) and absence (−CLOTR) of the CYP3A4 inhibitor, clotrimazole.

Drug	$P_{app,pig}$ Ex Vivo (10^{-6} cm/s)				Q_{DEP} (%) Q_{PERM} (%) (n) [a]					
	(−CLOTR)	(n)	(+CLOTR)	(n)	(−CLOTR)			(+CLOTR)		
Midazolam	0.183 ± 0.138	(4)	0.460 ± 0.070	(4)	8.06 ± 1.33	0.13 ± 0.09	(6)	7.49 ± 2.50	0.18 ± 0.08	(5)
Tamoxifen	0.124 ± 0.046	(3)	1.381 ± 1.080	(3)	1.82 ± 1.39	0.07 ± 0.07	(3)	1.82 ± 0.58	0.06 ± 0.06	(4)
Verapamil	0.008 ± 0.003	(4)	0.211 ± 0.071	(3)	1.88 ± 0.12	0.00 ± 0.00	(3)	3.00 ± 0.63	0.18 ± 0.07	(6)

[a] Number of replicates.

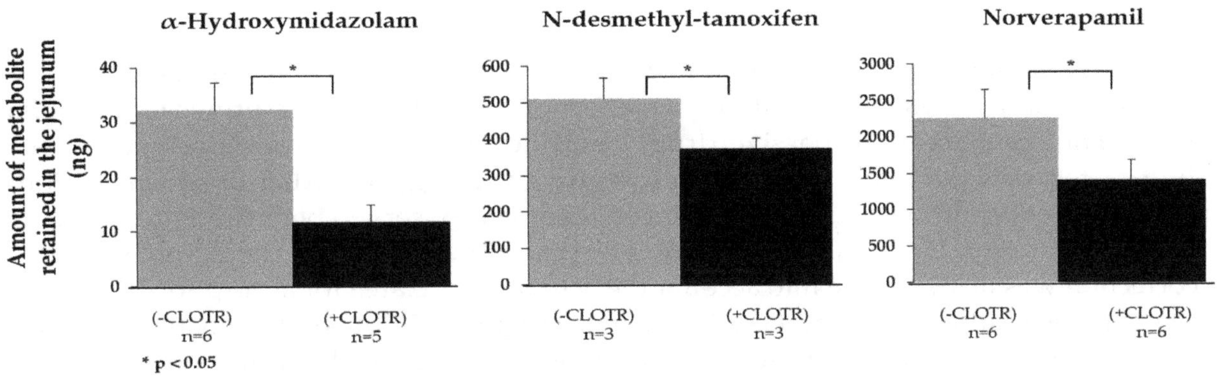

Figure 4. The enzymatic activity of CYP3A4 in the intestinal tissue was confirmed by investigating the transport of the CYP3A4 substrates midazolam, tamoxifen and verapamil (all prepared at a concentration of 100 μM in KBR) across the jejunum and quantification of the amounts (of their metabolites (α-hydroxymidazolam, N-desmethyl-tamoxifen and norverapamil) retained in the tissue in the presence (+CLOTR; 100 μM) or absence (−CLOTR) of the CYP3A4 inhibitor clotrimazole. Statistically significant differences were identified using the Student's t-test. (Mean ± SD; n = number of replicates).

3.5. Relative Contribution of Drug Deposition (Q_{DEP}) and Drug Permeation (Q_{PERM}) to the Transport Index (TI)

The values of Q_{DEP} and Q_{PERM} provide insight at a number of levels (Table 2). First, Q_{DEP} reports on the fraction of drugs that partitioned from the formulation in the donor compartment into the intestinal tissue but was unable to reach the receiver compartment within the timeframe of the permeation experiment. Thus, it is not taken into account in the calculations that measure the permeability coefficient and, hence, may contribute to the underestimation of intestinal absorption ex vivo. Second, the relative magnitudes of Q_{DEP} and Q_{PERM} reflect the effect of the drug physicochemical properties on molecular transport into and across the intestine (Tables 1 and 2). Highly lipophilic molecules, e.g., midazolam, tamoxifen and verapamil, used in the studies to investigate CYP3A4 activity showed a clear trend towards accumulation within the membrane. In a similar way, the moderately lipophilic character of ketoprofen and piroxicam may explain their retention within the intestinal tissue. Although the P-gp substrates, cimetidine and ranitidine, are significantly more polar, they demonstrated a selectivity for membrane accumulation over permeation; this was tentatively attributed to their capacity to form hydrogen bonds (HB): They both contained five HB acceptor groups in addition to multiple HB donor functions—three in the case of cimetidine and two for ranitidine. The relative values of Q_{DEP} and Q_{PERM} for metoprolol and, in particular, atenolol were more difficult to explain. In the case of metoprolol, a combination of modest lipophilicity and HB formation capacity (four HB acceptors and two HB donors) might be sufficient to account for its behavior. Atenolol was more polar but contained four HB acceptors and two HB donors. It was noted that most of the molecules with a propensity to accumulate were P-gp substrates, although whether and/or how this might influence retention is unclear at this point. Regional differences in the relative magnitudes of Q_{DEP} and Q_{PERM} were observed: The Q_{PERM}/Q_{DEP} ratio was significantly greater in the colon for antipyrine, cimetidine and metoprolol than in the small intestine.

In the case of the CYP3A4 substrates, the presence of clotrimazole only had a statistically significant effect on the Q_{DEP} and Q_{PERM} of verapamil ($p < 0.05$ and $p < 0.05$, respectively). As shown in Figure 4, during the permeation experiment, the metabolite norverapamil was formed, which is itself a strong CYP3A4 inhibitor [89]. CYP3A4 inhibition by clotrimazole in conjunction with norverapamil may have helped to increase the amount of verapamil in the tissue, which accumulated due to its lipophilicity.

4. Conclusions

The results demonstrated that viable porcine intestine ex vivo could be used in conjunction with an Ussing chamber system to evaluate the effect of physiological conditions on intestinal drug absorption. The comparison of passive drug absorption from KBR and with biorelevant media simulating fasted and fed states was a step forward in trying to predict drug absorption under more physiological conditions. An excellent correlation was observed between $P_{app,pig}$ and the drug permeability coefficient, $P_{eff,human}$, measured in vivo both in terms of the trend and absolute values once a correction was made to take into account the actual surface area for absorption in vivo [77]. The experiments investigating the differences in regional/segmental uptake demonstrated the potential of the model to aid in the rational design of formulations that enabled release in the region with the highest drug permeability. The advantages of using viable tissue were clearly shown in the studies illustrating the impact of P-gp transport and pre-systemic metabolism by CYP3A4 present in the gut wall. From an ethical standpoint, the technique had the advantage in that it did not require the sacrifice of any animals in the laboratory. Furthermore, healthy tissue was sourced from a large omnivorous mammal. In the next phase of the project, the aims are (i) to create a dynamic system that mimics molecular transit through the different compartments of the gastrointestinal tract and which enables the direct evaluation of oral drug dosage forms and (ii) to explore the potential applications in food and nutrition and the elucidation of active compounds present in complex formulations used in traditional medicine.

Author Contributions: Conceptualization, J.T., S.B., Y.N.K. and Y.E.A.; methodology, Y.E.A., J.T., S.B. and Y.N.K.; validation, Y.E.A.; formal analysis, Y.E.A. and Y.N.K.; investigation, Y.E.A.; resources, Y.N.K. and S.B.; writing—original draft preparation, Y.E.A. and Y.N.K.; visualization, Y.N.K. and Y.E.A.; supervision, Y.N.K. and Y.E.A.; project administration, Y.N.K. and Y.E.A.; funding acquisition, Y.N.K.

Acknowledgments: We are extremely grateful to the excellent staff from both slaughterhouses; without their support, this study would not have been possible.

References

1. Rogers, S.M.; Back, D.J.; Orme, M.L.E. Intestinal metabolism of ethinyloestradiol and paracetamol in vitro: Studies using Ussing chambers. *Br. J. Clin. Pharmacol.* **1987**, *23*, 727–734. [CrossRef] [PubMed]
2. Arnold, Y.E.; Imanidis, G.; Kuentz, M.T. Advancing in-vitro drug precipitation testing: New process monitoring tools and a kinetic nucleation and growth model. *J. Pharm. Pharmacol.* **2011**, *63*, 333–341. [CrossRef] [PubMed]
3. Cohen, J.L.; Hubert, B.B.; Leeson, L.J.; Rhodes, C.T.; Robinson, J.R.; Roseman, T.J.; Shefter, E. The development of USP dissolution and drug release standards. *Pharm. Res.* **1990**, *7*, 983–987. [CrossRef]
4. Minekus, M.; Marteau, P.; Havenaar, R.; Huis, J.H.J. A multicompartmental dynamic computer-controlled model simulating the stomach and small intestine. *Altern. Lab. Anim. ATLA* **1995**, *23*, 197–209.
5. Barker, R.; Abrahamsson, B.; Kruusmaegi, M. Application and validation of an advanced gastrointestinal in vitro model for the evaluation of drug product performance in pharmaceutical development. *J. Pharm. Sci.* **2014**, *103*, 3704–3712. [CrossRef]
6. Blanquet, S.; Zeijdner, E.; Beyssac, E.; Meunier, J.-P.; Denis, S.; Havenaar, R.; Alric, M. A dynamic artificial gastrointestinal system for studying the behavior of orally administered drug dosage forms under various physiological conditions. *Pharm. Res.* **2004**, *21*, 585–591. [CrossRef] [PubMed]
7. Arnold, Y.; Bravo Gonzalez, R.; Versace, H.; Kuentz, M. Comparison of different in vitro tests to assess oral lipid-based formulations using a poorly soluble acidic drug. *J. Drug Del. Sci. Technol.* **2010**, *20*, 143–148. [CrossRef]
8. Walter, E.; Janich, S.; Roessler, J.; Hilfinger, J.; Amidon, G. H29-MTX/Caco-2 cocultures as an in vitro model for the intestinal epithelium: In vitro-in vivo correlation with permeabiltiy data from rats and humans. *J. Pharm. Sci.* **1996**, *85*, 1070–1076. [CrossRef]
9. Hilgendorf, C.; Spahn-Langguth, H.; Regardh, C.; Lipka, E.; Amidon, G.; Langguth, P. Caco-2 versus Caco-2/HT29-MTX co-cultured cell lines: Permeabilities via diffusion, inside- and outside-directed carrier-mediated transport. *J. Pharm. Sci.* **2000**, *89*, 63–75. [CrossRef]

10. Araujo, F.; Sarmento, B. Towards the characterization of an in vitro triple co-culture intestine cell model for permeability studies. *Int. J. Pharm.* **2013**, *458*, 128–134. [CrossRef] [PubMed]
11. Lozoya-Agullo, I.; Araujo, F.; Gonzalez-Alvarez, I.; Merino-Sanjuan, M.; Gonzalez-Alvarez, M.; Bermejo, M.; Sarmento, B. Usefulness of Caco-2/HT29-MTX and Caco-2/HT29-MTX/Raji B coculture models to predict intestinal and colonic permeability compared to Caco-2 monoculture. *Mol. Pharm.* **2017**, *14*, 1264–1270. [CrossRef] [PubMed]
12. Wuyts, B.; Riethorst, D.; Brouwers, J.; Tack, J.; Annaert, P.; Augustijns, P. Evaluation of fasted satte human intestinal fluid as apical solvent system in the Caco-2 absoprtion model and comparison with FaSSIF. *Eur. J. Pharm. Sci.* **2015**, *67*, 126–135. [CrossRef]
13. Antoine, D.; Pellequer, Y.; Tempesta, C.; Lorscheidt, S.; Kettel, B.; Tamaddon, L.; Jannin, V.; Demarne, F.; Lamprecht, A.; Béduneau, A. Biorelevant media resistant co-culture model mimicking permeability of human intestine. *Int. J. Pharm.* **2015**, *481*, 27–36. [CrossRef]
14. Lozoya-Agullo, I.; Gonzalez-Alvarez, I.; Zur, M.; Fine-Shamir, N.; Cohen, Y.; Markovic, M.; Garrigues, T.M.; Dahan, A.; Gonzalez-Alvarez, M.; Merino-Sanjuan, M.; et al. Closed-loop Doluisio (colon, small intestine) and single-pass intestinal perfusion (colon, jejunum) in rat-biophysical model and predictions based on Caco-2. *Pharm. Res.* **2018**, *2018*, 2–23. [CrossRef]
15. Mani, V.; Hollis, J.H.; Gabler, N.K. Dietary oil composition differentially modulates intestinal endotoxin transport and postprandial endotoxemia. *Nutr. Metab.* **2013**, *10*, 1–9. [CrossRef]
16. Kansara, V.; Mitra, A.K. Evaluation of an ex vivo model implication for carrier-mediated retinal drug delivery. *Curr. Eye Res.* **2006**, *31*, 415–426. [CrossRef]
17. Eisenhut, M. Changes in ion transport in inflammatory disease. *J. Inflamm.* **2006**, *3*. [CrossRef]
18. Burshtein, G.; Friedman, M.; Greenberg, S.; Amnon, H. Transepithelial transport of a natural cholinesterase inhibitor, huperzine A, along the gastrointestinal tract: The role of ionization on absorption mechanism. *Planta Med.* **2013**, *79*, 259–265. [CrossRef]
19. Jin, L.; Boyd, B.J.; White, P.J.; Pennington, M.W.; Norton, R.S.; Nicolazzo, J.A. Buccal mucosal delivery of a potent peptide leads to therapeutically-relevant plasma concentrations for the treatment of autoimmune diseases. *J. Control. Release* **2015**, *199*, 37–44. [CrossRef]
20. Boudry, G. The Ussing chamber technique to evaluate alternatives to in-feed antibiotics for young pigs. *Anim. Res.* **2005**, *54*, 219–230. [CrossRef]
21. Ussing, H.H.; Zerahn, K. Active transport of sodium as the source of electric current in the short-circuited isolated frog skin. *Acta Physiol. Scand.* **1951**, *23*, 110–127. [CrossRef] [PubMed]
22. Wu-Pong, S.; Livesay, V.; Dvorchik, B.; Barr, W.H. Oligonucleotide transport in rat and human intestine Ussing chamber models. *Biopharm. Drug Dispos.* **1999**, *20*, 411–416. [CrossRef]
23. Nejdfors, P.; Ekelund, M.; Jeppson, B.; Weström, B.R. Mucosal in vitro permeability in the intestinal tract of the pig, the rat, and man: Species- and region-related differences. *Scand. J. Gastroenterol.* **2000**, *35*, 501–507. [PubMed]
24. Ungell, A.-L.; Nylander, S.; Bergstrand, S.; Sjöberg, A.; Lennernäs, H. Membrane transport of drugs in different regions of the intestinal tract of the rat. *J. Pharm. Sci.* **1998**, *87*, 360–366. [CrossRef]
25. Haslam, I.S.; O'Reilly, D.A.; Sherlock, D.J.; Kauser, A.; Womack, C.; Coleman, T. Pancreatoduodenectomy as a source of human small intestine for Ussing chamber investigations and comparative studies with rat tissue. *Biopharm. Drug Dispos.* **2011**, *32*, 210–221. [CrossRef]
26. Rozehnal, V.; Nakai, D.; Hoepner, U.; Fischer, T.; Kamiyama, E.; Takahashi, M.; Mueller, J. Human small intestinal and colonic tissue mounted in the Ussing chamber as a tool for characterizing the intestinal absorption of drugs. *Eur. J. Pharm. Sci.* **2012**, *46*, 367–373. [CrossRef] [PubMed]
27. Miyake, M.; Toguchi, H.; Nishibayashi, T.; Higaki, K.; Sugita, A.; Koganei, K.; Kamada, N.; Kitazume, M.T.; Hisamatsu, T.; Sato, T.; et al. Establishment of novel prediction system of intestinal absorption in humans using human intestinal tissue. *J. Pharm. Sci.* **2013**, *102*, 2564–2571. [CrossRef]
28. Sjöberg, A.; Lutz, M.; Tannergren, C.; Wingolf, C.; Borde, A.; Ungell, A.-L. Comprehensive study on regional human intestinal permeability and prediction of fraction absorbed of drugs using the Ussing chamber technique. *Eur. J. Pharm. Sci.* **2013**, *48*, 166–180. [CrossRef]
29. Söderholm, J.D.; Hedman, L.; Artursson, P.; Franzén, L.; Larsson, J.; Pantzar, N.; Permert, J.; Olaison, G. Integrity and metabolism of human ileal mucosa in vitro in the Ussing chamber. *Acta Physiol. Scand.* **1998**, *162*, 47–56. [CrossRef]

30. Menon, R.M.; Barr, W.H. Comparison of ceftibuten transport across Caco-2 cells and rat jejunum mounted on modified Ussing chambers. *Biopharm. Drug Dispos.* **2003**, *24*, 299–308. [CrossRef]
31. Kim, J.-S.; Mitchell, S.; Kijek, P.; Tsume, Y.; Hilfinger, J.; Amidon, G.L. The suitability of an in situ perfusion model for permeability determinations: Utility for BCS Class I biowaiver requests. *Mol. Pharm.* **2006**, *3*, 686–694. [CrossRef] [PubMed]
32. Lennernäs, H. Animal data: The contributions of the Ussing chamber and perfusion systems to predicting human oral drug delivery in vivo. *Adv. Drug Deliver. Rev.* **2007**, *59*, 1103–1120. [CrossRef]
33. Kararli, T.T. Comparison of the gastrointestinal anatomy, physiology, and biochemistry of humans and commonly used laboratory animals. *Biopharm. Drug Dispos.* **1995**, *16*, 351–380. [CrossRef] [PubMed]
34. Sjoegren, E.; Abrahamsson, B.; Augustijns, P.; Becker, D.; Bolger, M.B.; Brewster, M.; Brouwers, J.; Flanagan, T.; Harwood, M.; Heinen, C.; et al. In vivo methods for drug absorption—Comparative physiologies, model selection, correlation with in vitro methods (IVIC), and applications for formulation/API/excipient characterization including food effects. *Eur. J. Pharm. Sci.* **2014**, *57*, 99–151. [CrossRef] [PubMed]
35. Patterson, J.K.; Lei, X.G.; Miller, D.D. The pig as an experimental model for elucidation the mechanisms governing dietary influence on mineral absorption. *Exp. Bio. Med.* **2008**, *233*, 651–664. [CrossRef] [PubMed]
36. Musther, H.; Olivares-Morales, A.; Hatley, O.J.D.; Liu, B.; Hodjegan, A.R. Animal versus human oral drug bioavailability: Do they correlate? *Eur. J. Pharm. Sci.* **2014**, *57*, 280–291. [CrossRef] [PubMed]
37. Miller, E.; Ullrey, D. The pig as a model for human nutrition. *Ann. Rev. Nutr.* **1987**, *7*, 361–382. [CrossRef]
38. Witkamp, R.; Monshouwer, M. Pharmacokinetics in vivo and in vitro in swine. *Scan. J. Lab. Anim. Sci.* **1998**, *25*, 45–56.
39. Skaanild, M. Porcine cytochrome P450 and metabolism. *Curr. Pharm. Des.* **2006**, *12*, 1421–1427. [CrossRef] [PubMed]
40. Schrickx, J. *ABC-Transporters in the Pig*; Faculty of Veterinary Medicine, Utrecht University: Utrecht, The Netherlands, 2006.
41. Mouly, S.; Paine, M.F. P-glyocportein increases from proximal to distal regions of human small intestine. *Pharm. Res.* **2003**, *20*, 1595–1599. [CrossRef] [PubMed]
42. Tang, H.; Pak, Y.; Mayersohn, M. Protein expression pattern of p-glycoprotein along the gastrointestinal tract of the yucatan micropig. *J. Biochem. Mol. Toxicol.* **2004**, *18*, 18–22. [CrossRef] [PubMed]
43. Deusser, H.; Rogoll, D.; Scheppach, W.; Volk, A.; Melcher, R.; Richling, E. Gastrointestinal absorption and metabolism of apple polyphenols ex vivo by the pig intestinal mucosa in the Ussing chamber. *Biotechnol. J.* **2013**, *8*, 363–370. [CrossRef]
44. Erk, T.; Hauser, J.; Williamson, G.; Renouf, M.; Steiling, H.; Dionisi, F.; Richling, E. Structure- and dose-absorption relationships of coffee polyphenols. *Biofactors* **2013**, *40*, 103–112. [CrossRef]
45. Westerhout, J.; van de Steeg, A.; Grossouw, D.; Zeijdner, E.E.; Krul, C.A.M.; Verwei, M.; Wortelboer, H.M. A new approach to predict human intestinal absorption using porcine intestinal tissue and biorelevant matrices. *Eur. J. Pharm. Sci.* **2014**, *63*, 167–177. [CrossRef]
46. Neirinckx, E.; Vervaet, C.; Michiels, J.; De Smet, S.; Van den Broeck, W.; Remon, J.P.; De Backer, P.; Croubels, S. Feasibility of the Ussing chamber technique for the determination of in vitro jejunal permeability of passively absorbed compounds in different animal species. *J. Vet. Pharmacol. Therap.* **2010**, *34*, 290–297. [CrossRef]
47. Herrmann, J.; Hermes, R.; Breves, G. Transepithelial transport and intraepithelial metabolism of short-chain fatty acids (SCFA) in the porcine proximal colon are influenced by SCFA concentration and luminal pH. *Comp. Biochem. Physiol. A Mol. Integr. Physiol.* **2011**, *158*, 169–176. [CrossRef]
48. Lampen, A.; Zhang, Y.; Hackbarth, I.; Benet, L.Z.; Sewig, K.-F.; Christians, U. Metabolism and transport of the macrolide immunosuppressant sirolimus in the small intestine. *J. Pharmcol. Exp. Ther.* **1998**, *285*, 1104–1112.
49. Lampen, A.; Christians, U.; Gonschior, A.-K.; Bader, A.; Hackbarth, I.; von Engelhardt, W.; Sewing, K.-F. Metabolism of the macrolide immunosuppressant, tacrolimus, by the pig gut mucosa in the Ussing chamber. *Br. J. Pharmacol.* **1996**, *117*, 1730–1734. [CrossRef]
50. Aucamp, M.; Odendaal, R.; Wilna, L.; Hamman, J. Amorphous azithromycin with improved aqueous solubility and intestinal membrane permeability. *Drug Dev. Ind. Pharm.* **2015**, *41*, 1100–1108. [CrossRef]
51. Atlabachew, M.; Combrinck, S.; Viljoen, A.M.; Hamman, J.H.; Gouws, C. Isolation and in vitro permeation of phenylpropylamino alkaloids from Khat (*Catha edulis*) across oral and intestinal mucosal tissues. *J. Ethnopharmacol.* **2016**, *194*, 307–315. [CrossRef]

52. De Bruyn, S.; Willers, C.; Steyn, D.; Steenekamp, J.; Hamman, J. Development and evaluation of double-phase multiple-unit dosage form for enhanced insulin intestinal delivery. *Drug Deliv. Lett.* **2018**, *8*, 52–60. [CrossRef]
53. Gerber, W.; Hamman, J.H.; Steyn, J.D. Excipient-drug pharmacokinetic interactions: Effect of disintegrants on efflux across excised pig intestinal tissues. *J. Food Drug Anal.* **2018**, *26*, S115–S124. [CrossRef] [PubMed]
54. Pietzonka, P.; Walter, E.; Duda-Johner, S.; Langguth, P.; Merkle, H.P. Compromised integrity of excised porcine intestinal epithelium obtained from the abattoir affects the outcome of in vitro particle uptake studies. *Eur. J. Pharm. Sci.* **2002**, *15*, 39–47. [CrossRef]
55. Shikanga, E.A.; Hamman, J.H.; Chen, W.; Combrinck, S.; Gericke, N.; Viljoen, A.M. In vitro permeation of mesembrine alkaloids from *Sceletium tortuosum* across porcine buccal, sublingual, and intestinal mucosa. *Planta Med.* **2012**, *78*, 260–268. [CrossRef] [PubMed]
56. Hoegman, M.; Moerk, A.-C.; Roomans, G.M. Hypertonic saline increases tight junction permeability in airway epithelium. *Eur. Respir. J.* **2002**, *20*, 1444–1448. [CrossRef]
57. Clark, L.L. A guide to Ussing chamber studies of mouse intestine. *Am. J. Physiol. Gastrointest. Liver Physiol.* **2009**, *296*, G1151–G1166. [CrossRef] [PubMed]
58. Jantratid, E.; Niels, J.; Reppas, C.; Dressman, J.B. Dissolution media simulating conditions in the proximal human gastrointestinal tract: An update. *Pharm. Res.* **2008**, *25*, 1663–1676. [CrossRef] [PubMed]
59. Winiwarter, S.; Bonham, N.M.; Ax, F.; Hallberg, A.; Lennernäs, H.; Karlén, A. Correlation of human jejunal permeability (in vivo) of drugs with experimentally and theoretically derived parameters. A multivariate data analysis approach. *J. Med. Chem.* **1998**, *41*, 4934–4949. [CrossRef]
60. Sarti, F.; Müller, C.; Iqbal, J.; Perera, G.; Laffleur, F.; Bernkop-Schnürch, A. Development and in vivo evaluation of an oral vitamin B12 delivery system. *Eur. J. Pharm. Biopharm.* **2013**, *84*, 132–137. [CrossRef]
61. Zhang, W.; Ramamoorthy, Y.; Kilicarslan, T.; Nolte, H.; Tyndale, R.F.; Sellers, E.M. Inhibition of cytochromes P450 by antifungal imidazole derivatives. *Drug Metab. Dispos.* **2002**, *30*, 314–318. [CrossRef]
62. Artursson, P. Epithelial transport of drugs in cell culture. I: A model for studying the passive diffusion of drugs over intestinal absorbtive (Caco-2) cells. *J. Pharm. Sci.* **1990**, *79*, 476–482. [CrossRef] [PubMed]
63. Cazares-Delgadillo, J.; Naik, A.; Ganem-Rondero, A.; Quintanar-Guerrero, D.; Kalia, Y. Transdermal delivery of Cytochrome C—A 12.4 kDa protein-across intact skin by constant-current iontophoresis. *Pharm. Res.* **2007**, *24*, 1360–1368. [CrossRef] [PubMed]
64. Yu, J.; Kalaria, D.R.; Kalia, Y.N. Erbium: YAG fractional laser ablation for the percutaneous delivery of intact functional therapeutic antibodies. *J. Control. Release* **2011**, *156*, 53–59. [CrossRef]
65. Lapteva, M.; Mondon, K.; Moller, M.; Gurny, R.; Kalia, Y.N. Polymeric micelle nanocarriers for the cutaneous delivery of tacrolimus: A targeted approach for the treatment of psoriasis. *Mol. Pharm.* **2014**, *11*, 2989–3001. [CrossRef] [PubMed]
66. Chen, Y.; Kalia, Y.N. Short-duration ocular iontophoresis of ionaziable aciclovir prodrugs: A new approach to treat herpes simplex infections in the anterior and posterior segments of the eye. *Int. J. Pharm.* **2018**, *536*, 292–300. [CrossRef]
67. Miyake, M.; Kondo, S.; Koga, T.; Yoda, N.; Nakazato, S.; Emoto, C.; Mukai, T.; Toguchi, H. Evaluation of intestinal metabolism and absorption using Ussing chamber system, equipped with intestinal tissue from rats and dogs. *Eur. J. Pharm. Biopharm.* **2018**, *122*, 49–53. [CrossRef]
68. Bachhav, Y.G.; Heinrich, A.; Kalia, Y.N. Using laser microporation to improve transdermal deliveriy of diclofenac: Increasing bioavailability and the range of therapeutic applications. *Eur. J. Pharm. Biopharm.* **2011**, *78*, 408–414. [CrossRef]
69. Kalaria, D.R.; Patel, P.; Merino, V.; Patravale, V.B.; Kalia, Y.N. Controlled iontophoretic transport of huperzine A across skin in vitro and in vivo: Effect of delivery conditions and comparison of pharmacokinetic models. *Mol. Pharm.* **2013**, *10*, 4322–4329. [CrossRef]
70. Kalaria, D.R.; Patel, P.; Merino, V.; Patravale, V.B.; Kalia, Y.N. Controlled iontophoretic delivery of pramipexole: Electrotransport kinetics in vitro and in vivo. *Eur. J. Pharm. Biopharm.* **2014**, *88*, 56–63. [CrossRef]
71. Dressman, J.B.; Amidon, G.L.; Reppas, C.; Shah, V.P. Dissolution testing as a prognostic tool for oral drug absorption: Immediate release dosage forms. *Pharm. Res.* **1998**, *15*, 11–22. [CrossRef]
72. Ingels, F.; Deferme, S.; Destexhe, E.; Oth, M.; Van den Mooter, G.; Augustijns, P. Simulated intestinal fluid as transport medium in the Caco-2 cell culture model. *Int. J. Pharm.* **2002**, *232*, 183–192. [CrossRef]
73. Patel, N.; Forbes, B.; Eskola, S.; Murray, J. Use of simulated intestinal fluids with Caco-2 cells. *Drug Dev. Ind. Pharm.* **2006**, *32*, 151–161. [CrossRef] [PubMed]

74. Lind, M.L.; Jacobsen, J.; Holm, R.; Müllertz, A. Development of simulated intestinal fluids containing nutrients as transport media in the Caco-2 cell culture model: Assessment of cell viability, monolayer integrity and transport of poorly aqueous soluble drug and a substrate of efflux mechanisms. *Eur. J. Pharm. Sci.* **2007**, *32*, 261–270. [CrossRef] [PubMed]
75. Markopoulos, C.; Thoenen, F.; Preisig, D.; Symillides, M.; Vertzoni, M.; Parrott, N.; Reppas, C.; Imanidis, G. Biorelevant media for transport experiments in the Caco-2 model to evaluate drug absorption in the fasted and the fed state and their usefulness. *Eur. J. Pharm. Biopharm.* **2014**, *86*, 438–448. [CrossRef] [PubMed]
76. Knutson, L.; Odlind, B.; Hällgren, R. A new technique for segmental jejunal perfusion in man. *Am. J. Gastroenterol.* **1989**, *84*, 1278–1284.
77. Olivares-Morales, A.; Lennernaes, H.; Aarons, L.; Rostami-Hodjegan, A. Translating human effective jejunal intestinal permeability to surface-dependent intrinsic permeability: A pragmatic method for a more mechanistic prediction of regional oral drug absorption. *AAPS J.* **2015**, *17*, 1177–1192. [CrossRef]
78. Lennernäs, H. Human intestinal permeability. *J. Pharm. Sci.* **1998**, *87*, 403–410. [CrossRef]
79. Miller, J.M.; Beig, A.; Krieg, B.J.; Carr, R.A.; Borchardt, T.B.; Amidon, G.E.; Amidon, G.L.; Dahan, A. The solubility-permeability interplay: Mechanistic modeling and predicitive application of the impact of micellar solubilization on intestinal permeation. *Mol. Pharm.* **2011**, *8*, 1848–1856. [CrossRef]
80. Yano, K.; Masaoka, Y.; Kataoka, M.; Sakuma, S.; Yamashita, S. Mechanisms of membrane transport of poorly soluble drugs: Role of micelles in oral absorption processes. *J. Pharm. Sci.* **2010**, *99*, 1336–1345. [CrossRef]
81. Tannergren, C.; Bergendal, A.; Lennernäs, H.; Abrahamsson, B. Toward an increased understanding of the barriers to colonic drug absorption in humans: Implication for early controlled release candidate assessment. *Mol. Pharm.* **2009**, *6*, 60–73. [CrossRef]
82. Lennernäs, H.; Palm, K.; Fagerholm, U.; Artursson, P. Comparison between active and passive drug transport in human intestinal epithelial (Caco-2) cells in vitro and human jejunum in vivo. *Int. J. Pharm.* **1996**, *127*, 103–107. [CrossRef]
83. Collett, A.; Higgs, N.B.; Sims, M.; Rowland, M.; Warhurst, G. Modulation of the permeability of H_2 receptor antagonists cimetidine and ranitidine by p-glycoprotein in rat intestine and the human colonic cell line Caco-2. *J. Pharmacol. Exp. Ther.* **1999**, *288*, 171–178. [PubMed]
84. Dahlgren, D.; Roos, C.; Sjögren, E.; Lennernäs, H. Direct in vivo human intestinal permeability (Peff) determined with different clinical perfusion and intubation methods. *J. Pharm. Sci.* **2015**, *104*, 2702–2726. [CrossRef]
85. Lennernäs, H. Regional intestinal drug permeation: Biopharmaceutics and drug development. *Eur. J. Pharm. Sci.* **2014**, *57*, 333–341. [CrossRef] [PubMed]
86. Ashmawy, S.M.; El-Gizawy, S.A.; El Maghraby, G.M.; Osman, M.A. Regional difference in intestinal drug absorption as a measure for the potential effect of P-glycoprotein efflux transporters. *J. Pharm. Pharmacol.* **2019**, *71*, 362–370. [CrossRef] [PubMed]
87. Cao, X.; Gibbs, S.T.; Fang, L.; Miller, H.A.; Landowski, C.P.; Shin, H.-C.; Lennernas, H.; Zhing, Y.; Amidon, G.L.; Yu, L.X.; et al. Why is it challenging to predict intestinal drug absorption and oral bioavailability in human using rat model. *Pharm. Res.* **2006**, *28*, 1675–1686. [CrossRef] [PubMed]
88. Salomon, J.J.; Hagos, Y.; Petzke, S.; Kühne, A.; Gausterer, J.C.; Hosoya, K.-I.; Ehrhardt, C. Beta-2 adrenergic agonists are substrates and inhibitors of human organic cation transporter 1. *Mol. Pharm.* **2015**, *12*, 2633–2641. [CrossRef] [PubMed]
89. Wang, Y.-H.; Jones, D.R.; Hall, S.D. Differential mechanism-based inhibition of CYP3A4 and CYP3A5 by verapamil. *Drug Metab. Dispos.* **2005**, *33*, 664–671. [CrossRef] [PubMed]

8

Exploring Bioequivalence of Dexketoprofen Trometamol Drug Products with the Gastrointestinal Simulator (GIS) and Precipitation Pathways Analyses

Marival Bermejo [1,2,*], Gislaine Kuminek [1], Jozef Al-Gousous [1,3], Alejandro Ruiz-Picazo [2], Yasuhiro Tsume [1,4], Alfredo Garcia-Arieta [5], Isabel González-Alvarez [2], Bart Hens [1,6], Deanna Mudie [1,7], Gregory E. Amidon [1], Nair Rodriguez-Hornedo [1] and Gordon L. Amidon [1]

1 Department of Pharmaceutical Sciences, College of Pharmacy, University of Michigan, Ann Arbor, MI 48109, USA; gkuminek@umich.edu (G.K.); jalgouso@umich.edu (J.A.-G.); ytsume@umich.edu (Y.T.); barthens@umich.edu (B.H.); deanna.mudie@lonza.com (D.M.); geamidon@umich.edu (G.E.A.); nrh@umich.edu (N.R.-H.); glamidon@umich.edu (G.L.A.)

2 Department Engineering Pharmacy Section, Miguel Hernandez University, San Juan de Alicante, 03550 Alicante, Spain; alejandroruizpicazo@gmail.com (A.R.-P.); isabel.gonzalez@goumh.umh.es (I.G.-A.)

3 Department of Biopharmaceutics and Pharmaceutical Technology, Johannes Gutenberg Universität Mainz, D-55099 Mainz, Germany

4 Merck and Co., Inc., 126 E Lincoln Ave, Rahway, NJ 07065, USA

5 Service on Pharmacokinetics and Generic Medicines, Division of Pharmacology and Clinical Evaluation, Department of Human Use Medicines, Spanish Agency for Medicines and Health Care Products, 28022 Madrid, Spain; agarciaa@aemps.es

6 Department of Pharmaceutical and Pharmacological Sciences, KU Leuven, Herestraat 49, 3000 Leuven, Belgium

7 Drug Product Development and Innovation, Lonza Pharma and Biotech, Bend, OR 97703, USA

* Correspondence: mbermejo@goumh.umh.es

Abstract: The present work aimed to explain the differences in oral performance in fasted humans who were categorized into groups based on the three different drug product formulations of dexketoprofen trometamol (DKT) salt—Using a combination of in vitro techniques and pharmacokinetic analysis. The non-bioequivalence (non-BE) tablet group achieved higher plasma C_{max} and area under the curve (AUC) than the reference and BE tablets groups, with only one difference in tablet composition, which was the presence of calcium monohydrogen phosphate, an alkalinizing excipient, in the tablet core of the non-BE formulation. Concentration profiles determined using a gastrointestinal simulator (GIS) apparatus designed with 0.01 N hydrochloric acid and 34 mM sodium chloride as the gastric medium and fasted state simulated intestinal fluids (FaSSIF-v1) as the intestinal medium showed a faster rate and a higher extent of dissolution of the non-BE product compared to the BE and reference products. These in vitro profiles mirrored the fraction doses absorbed in vivo obtained from deconvoluted plasma concentration–time profiles. However, when sodium chloride was not included in the gastric medium and phosphate buffer without bile salts and phospholipids were used as the intestinal medium, the three products exhibited nearly identical concentration profiles. Microscopic examination of DKT salt dissolution in the gastric medium containing sodium chloride identified that when calcium phosphate was present, the DKT dissolved without conversion to the less soluble free acid, which was consistent with the higher drug exposure of the non-BE formulation. In the absence of calcium phosphate, however, dexketoprofen trometamol salt dissolution began with a nano-phase formation that grew to a liquid–liquid phase separation (LLPS) and formed the less soluble free acid crystals. This phenomenon was dependent on the salt/excipient concentrations and the presence of free acid crystals in the salt phase. This work demonstrated the importance of excipients and purity of salt phase on the evolution and rate of salt disproportionation pathways. Moreover, the presented data clearly showed the usefulness of the GIS apparatus as a discriminating tool that could highlight the differences in formulation behavior when utilizing physiologically-relevant media and experimental conditions in combination with microscopy imaging.

Keywords: gastrointestinal absorption; dexketoprofen; gastrointestinal simulator; microscopy imaging; liquid–liquid phase separation; oral absorption; in vitro dissolution

---

1. Introduction

The development of generic oral drug products containing dexketoprofen trometamol (DKT, weak acid salt, Biopharmaceutics Classification System (BCS) class 1 drug) is challenging as the reference product does not dissolve rapidly. Since the dissolution of the reference product is not complete (<85%) in 30 min in the paddle apparatus at 50 rotations per minute (rpm) in any of the Biopharmaceutics Classification System's (BCS) buffer media, a biowaiver approach is currently not permitted [1,2].

In Spain, three out of four formulations of DKT tablets failed the first in vivo bioequivalence (BE) study [3]. These products were previously tested with the European Medicines Agency (EMA) dissolution method requested for biowaiver applications, i.e., performing dissolution tests in USP-2 apparatus at 50 rpm with different buffers at pH 1.2, 4.5, and 6.8. Garcia-Arieta and co-workers showed the relevance of the agitation rate (50 rpm versus 75 rpm) on the dissolution profile outcomes [3]. Dissolution profiles of one DKT product using USP apparatus 2 (pH 1.2, 4.5, and 6.8) exhibited profiles ($f2 < 50$) that were not similar to in vivo BE. Another product exhibited in vitro BE ($f2 > 50$) but failed the in vivo BE study. Therefore, the USP apparatus 2 did not reflect the in vivo BE outcome.

The aim of this work was to determine the reasons for the differences in dissolution behavior between bioequivalent (BE) and non-bioequivalent (non-BE) DKT products. First, a physiologically-relevant, multi-compartmental dissolution apparatus, the gastrointestinal simulator (GIS), was evaluated to ascertain whether it could reflect the in vivo BE outcomes. Both the DKT products as well as the reference product were studied in the GIS. In the second step, salt to free acid precipitation pathways during dissolution of DKT were examined by inverted microscopy to identify the factors that influenced drug precipitation.

2. Materials and Methods

2.1. Chemicals

Three different formulations were tested in the GIS and USP-2 apparatus: the reference Spanish marketed product (Enantyum®, Laboratorios Menarini S.A., Barcelona, Spain) and two generic drug products. Acetonitrile was obtained from VWR International (West Chester, PA, USA). Methanol (MeOH), HCl, and trifluoroacetic acid (TFA) were purchased from Fisher Scientific (Pittsburgh, PA, USA). NaOH, NaCl, and $NaH_2PO_4.H_2O$ were received from Sigma-Aldrich (St. Louis, MO, USA). Purified water (i.e., filtrated and deionized) was used in the analysis methods and in dissolution studies to prepare the dissolution media (Millipore, Billerica, MA, USA). Simulated intestinal fluid (SIF) powder was obtained from Biorelevant (Croydon, UK).

Table 1 represents the qualitative composition for each formulation in terms of excipients and coating material.

The main difference between both test products is that there is calcium phosphate in the tablet core of the non-BE product.

Table 1. Qualitative differential composition of the reference marketed drug product and the test products. The ingredients in bold are the added excipients to the core or the coating of the tablet for both test products, which was not presented in the reference marketed drug product.

Dexketoprofen 25 mg (as Dexketoprofen Trometamol 36.9 mg) Film-Coated tablets	Qualitative Composition of Excipients
Reference marketed drug product (Enantyum®)	Core: microcrystalline cellulose, maize starch, glycerol distearate, sodium starch glycolate Coating: hypromellose, titanium dioxide, polyethylene glycol (PEG) 600, and propylene glycol
Test product (bioequivalence (BE))	Core: microcrystalline cellulose, maize starch, glycerol distearate, sodium starch glycolate, **magnesium stearate and colloidal silica** * Coating: hypromellose, titanium dioxide, polyethylene glycol (PEG) 600, propylene glycol, **macrogol 6000 and talc**
Test product failing BE study (Non-BE)	Core: microcrystalline cellulose, maize starch, glycerol distearate, sodium starch glycolate, **magnesium stearate, colloidal silica and calcium monohydrogen phosphate** Coating: hypromellose, titanium dioxide, polyethylene glycol (PEG) 600, and propylene glycol, **macrogol 6000 and talc**

* The ingredients that listed in bold in Table 1 represent the differences between the test and reference products. These excipients were not included in the marketed reference product.

2.2. Design of the In Vitro Dissolution Studies Performed with the GIS

The GIS is a three-compartmental dissolution device, which consists of (i) a gastric chamber ($GIS_{stomach}$), (ii) a duodenal chamber ($GIS_{duodenum}$), and (iii) a jejunal chamber ($GIS_{jejunum}$). The design of the GIS is depicted in Figure 1.

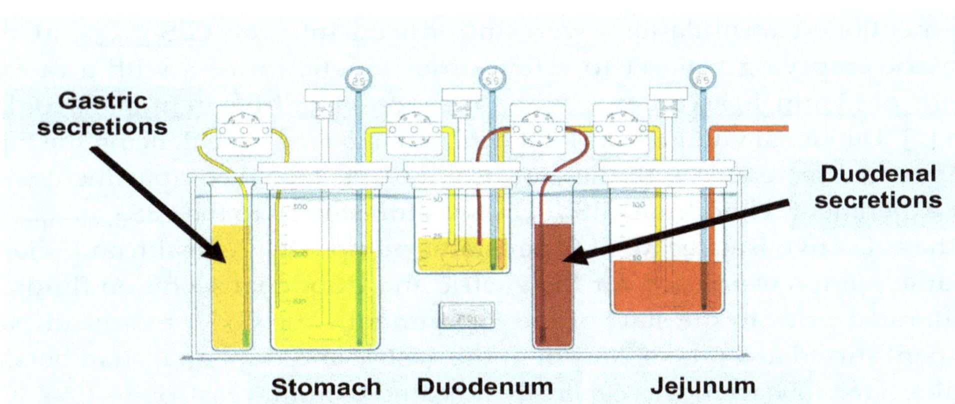

Figure 1. Setup and design of the gastrointestinal simulator (GIS) that was applied to test the different formulations of dexketoprofen trometamol (DKT) in fasted state conditions.

The different dissolution protocols that were applied to test the different formulations in the multicompartmental GIS device are shown in Tables 2 and 3. Table 2 represents the dissolution experiments that were performed in the absence of NaCl (i.e., Protocol 1). The gastric chamber contained simulated gastric fluid (SGF) and the duodenal compartment contained phosphate buffer, pH 6.8 (50 mM). We will refer to this test condition as the standard dissolution "Protocol 1" throughout the manuscript. To explore the impact of endogenous constituents present in the stomach (i.e., NaCl) and in the small intestine (i.e., bile salts and phospholipids), Protocol 2 was developed. In that case, the impact of NaCl on the conversion from salt to free acid could be investigated in the gastric compartment (i.e., acidic pH), and how the created solution concentrations will further behave in the duodenal compartment in a more biorelevant setting. Table 3 represents a higher level of biorelevant dissolution testing by using SGF in the gastric compartment in the presence of NaCl. The duodenal compartment contains fasted state simulated intestinal fluid (FaSSIF-v1). We will refer to this test condition as the standard dissolution "Protocol 2" throughout the manuscript.

Table 2. Overview of dissolution media, initial volumes, and secretion rates applied in the gastrointestinal simulator (GIS) device for the first set of standard dissolution experiments (i.e., standard dissolution settings). The jejunal compartment was empty at the start of the experiment.

Fasted State Test Condition Protocol 1	$GIS_{stomach}$	$GIS_{duodenum}$
Dissolution media	Simulated gastric fluid (SGF), pH 2.0, 0.01 M HCl	Phosphate buffer, pH 6.8–50 mM
Initial volume	50 mL SGF + 250 mL of tap water	50 mL
Secretions	1 mL/min of SGF	1 mL/min of phosphate buffer, pH 6.8–100 mM

Table 3. Overview of dissolution media, initial volumes, and secretion rates applied in the GIS device for the second set of dissolution experiments with a higher level of biorelevance by adding NaCl to SGF and by adding sodium taurocholate and lecithin to the phosphate buffer in order to obtain fasted state simulated intestinal fluids (FaSSIF-v1). The jejunal compartment was empty at the start of the experiment.

Fasted State Test Condition Protocol 2	$GIS_{stomach}$	$GIS_{duodenum}$
Dissolution media	Simulated gastric fluid (SGF), pH 2.0, 0.01 M HCl + 34.2 mM NaCl	FaSSIF-v1 (pH 6.5)
Initial volume	50 mL SGF + 250 mL of tap water	50 mL
Secretions	1 mL/min of SGF	1 mL/min of 4 times concentrated FaSSIF-v1 (4x FaSSIF-v1)

The above-mentioned formulations were introduced into the $GIS_{stomach}$ at the start of the experiment. Gastric emptying was set to a first-order kinetic process with a rate corresponding to a gastric half-life of 13 min, in accordance with the reported half-life in humans for liquids, ranging from 4 to 13 min [5]. Duodenal volume was kept constant at 50 mL by balancing the input (i.e., gastric emptying and duodenal secretion) with the output flow. The jejunal compartment was empty at the beginning of the experiment. Fluid from $GIS_{stomach}$ was transferred to the $GIS_{duodenum}$ and then to the $GIS_{jejunum}$ with the aid of two Ismatec REGLO peristaltic pumps (IDEX Health and Science, Glattbrugg, Switzerland). Same pumps were used for the gastric and duodenal secretion fluids. All peristaltic pumps were calibrated prior to the start of the experiment. The CM-1 overhead paddles (Muscle Corp., Osaka, Japan) stirred at a rate of 20 rpm in the gastric and duodenal chambers. For every 25 s, a high-speed, quick burst (500 rpm) was cyclically repeated to mimic gastrointestinal (GI) contractions and to homogenize the compartment facilitating the solid particle transfer from one chamber to the next one. The jejunal chamber was stirred with a magnetic bar at an approximate rate of 50 rpm. All experiments were performed at 37 °C. After 60 min, pumps were shut down as the gastric content was emptied. Concentrations in the $GIS_{duodenum}$ and $GIS_{jejunum}$ were still measured up to 120 min. Samples were withdrawn from the GIS compartments at predetermined time-points up to 120 min in order to measure the dissolved amount of DKT. The pumps and overhead paddles were controlled by an in-house computer software program. Solution concentrations were determined by centrifuging 300 μL of the withdrawn sample for 1 min at a speed of 17,000 *g* (AccuSpin Micro 17, Fisher Scientific, Pittsburgh, PA, USA). After centrifugation, 100 μL of the supernatant was diluted 1:1 with MeOH, and the MeOH sample was diluted 1:1 again with 0.1 N HCl and transferred to high performance liquid chromatography (HPLC) capped vials. All obtained samples were analyzed by HPLC (see below Section 2.8).

2.3. Design of the In Vitro Dissolution Studies Performed with USP-2

To investigate the impact of each region of the human GI tract separately, single-compartmental dissolution studies were performed. Dissolution studies in the USP-2 (paddle) apparatus were performed at 37 °C and 30 rpm in 500 mL of fluid. Three tablets of each formulation were tested in four different media: (1) FaSSIF-v1 at pH 6.5; (2) 0.01 N HCl (pH 2); (3) 0.01 N HCl + 34 mM NaCl; and (4) 0.01 N HCl + 135 mM. The concentrations of Na^+ and Cl^- measured in human gastric fluids are equal to 68 ± 29 mM and 102 ± 28 mM, respectively [6]. Samples of 500 µL were taken and immediately centrifuged and diluted as described previously.

2.4. In Silico Deconvolution to Obtain In Vivo Bioavailability Input Rate

Intravenous pharmacokinetic data were obtained from Valles and co-workers [7]. A two-compartmental pharmacokinetic (PK) open model was fitted to the data to get DKT disposition constants as depicted in Table 4.

Table 4. Disposition parameters of DKT for a two-compartmental pharmacokinetic (PK) model: V1 represents the central compartment volume; K_{10} represents a first-order elimination rate constant; K_{12} and K_{21} reflect the two rate constants distributing the drug between the peripheral and central compartment, respectively.

Parameter	Unit	Value	Standard Error	CV%
V_1	mL	3549.53	201.23	5.67
K_{10}	1/h	1.64	0.08	5.14
K_{12}	1/h	0.93	0.13	14.34
K_{21}	1/h	0.96	0.09	8.91

PK parameters were used to apply Loo–Riegelman mass balance deconvolution method in order to obtain the plots of bioavailable fractions versus time profile of all the assayed formulations. As oral plasma data were obtained from different BE studies, the plasma concentration–time profiles for all test formulations were normalized using the reference formulations ratios at each time point between both BE studies [8,9]. Similar normalization results were obtained by using the area under the curve (AUC) references ratios (data not shown).

2.5. Description of the Two-Step In Vitro–In Vivo Correlation (IVIVC)

Fractions dissolved in jejunal chambers of each formulation were used to develop the two-step IVIVC. To estimate the fractions dissolved, the maximum amount of DKT dissolved among the three formulations was used to transform amounts into fractions. Bioavailable fractions obtained by Loo–Riegelman method of each formulation at each time point versus the fractions dissolved of the corresponding formulation at the same time points were represented. For non-coincident sampling times in vitro versus in vivo, the corresponding dissolved or absorbed fractions were estimated by linear interpolation between the previous and next time point. The obtained IVIVC relationship was internally validated—theoretical fractions absorbed were calculated from the experimental fractions dissolved by using the IVIVC equation. The fractions absorbed were back-transformed toward concentrations by applying Equation (1) [10].

$$C_T = \frac{(X_A)_T}{V_c} - \frac{(X_P)_{T-1}}{V_c} e^{-K_{21}\Delta t} + C_{T-1}K_{12}\frac{\Delta t}{2} - C_{T-1}\frac{K_{12}}{K_{21}}1 - e^{-K_{21}\Delta t} - C_{T-1}K_{el}\frac{\Delta t}{2} \\ -AUC_{T-1}\frac{K_{el}}{1} + K_{12}\frac{\Delta t}{2} + K_{el}\frac{\Delta t}{2} \quad (1)$$

where C_T is the plasma concentration at time t; C_{T-1} is the plasma concentration at the previous time point $(T-1)$; $(X_A)_T$ is the absorbed amount at time t; $(X_P)_{T-1}$ is the amount in the peripheral compartment at the previous sampling time; Δt is the time interval between two consecutive sampling times; V_c is the central compartment volume; K_{12} and K_{21} are the distribution constants and K_{el}

the elimination rate constant from the central compartment. The peripheral "concentrations" were estimated with Equation (2) [11]:

$$P_t = K_{12} \cdot e^{-K_{21} \cdot t} \cdot \int_0^t C \cdot e^{K_{21} \cdot t} \partial t \quad (2)$$

where K_{12} and K_{21} are the values obtained previously from literature in Table 4.

The predicted plasma levels were used to estimate plasma C_{max} and AUC predicted values to be compared with the experimental ones and to estimate the relative prediction error (Equation (3)):

$$RE\% = 100 \times \left(\frac{experimental\ value - predicted\ value}{experimental\ value} \right) \quad (3)$$

2.6. Evaluation of DKT to Free Acid Conversion Pathways/Kinetics During Salt Dissolution

DKT to free acid conversion was studied in situ by optical microscopy. The studies were conducted at room temperature (22–23 °C) using an inverted optical microscope (Leica DMi8, Wetzlar, Germany) and 10×, 20×, or 40× magnification objective lenses. An inverted microscope has the advantage of a long focal length that allows examination of the phases formed during dissolution without having to remove the solution. Two concentration levels of both DKT and excipients were studied by varying the amount of DKT and excipients added to 96-well plates followed by the addition of 300 µL of hydrochloric acid (pH 2 (0.01 M) and 34.2 mM NaCl) with pre-dissolved tablet excipients. The influence of excipients was determined by dissolving formulation excipients in the dissolution media prior to DKT salt addition. The high concentration level (C_H) corresponds to 685 ± 23 µg of salt added to a 300 µL aliquot of a solution of 1 tablet dissolved in 20 mL, whereas the low concentration (C_L) corresponds to 38 ± 1 µg of salt added to a 300 µL aliquot of 1 tablet dissolved in 300 mL. From that point of view, the high concentration (C_H) is 18 times higher than the low concentration (C_L).

Brightfield images were collected with a Leica DMC2900 camera controlled with LAS v4.7 software (Leica Microsystems, Wetzlar, Germany). Solid particles of the free acid were added at two different levels, representing <3% (*w/w*) and 3% (*w/w*) relative to the total amount of salt present in the well. In that way, the influence of salt purity on drug precipitation could be determined.

2.7. Solubility and pH_{max} Determination

Drug solubility was measured by adding the DKT to solutions at various pH values and stirring at 37 °C for 24 h. The pH was adjusted by adding HCl or NaOH to the solutions. Solubility values were used to calculate the salt solubility product, K_{sp}, according to the following equation

$$K_{sp} = [DK^-][TH^+] \quad (4)$$

where $[DK^-]$ represent the concentration of ionized drug and $[TH^+]$ represents the concentration of counterion. The pH_{max} was calculated from the intersection of the DKT and free acid solubility curves generated according to equations presented in the results section. The pH_{max} refers to the pH where both the DKT and free acid have equal solubilities.

2.8. Concentration Analysis of DKT by HPLC

DKT concentrations in the samples were measured by HPLC-UV (Hewlett Packard series 1100 HPLC Pump combined with Agilent Technologies 1200 Series Autosampler). A volume of 75 µL was injected into the HPLC system (Waters 515 HPLC Pump with Waters 717 Autosampler). DKT was detected with an UV lamp at 262 nm (Water 996 Photodiode Array Detector). The mobile phase consisted of 60:40 mixture of acetonitrile and purified water A (both containing 0.1% TFA). Stationary phase was a C-18 Agilent Eclipse XDB (4.6 × 150 mm; 3.5 µm). Elution flow was 1 mL/min and retention time for DKT was 3.95 min. Calibration curves were made in mobile phase based on a stock solution of DKT in methanol. Linearity was observed between 1.5 µg/mL and 300 µg/mL covering all the experimental sample values. The observed peaks were integrated using Millenium software (Agilent Technologies, County of Santa Clara, CA, USA). The developed analytical method met the standards for precision and accuracy.

2.9. Data Analysis and Presentation

Dissolution profiles of DKT in all GIS compartments were plotted either as drug concentration or mass of drug versus time (average ± standard deviation; n = 4). Dissolution profiles from USP-2 experiments were represented as the fraction dose dissolved versus time (average n = 3).

3. Results and Discussion

3.1. Solubilities and Solution Stabilities of DKT and Free Acid Solid Forms as a Function of pH

Dexketoprofen is a lipophilic (LogP 3.61) weak acid with pK_a of 4.02 at 37 °C [12,13]. The DKT salt was developed to enhance its solubility over the free acid and improve dissolution in the GI tract. Salt formation is a well-known strategy to increase the solubility of either lipophilic weak acids or bases in order to improve oral absorption. Nevertheless, the expected benefits of forming a salt may not work if the level of supersaturation leads to drug precipitation to the free acid or base, thereby reducing the drug exposure levels for absorption [14–16]. The "supersaturation/precipitation interactive process" depends on the characteristics of the weak acid or base and, not unimportant, on the dissolution study design with respect to media composition and hydrodynamics that will determine the bulk and interfacial pH around the dissolving particles.

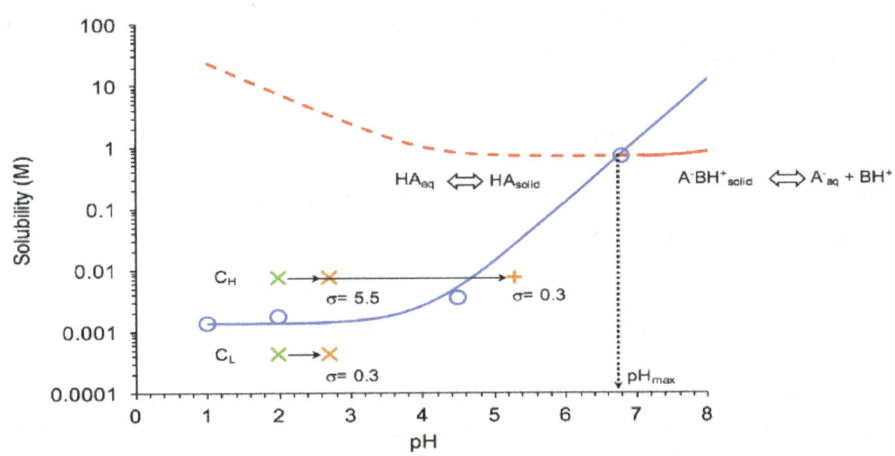

Figure 2. Solubility—pH dependence of free acid and DKT salt indicating the stability regions for salt and free acid solid-state forms and the conditions under which dissolution-precipitation microscopy studies were carried out. Salt has a pH_{max} of 6.7 below which supersaturation with respect to free acid can occur. Two salt concentrations were studied: C_L represents the low dose concentration. C_H represents a higher concentration of 18x C_L, as described in the Materials and Methods section. Arrows represent the pH changes that different salt formulations experienced. Green X represents initial concentration and pH. As the salt dissolves, the bulk pH increased to 2.7 ± 0.2 (orange X) for the bioequivalence (BE) and reference formulation excipients, whereas the pH increased up to 5.3 (orange+) for the non-bioequivalence (non-BE) formulation excipients. Solubility curve for salt (red line) was calculated from Equation (6), using K_{sp} and $pK_{a,DK}$ reported in the text and $pK_{a,T}$ = 8.1 [17]. The free acid solubility curve (blue line) was calculated according to Equation (7). Open circles represent DK measured solubilities at 37 °C. The dashed red line represents supersaturated conditions with respect to DK if solutions are saturated with salt.

The influence of pH on the stability of the DKT salt and DK free acid was determined by examining the solubility-pH profiles presented in Figure 2. These results show that DKT salt has a pH_{max} at

6.7, where both salt and free acid have equal solubilities; thus, both phases are stable. Below pH_{max}, the salt is more soluble than the free acid, and generates supersaturation with respect to the acid. Supersaturation is expressed as the ratio of salt to free acid solubility, $S_{salt}/S_{acid/intrinsic}$. The lower the pH below pH_{max}, the higher is the supersaturation that the salt may generate, and the higher is the driving force for salt to free acid conversion. On the other hand, the salt is stable at $pH \geq pH_{max}$.

Given the salt solubility at pH_{max} and the free acid S_0 values, supersaturation with respect to free acid can be very high (>500) causing drug precipitation and depletion of drug concentration levels. Salt to drug conversions were examined by microscopy at two salt concentrations, one equivalent to the dose and one higher, as indicated in the graph. Although at C_L the bulk solution is undersaturated with respect to free acid, the salt particles can exhibit supersaturation at the salt/liquid interface as this region is saturated with respect to salt. The solubility−pH profiles for the salt and the free acid were generated according to equations derived from the solution chemistry equilibria. For the salt, the equilibrium reaction is

$$DK^-TH^+ \overset{K_{sp}}{\leftrightarrow} DK^- + TH^+ \tag{5}$$

The equilibrium constant for this reaction is the salt solubility product (K_{sp}) given by Equation (4). K_{sp} of DKT was determined to be 4.96×10^{-1} M^2, from the measured $[DK^-]$ or salt solubility, $S_{salt} = 7.04 \times 10^{-1}$ M at pH 6.8. While K_{sp} is constant with pH, salt solubility is not, and its dependence on pH is given (assuming no precipitation of protonated dexketoprofen and no solubility-limiting effect by other ions in the medium) by

$$S_{salt} = \sqrt{K_{sp}\left(1 + 10^{pK_{a,DK} - pH}\right)\left(1 + 10^{pH - pK_{a,T}}\right)} \tag{6}$$

where $K_{a,DK}$ and $K_{a,T}$ are the acid and base dissociation constants of the salt constituents. For the free acid, the solubility in terms of pH is expressed by

$$S_{acid} = S_0\left(1 + 10^{pH - pK_{a,DK}}\right) \tag{7}$$

where S_0 is the intrinsic solubility of the free acid, determined to be 1.36×10^{-3} M. The pH_{max} was also calculated applying the following equation:

$$pH_{max} = pK_{a,DK} + log\frac{\sqrt{K_{sp}}}{S_0} \tag{8}$$

obtained by solving Equations (6) and (7) for pH when $S_{salt} = S_{acid}$ at $pK_{a,DT} < pH < pK_{a,T}$, under conditions where both drug and counterion are fully ionized. The pH_{max} value of 6.7 obtained by this equation is equal to that obtained graphically because trometamol is still almost completely ionized at this pH.

3.2. Formulation Performance of the DKT Formulations in the GIS with Protocols 1 and 2

Since the GIS can incorporate the dynamic shift in fluid pH and composition as the dosage form transits from the stomach to the intestine, it has previously shown utility in predicting the in vivo performance of weak bases [4,18–22]. In this study, GIS dissolution experiments were performed using two different protocols, representing two different medium compositions in the gastric and intestinal compartments. Whereas Protocol 1 contained SGF in the gastric compartment and pH 6.8 phosphate buffer in the intestinal compartments, in Protocol 2, sodium chloride was added to SGF in the gastric compartment and FaSSIF-v1 was added to the intestinal compartment. Figures 3 and 4 include the observed solution DKT concentrations as a function of time for the three different formulations as tested in the GIS device, applying Protocol 1 and Protocol 2, respectively.

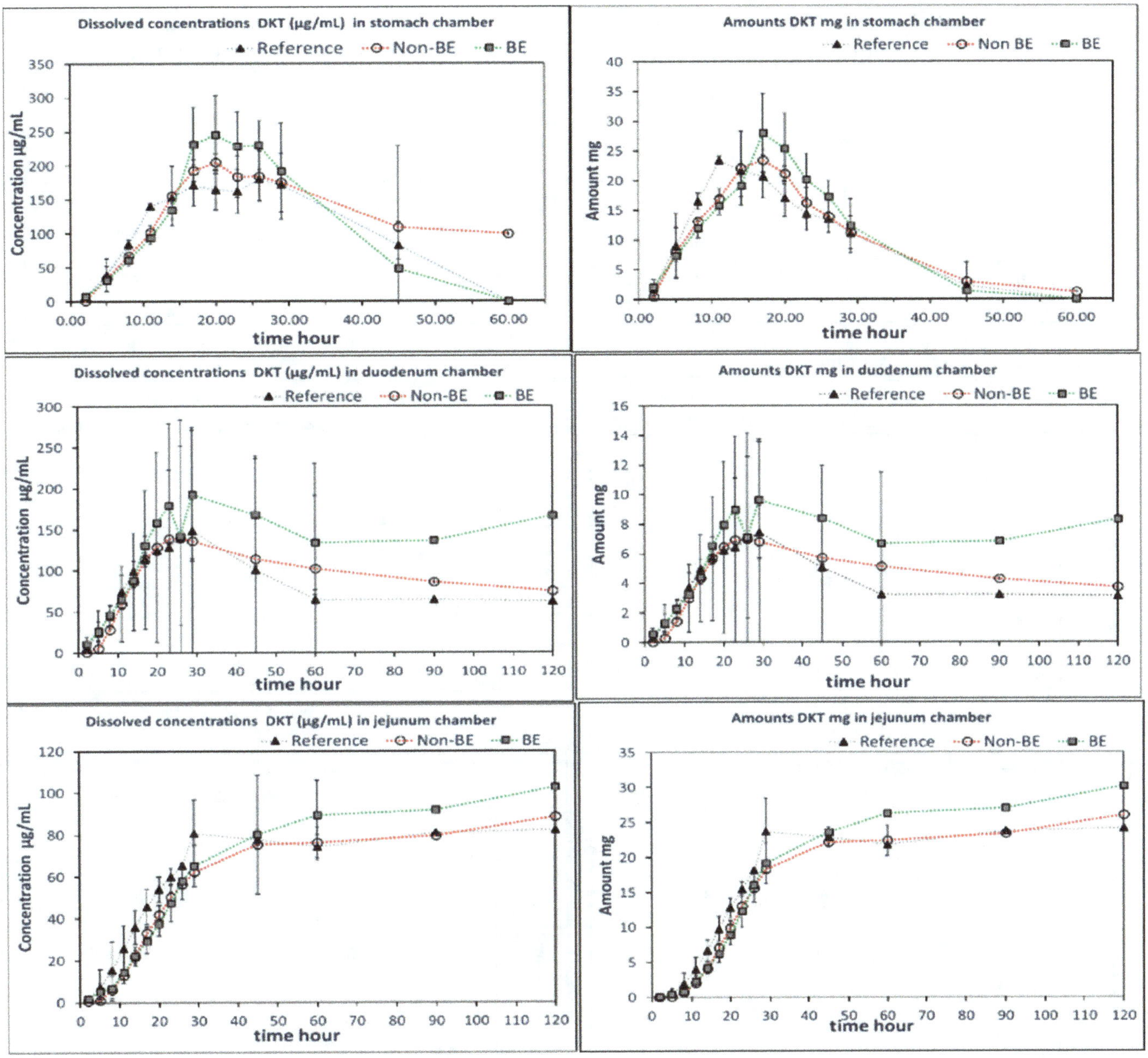

Figure 3. DKT concentrations (**left panels**) and amounts in solution (**right panels**) in the $GIS_{stomach}$, $GIS_{duodenum}$, and $GIS_{jejunum}$ vessels obtained with Protocol 1 with HCl 0.01M in $GIS_{stomach}$ and phosphate buffer 50 mM (pH 6.8) in the duodenal chamber (n = 3). Standard deviations overlap over the three profiles and they are not shown. Dotted lines are included to facilitate visual profile comparison.

Remarkably, differences in dissolution behavior were observed in the gastric compartment of the GIS apparatus in the presence and absence of NaCl. When NaCl was absent from the gastric medium (Protocol 1), the gastric dissolution profiles did not discriminate between the three formulations. However, when NaCl was added to the gastric medium (Protocol 2), differentiation was observed between the formulations, whereby the non-BE formulation dissolved earlier and to a great extent, as was observed in vivo (deconvoluted profiles). The addition of NaCl to SGF resulted in observed differences in the disintegration behavior in the gastric chamber as discussed further in the next section.

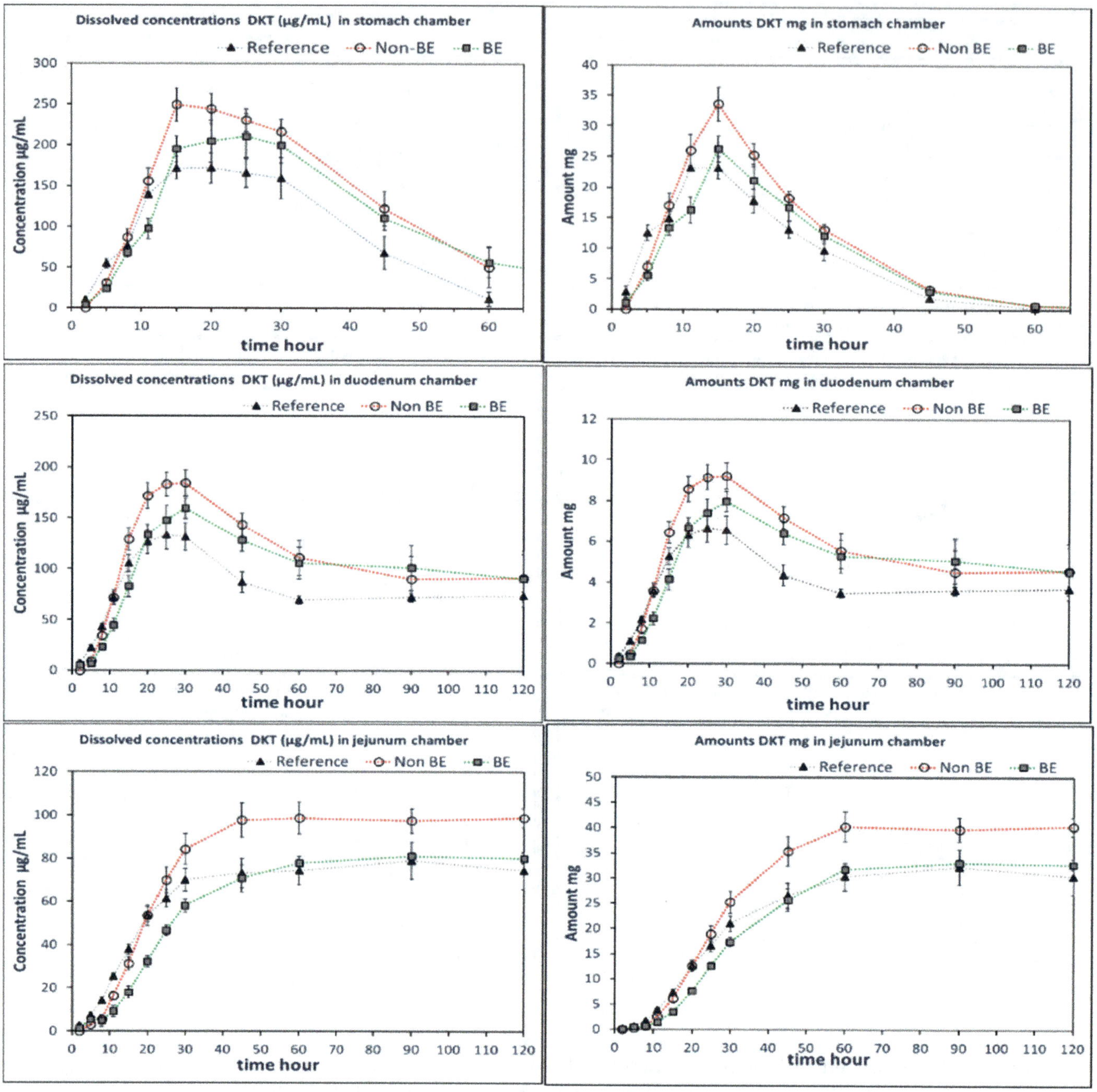

Figure 4. DKT concentrations (**left panels**) and amounts in solution (**right panels**) in the $GIS_{stomach}$, $GIS_{duodenum}$, and $GIS_{jejunum}$ vessels obtained with Protocol 2 with NaCl in $GIS_{stomach}$ at 34 mM and FaSSIF-v1 in the duodenal chamber. Experimental data were shown as mean ± SD (n = 4). Dotted lines are included to facilitate visual profile comparison.

The differences in dissolution rates across the three formulations as observed in the $GIS_{stomach}$ with Protocol 2 were maintained after the transfer to the duodenal chamber. Finally, the $GIS_{jejunum}$ accumulated the differences and the jejunum cumulative dissolution profiles of the three assayed formulations followed the same trend as the oral fractions absorbed obtained from deconvolution of plasma profiles, as depicted in Figure 5.

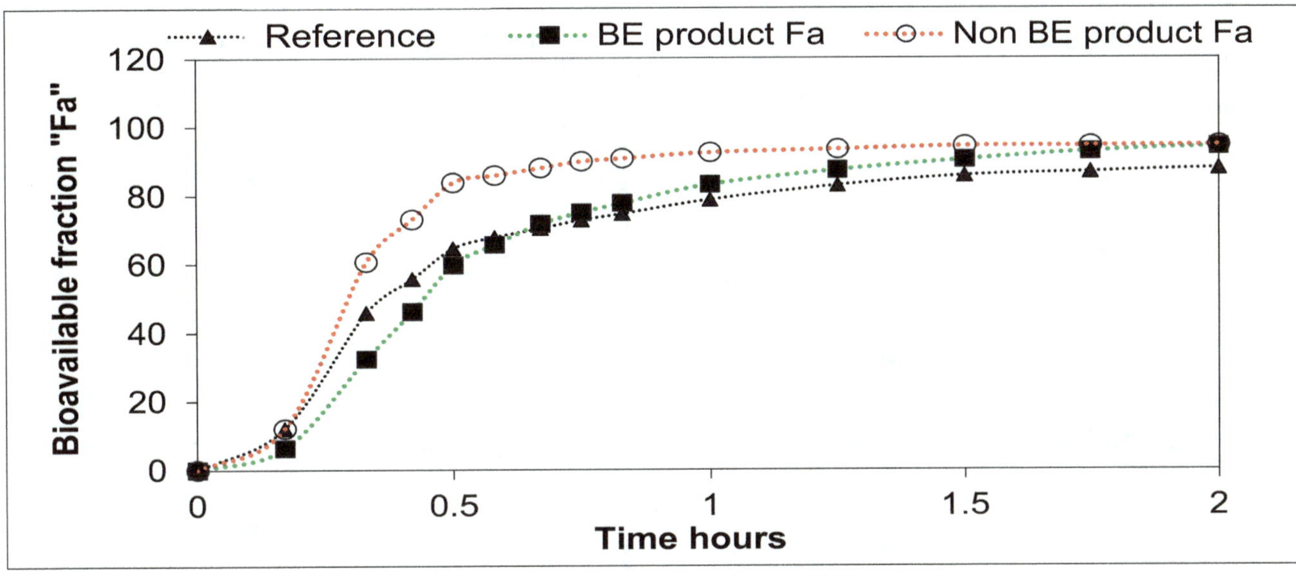

Figure 5. Bioavailable DKT fractions obtained from plasma levels through Loo–Riegelman deconvolution.

Measured DKT concentrations in the $GIS_{stomach}$ were the result of the balance between the supersaturation factor of DKT promoted by the salt and the precipitation of the free acid. That balance evolved differently in the presence or in the absence of NaCl. Potential reasons for these observations are the differences in solubility of sodium dexketoprofen versus the trometamol salt and the increased solubility of calcium monohydrogen phosphate in the presence of NaCl. After transfer to the duodenal chamber, a reflection of the gastric dissolution profiles was observed in the FaSSIF-v1 media, using Protocol 2. In Protocol 1, no differences between dissolution profiles were observed in the duodenal chamber. It could be due to the fact that the three formulations already behaved similarly in the $GIS_{stomach}$ but, on the other hand, the higher buffer strength of the 50 mM phosphate buffer used in Protocol 1 readily promoted DKT dissolution hiding the effect of calcium phosphate on solid surface pH.

As for why did the differences between the studied formulations appear with Protocol 2 but not Protocol 1, the USP paddle dissolution results in FaSSIF-v1, shown in Figure 6, indicate that the incorporation of NaCl into the simulated gastric fluid rather than the use of FaSSIF-v1 is the primary reason. This is rather intriguing due to the low NaCl molarity present in the $GIS_{stomach}$ owing to the six-fold dilution with water. Applying the ionic strength and activity coefficient calculations shows that any effect on the DKT and/or calcium phosphate behavior would be marginal at those NaCl concentrations. Our current hypotheses for possible causes have not yet been experimentally tested. Therefore, additional future studies are planned to investigate the possible causes behind this effect.

3.3. The Impact of NaCl on Disintegration and Dissolution

Results of the dissolution experiments in the USP-2 apparatus using four different media (FaSSIF-v1 at pH 6.5; 0.01 N HCl (pH 2); 0.01 N HCl + 34 mM NaCl; and 0.01 N HCl + 135 mM), which were designed to explore the impact of NaCl on formulation disintegration/drug dissolution, are depicted in Figure 6. The different concentrations of NaCl cover the observed values as observed in the human stomach [6].

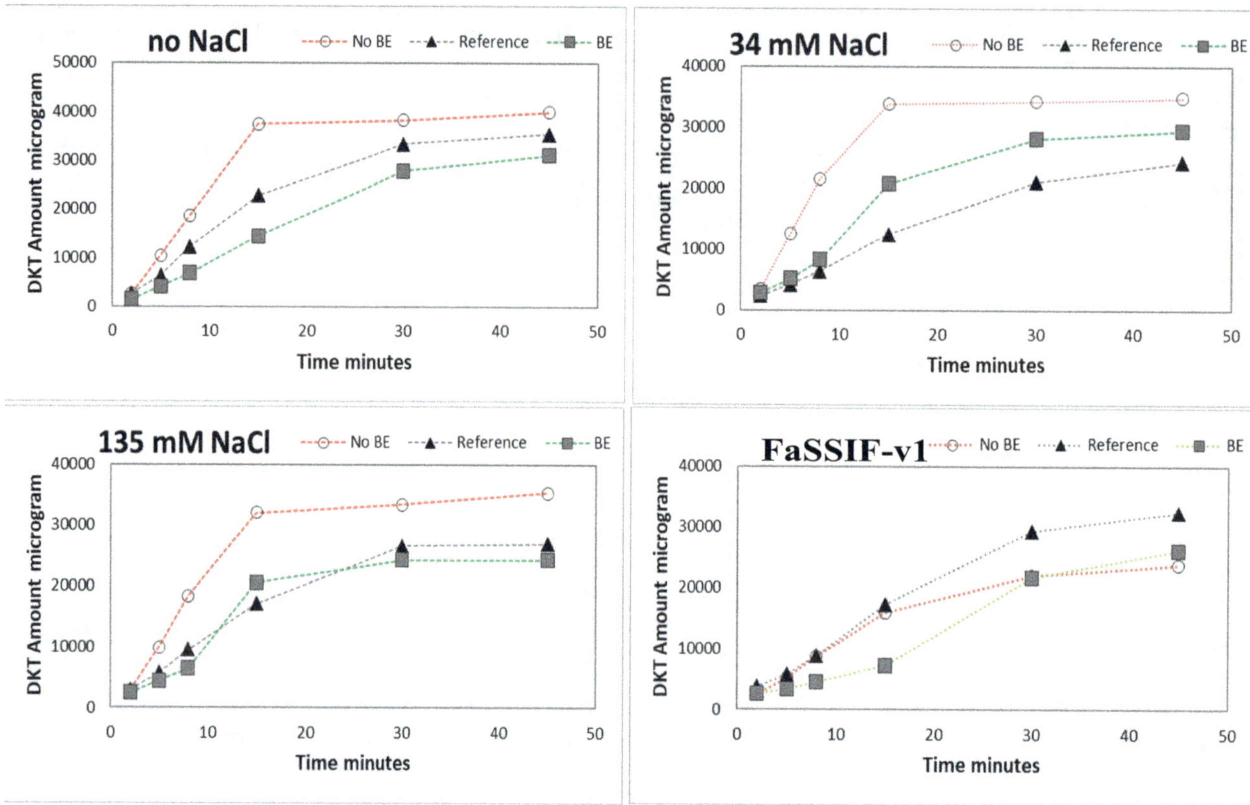

Figure 6. Amounts of DKT in micrograms dissolved in USP-2 apparatus (500 mL; 50 rpm) in acidic media (HCl 0.01M pH = 2) at different levels of NaCl content and in FaSSIF-v1 media. Data are presented as means ($n = 3$).

The presence of NaCl mainly affected the disintegration and dissolution process of the non-BE formulation resulting in an enhanced dissolution rate in the presence of NaCl, which was not observed for the BE-formulation and the reference drug product. While performing these dissolution experiments, remarkable differences in disintegration behavior could also be observed between the non-BE formulations and the other two formulations.

The faster dissolution of DKT from the non-BE formulation compared to the other formulations under Protocol 2 is most likely related to the high content of calcium phosphate in the tablet core of the non-BE formulation, which is not present in the other formulations. This high level of calcium phosphate in the tablet core of the non-BE formulation can increase the pH at the solid surface accelerating the dissolution of DKT and also facilitating tablet disintegration. Modulation of microenvironmental pH has been shown as an effective strategy to modulate the dissolution rate of GDC-0810, a weak acid of an oral anticancer drug, by using sodium bicarbonate to change solid surface pH [23]. This same strategy of using pH-modifiers has been proposed as a release modulating mechanism in solid dispersions [24] and other immediate-release dosage forms [25]. Solid surface pH data was not obtained in these dissolution experiments and bulk pH values of the media during dissolution experiments were available only in $GIS_{stomach}$ at 13 min with Protocol 2. At that time, the non-BE formulation containing calcium phosphate presented a pH of 3.5, 1 unit higher than the pH of the reference and BE formulation that was approximately 2.5. Calcium phosphate can increase the pH at the solid surface of the drug-excipients particles, then increasing DKT solubility, and consequently decreasing the degree of supersaturation, which will, subsequently, prevent or reduce the precipitation gradient [25]. Besides calcium phosphate, FaSSIF-v1 surfactants seem to play a major role in the supersaturation/free acid precipitation balance as it has been reported for other ionizable compounds [26–28].

3.4. In Vitro–In Vivo Correlations (IVIVC) for the Different Drug Products

When fractions absorbed of the three formulations were plotted against the fractions dissolved in jejunal chamber when Protocol 2 was applied, a single relationship was obtained, indicating dissolution was the limiting factor for DKT systemic input (Figure 7).

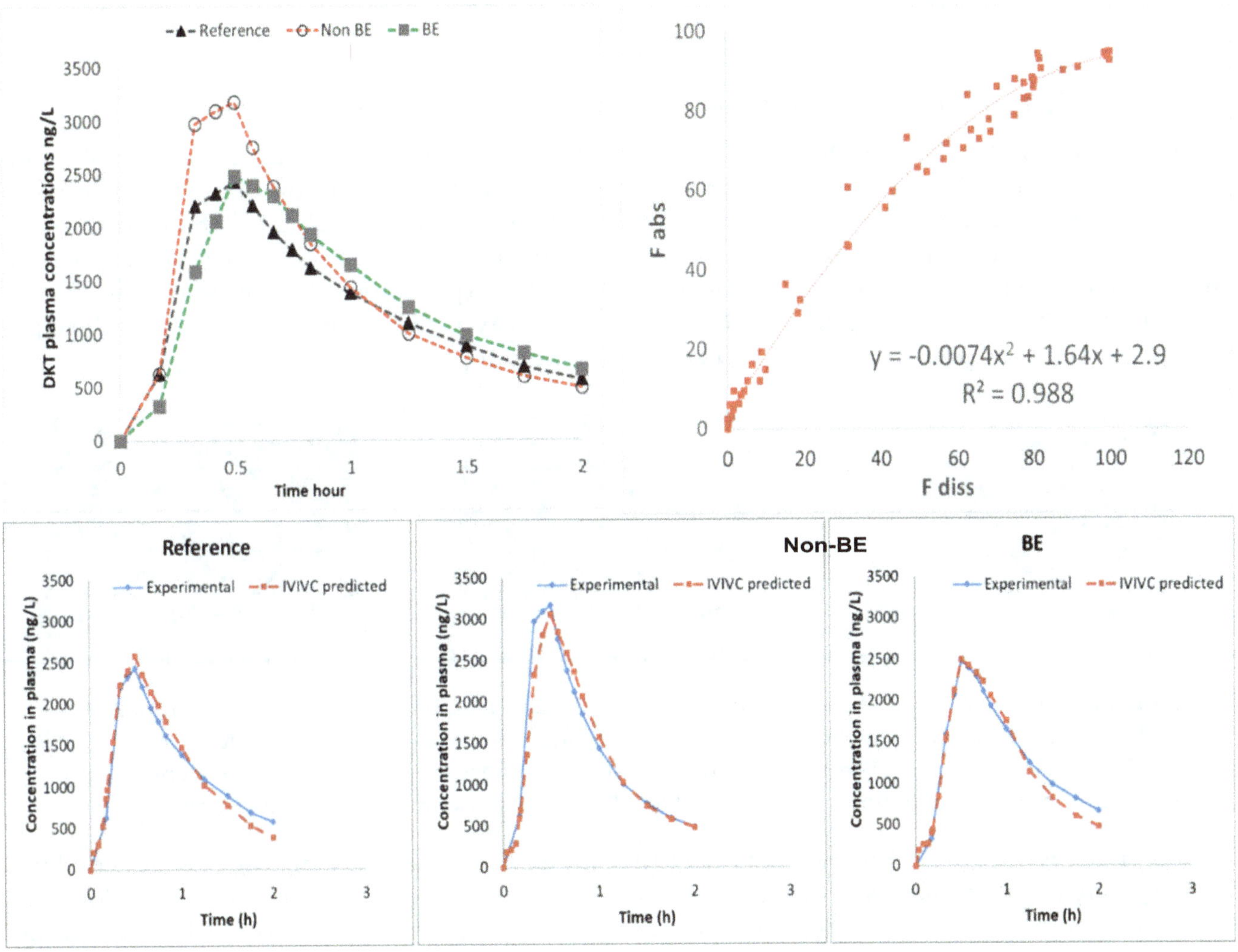

Figure 7. Invitro–invivo correlation (IVIVC) level A. (**Top left plot**) Human plasma levels of DKT after oral administration of the reference product (Enantyum®) and two test formulations from two BE trials. Concentrations of test products were normalized using the ratio of reference concentrations. Plasma levels are shown up to 2 h to highlight C_{max} differences. (**Top right plot**) Non-linear IVIVC plotting fraction absorbed versus fraction dissolved. (**Bottom plots**) Internal validation through prediction of plasma levels for each formulation.

Nevertheless, the obtained relationship is not linear but curved due to a time-scale shift from in vivo to in vitro. In vivo dissolution and, consequently, absorption is faster than what was simulated in vitro. A time-scaling approach was not considered to be necessary as the time shift was less than 30 min and the non-linear equation presented a good predictive performance. The reason for the slight time shift could be the fact that jejunal dissolved amounts were used while in vivo dissolution/absorption from duodenum can play a relevant/significant role. The internal validation of the obtained IVIVC was done by estimating fractions absorbed from the experimental dissolved ones using the obtained non-linear equation and then back-transforming fractions absorbed in plasma levels. Relative prediction errors of plasma C_{max} and AUC were lower than 10% for all the formulations (Table 5).

Table 5. Experimental and predicted plasma C_{max} and area under the curve (AUC) values for all DKT formulations and relative prediction errors.

	C_{max} Exp ng/L	C_{max} Pred ng/L	RE%	AUC Exp ng/L*h	AUC Pred ng/L*h	RE%
Reference	2430.6	2576.3	−5.99	2497.3	2520	−0.92
Non-BE	3177.3	3062.5	3.61	2785.7	2739	1.69
BE	2478.5	2491.9	−0.54	2626	2538	3.35
Average			3.38			1.98

3.5. Differences between Drug Salt to Free Acid Conversions for BE and non-BE Formulations

Drug exposure levels are influenced by the kinetics of salt dissolution and drug precipitation as well as the evolution of drug phases. Microscopic examination of salt dissolution in pH 2 identified two main pathways depending on the formulation excipients: (1) salt dissolved without conversion in the presence of calcium phosphate as one of the excipients (non-BE formulation), (2) salt dissolution formed a nano-phase that grew to spherical and island morphologies that converted to free acid crystals (Figure 8). The time course of the second pathway was dependent on the salt/excipient concentration and the presence of free acid crystals in the salt phase.

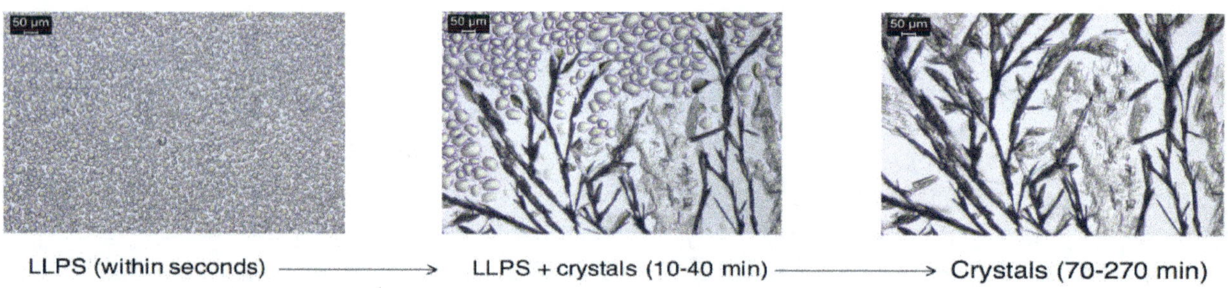

Figure 8. Diagram showing the DKT transformations to DK drug phases during dissolution. A more soluble drug phase appears first as liquid–liquid phase separation (LLPS), followed by a less soluble crystalline phase. The kinetics and pathways of these transformations are dependent on salt concentration, formulation excipients and level of drug phase impurity in the salt phase.

Shown in Figure 8 is the precipitated phase that appears as non-coalescing drops suspended in the dissolution media. This phase surrounds the fast dissolving salt particles, within seconds. Conversion of this fine precipitate to drug crystals was observed after 2 min or longer (up to 1 h) depending on initial salt concentration, formulation excipients, and presence of drug impurity in salt.

The massive phase separation appears initially hazy as its size is in the submicron range and below the level of detection of the microscope. This phenomenon has been referred to as spinodal, oiling out, or liquid–liquid phase separation (LLPS), consistent with that observed for other weakly basic drugs under high supersaturations, such as ritonavir [29–33]. The supersaturations with respect to drug, generated at the surface of the dissolving DKT salt particles are very high (>500 at pH 2) based on the solubilities of the salt and drug forms shown in Figure 2. While the interfacial pH was not evaluated, the surface of the dissolving salt is saturated with respect to the salt and generates much higher supersaturations than those in the bulk dissolution media. In fact, the appearance of LLPS occurred even when the bulk solution was below the drug solubility ($\sigma = 0.3$) (Figure 2).

Table 6 summarizes DKT transformations to drug phases during dissolution. Observed dissolution of all phases initially or after the appearance of LLPS and drug crystals is consistent with undersaturated drug conditions in the bulk solution at dose concentration (C_L). Non-BE formulation excipients in the media at higher concentrations (C_H) increased pH to 5.3, and no precipitation was observed as the solution concentration is below salt and drug solubility. This is most probably because of the neutralization of HCl by the large level of calcium phosphate present. REF and BE formulation excipients exhibited different conversion behavior at C_H; LLPS formed and crystallized after 10–30 min.

The presence of drug crystals as impurity (less than or equal to 3%) in the salt phase led to the faster conversion of LLPS to less soluble drug crystals, i.e., faster drug crystallization and LLPS dissolution. Faster conversion rates result in lower drug exposure levels.

It is important to consider that concentration levels varied for both salt and excipients, as the excipient concentrations were varied by diluting the dissolved tablet prior to adding the salt. Therefore, the different behavior of the high concentration of excipients with the non-BE shows the key role of alkalinizing excipients on stabilizing the salt, as the pH approaches the pH_{max}.

Furthermore, the dilution of the gastric fluid by water in the $GIS_{stomach}$ of the GIS setup explains the C_H results better matching the trend of the GIS data than the C_L results. This is because the lower HCl concentrations caused by dilution were not sufficient to eliminate the pH differences caused by the presence of calcium phosphate in the non-BE formulation. This gave rise to an end effect similar to the high calcium phosphate levels under C_H conditions being able to effectively neutralize the 0.01 M HCl. This is supported by the aforementioned observation of higher pH value in the $GIS_{stomach}$ for the non-BE formulation compared to the reference one, which is more in line with the C_H than with the C_L results.

Table 6. Evolution of drug phases during DKT dissolution in different formulation conditions.

Formulation	Condition	LLPS	Crystal	Full Dissolution	Final pH
Non-BE	C_H [b]	–	–	+ [a]	5.3
	C_L [c]	+	–	+(80 min)	2.8
	C_L + DK solid [d]	+	+	+(>7 h)	2.9
BE	C_H	++	++	NA	2.9
	C_L	+	–	+(90 min)	2.6
	C_L + DK solid	+	+	+(>4 h)	2.8
REF	C_H	++	++	NA	2.9
	C_L	+	–	+(60 min)	2.6
	C_L + DK solid	+	+	+(>2 h)	2.7
Salt in buffer no excipients	C_H	++	++	NA	2.7
	C_L	+	–	+(85 min)	2.7
	C_H + DK solid	++	++	–	2.7

[a] within seconds; [b] C_L, low concentration, dose in 300 mL solution (total drug concentration = 4.3×10^{-4} M); [c] C_H, high concentration = 18 × C_L (total drug concentration = 7.7×10^{-3} M); [d] DK solid, represents less than or equal to 3% free acid drug as impurity in the salt phase; and NA, not applicable as C_H at this final pH is above free acid solubility.

4. Conclusions and Future Directions

Differences in dissolution behavior between the BE and non-BE DKT products are a result of drug salt to free acid phase conversion rates and mechanisms. In this case, the presence of an alkalinizing excipient in a tablet formulation of a salt of a weakly acidic drug suppresses salt disproportionation as pH approaches pH_{max}, leading to a higher extent of drug dissolved and failing BE requirements. This is a case where salt disproportionation appears to modulate the behavior of a highly soluble salt in a favorable way by the formation of a transient phase prior to crystallization of the less soluble free acid. Rates of formation of less-soluble drug phases, LLPS, and crystal forms during DKT salt dissolution are dependent on the excipients, dissolution pH, and presence of DK free acid as an impurity in the salt. Excipients that increase pH (calcium phosphate) decreased free acid precipitation and enhanced dissolved levels of drug in the non-BE formulation. The BE product was associated with a faster conversion to KT crystals, whereas non-BE product experienced less drug precipitation under the same condition. Generic and non-generic DKT formulations were discriminated in vitro in the GIS device by adding NaCl to SGF and using FaSSIF-v1 media in the duodenum compartment. However, the relevant GI variables for the development of "In Vivo Product Predictive Dissolution Methods" need to be adapted to each compound. The selection of particular dissolution conditions as media and secretion fluids composition for the GIS device will depend on (i) the BCS profile of the drug, (ii) its ionization characteristics, and (iii) its formulation characteristics (e.g., presence of calcium monohydrogenphosphate). The ionic strength impact as well as the surfactants effects on the supersaturation/precipitation balance needs to be further investigated.

Author Contributions: M.B., G.K., J.A.-G., I.G.-A., G.E.A, N.R.-H. and G.L.A. designed and experimentally conducted the in vitro experiments. B.H., Y.T., D.M., A.G.-A. and A.R.-P. contributed to the writing of this manuscript and the analyses and interpretation of the data.

Acknowledgments: The pharmaceutical companies that allowed the anonymous publication of the data included in these generic pharmaceutical developments are acknowledged.

Abbreviation

DKT	dexketoprofen trometamol
DK	dexketoprofen
FaSSIF-v1	fasted state simulated intestinal fluids version 1
SGF	simulated gastric fluids
HPLC	high-performance liquid chromatography
LLPS	liquid–liquid phase separation
PK	pharmacokinetics
GIS	gastrointestinal simulator
USP	United States Pharmacopeia
GI	gastrointestinal
BE	bioequivalence
AUC	area under the curve
C_{max}	maximal concentration
C_H	high concentration of DKT
C_L	low concentration of DKT
IVIVC	in vitro–in vivo correlation
REF	reference listed drug product
Non-BE	non-bioequivalent
S_{salt}	Solubility of the salt form of dexketoprofen (i.e., dexketoprofen trometamol)
S_{acid}	Solubility of the salt form of dexketoprofen
NaCl	sodium chloride
S_0	intrinsic solubility of dexketoprofen
pH_{max}	the pH_{max} refers to the pH where both the DKT and free acid have equal solubilities.
K_{sp}	salt solubility product
TH^+	positively ionized trometamol
$GIS_{stomach}$	gastrointestinal simulator gastric chamber
$GIS_{duodenum}$	gastrointestinal simulator duodenal chamber
$GIS_{jejunum}$	gastrointestinal simulator jejunal chamber
F_a	fraction absorbed
HA	acid form
A^-	negative ionized acid form
BH	protonated basic form
RE%	relative prediction error in percentage
EMA	European Medicines Agency
BCS	biopharmaceutics classification system
NaOH	sodium hydroxide
HCl	hydrochloric acid
TFA	trifluoracetic acid

References

1. Cardot, J.-M.; Garcia Arieta, A.; Paixao, P.; Tasevska, I.; Davit, B. Implementing the Biopharmaceutics Classification System in Drug Development: Reconciling Similarities, Differences, and Shared Challenges in the EMA and US-FDA-Recommended Approaches. *AAPS J.* **2016**, *18*, 1039–1046. [CrossRef] [PubMed]
2. Davit, B.M.; Kanfer, I.; Tsang, Y.C.; Cardot, J.-M. BCS Biowaivers: Similarities and Differences Among EMA, FDA, and WHO Requirements. *AAPS J.* **2016**, *18*, 612–618. [CrossRef] [PubMed]
3. Garcia-Arieta, A.; Gordon, J.; Gwaza, L.; Mangas-Sanjuan, V.; Álvarez, C.; Torrado, J.J. Agitation Rate and Time for Complete Dissolution in BCS Biowaivers Based on Investigation of a BCS Biowaiver for Dexketoprofen Tablets. *Mol. Pharm.* **2015**, *12*, 3194–3201. [CrossRef] [PubMed]
4. Hens, B.; Bermejo, M.; Tsume, Y.; Gonzalez-Alvarez, I.; Ruan, H.; Matsui, K.; Amidon, G.E.; Cavanagh, K.; Kuminek, G.; Benninghoff, G.; et al. Evaluation and optimized selection of supersaturating drug delivery systems of posaconazole (BCS class 2b) in the gastrointestinal simulator (GIS): An in vitro-in silico-in vivo approach. *Eur. J. Pharm. Sci.* **2018**, *15*, 258–269. [CrossRef] [PubMed]
5. Hens, B.; Brouwers, J.; Anneveld, B.; Corsetti, M.; Symillides, M.; Vertzoni, M.; Reppas, C.; Turner, D.B.; Augustijns, P. Gastrointestinal transfer: In vivo evaluation and implementation in in vitro and in silico predictive tools. *Eur. J. Pharm. Sci.* **2014**, *63*, 233–242. [CrossRef] [PubMed]
6. Lindahl, A.; Ungell, A.L.; Knutson, L.; Lennernäs, H. Characterization of fluids from the stomach and proximal jejunum in men and women. *Pharm. Res.* **1997**, *14*, 497–502. [CrossRef] [PubMed]
7. Valles, J.; Artigas, R.; Crea, A.; Muller, F.; Paredes, I.; Zapata, A.; Capriati, A. Clinical pharmacokinetics of parenteral dexketoprofen trometamol in healthy subjects. *Methods Find. Exp. Clin. Pharmacol.* **2006**, *28*, 7–12. [PubMed]
8. Ruiz Picazo, A.; Martinez-Martinez, M.T.; Colón-Useche, S.; Iriarte, R.; Sánchez-Dengra, B.; González-Álvarez, M.; García-Arieta, A.; González-Álvarez, I.; Bermejo, M. In Vitro Dissolution as a Tool for Formulation Selection: Telmisartan Two-Step IVIVC. *Mol. Pharm.* **2018**, *15*, 2307–2315. [CrossRef] [PubMed]
9. González-García, I.; Mangas-Sanjuan, V.; Merino-Sanjuán, M.; Álvarez-Álvarez, C.; Díaz-Garzón Marco, J.; Rodríguez-Bonnín, M.A.; Langguth, T.; Torrado-Durán, J.J.; Langguth, P.; García-Arieta, A.; et al. IVIVC approach based on carbamazepine bioequivalence studies combination. *Pharmazie* **2017**, *72*, 449–455. [PubMed]
10. Humbert, H.; Cabiac, M.D.; Bosshardt, H. In vitro-in vivo correlation of a modified-release oral form of ketotifen: In vitro dissolution rate specification. *J. Pharm. Sci.* **1994**, *83*, 131–136. [CrossRef] [PubMed]
11. Wagner, J.G. Pharmacokinetic absorption plots from oral data alone or oral/intravenous data and an exact Loo-Riegelman equation. *J. Pharm. Sci.* **1983**, *72*, 838–842. [CrossRef] [PubMed]
12. Avdeef, A.; Tsinman, O. Miniaturized rotating disk intrinsic dissolution rate measurement: Effects of buffer capacity in comparisons to traditional wood's apparatus. *Pharm. Res.* **2008**, *25*, 2613–2627. [CrossRef] [PubMed]
13. ChemAxon—Software Solutions and Services for Chemistry and Biology. Available online: https://chemaxon.com/products/calculators-and-predictors#logp_logd (accessed on 5 February 2019).
14. Patel, M.A.; Luthra, S.; Shamblin, S.L.; Arora, K.K.; Krzyzaniak, J.F.; Taylor, L.S. Effect of excipient properties, water activity, and water content on the disproportionation of a pharmaceutical salt. *Int. J. Pharm.* **2018**, *546*, 226–234. [CrossRef] [PubMed]
15. Thakral, N.K.; Kelly, R.C. Salt disproportionation: A material science perspective. *Int. J. Pharm.* **2017**, *520*, 228–240. [CrossRef] [PubMed]
16. Thakral, N.K.; Behme, R.J.; Aburub, A.; Peterson, J.A.; Woods, T.A.; Diseroad, B.A.; Suryanarayanan, R.; Stephenson, G.A. Salt Disproportionation in the Solid State: Role of Solubility and Counterion Volatility. *Mol. Pharm.* **2016**, *13*, 4141–4151. [CrossRef] [PubMed]
17. Morgan, M.E.; Liu, K.; Anderson, B.D. Microscale Titrimetric and Spectrophotometric Methods for Determination of Ionization Constants and Partition Coefficients of New Drug Candidates. *J. Pharm. Sci.* **1998**, *87*, 238–245. [CrossRef] [PubMed]
18. Matsui, K.; Tsume, Y.; Amidon, G.E.; Amidon, G.L. The Evaluation of In Vitro Drug Dissolution of Commercially Available Oral Dosage Forms for Itraconazole in Gastrointestinal Simulator with Biorelevant Media. *J. Pharm. Sci.* **2016**, *105*, 2804–2814. [CrossRef] [PubMed]

19. Matsui, K.; Tsume, Y.; Amidon, G.E.; Amidon, G.L. In Vitro Dissolution of Fluconazole and Dipyridamole in Gastrointestinal Simulator (GIS), Predicting in Vivo Dissolution and Drug-Drug Interaction Caused by Acid-Reducing Agents. *Mol. Pharm.* **2015**, *12*, 2418–2428. [CrossRef] [PubMed]
20. Matsui, K.; Tsume, Y.; Takeuchi, S.; Searls, A.; Amidon, G.L. Utilization of Gastrointestinal Simulator, an in Vivo Predictive Dissolution Methodology, Coupled with Computational Approach To Forecast Oral Absorption of Dipyridamole. *Mol. Pharm.* **2017**, *14*, 1181–1189. [CrossRef] [PubMed]
21. Tsume, Y.; Takeuchi, S.; Matsui, K.; Amidon, G.E.; Amidon, G.L. In vitro dissolution methodology, mini-Gastrointestinal Simulator (mGIS), predicts better in vivo dissolution of a weak base drug, dasatinib. *Eur. J. Pharm. Sci.* **2015**, *76*, 203–212. [CrossRef] [PubMed]
22. Tsume, Y.; Igawa, N.; Drelich, A.J.; Amidon, G.E.; Amidon, G.L. The combination of GIS and biphasic to better predict in vivo dissolution of BCS class IIb drugs, ketoconazole and raloxifene. *J. Pharm. Sci.* **2017**, *107*, 307–316. [CrossRef] [PubMed]
23. Hou, H.H.; Jia, W.; Liu, L.; Cheeti, S.; Li, J.; Nauka, E.; Nagapudi, K. Effect of Microenvironmental pH Modulation on the Dissolution Rate and Oral Absorption of the Salt of a Weak Acid—Case Study of GDC-0810. *Pharm. Res.* **2018**, *35*, 37. [CrossRef] [PubMed]
24. Tran, P.H.-L.; Tran, T.T.-D.; Lee, K.-H.; Kim, D.-J.; Lee, B.-J. Dissolution-modulating mechanism of pH modifiers in solid dispersion containing weakly acidic or basic drugs with poor water solubility. *Expert Opin. Drug Deliv.* **2010**, *7*, 647–661. [CrossRef] [PubMed]
25. Badawy, S.I.F.; Hussain, M.A. Microenvironmental pH Modulation in Solid Dosage Forms. *J. Pharm. Sci.* **2007**, *96*, 948–959. [CrossRef] [PubMed]
26. Indulkar, A.S.; Gao, Y.; Raina, S.A.; Zhang, G.G.Z.; Taylor, L.S. Crystallization from Supersaturated Solutions: Role of Lecithin and Composite Simulated Intestinal Fluid. *Pharm. Res.* **2018**, *35*, 158. [CrossRef] [PubMed]
27. Indulkar, A.S.; Mo, H.; Gao, Y.; Raina, S.A.; Zhang, G.G.Z.; Taylor, L.S. Impact of Micellar Surfactant on Supersaturation and Insight into Solubilization Mechanisms in Supersaturated Solutions of Atazanavir. *Pharm. Res.* **2017**, *34*, 1276–1295. [CrossRef] [PubMed]
28. Bevernage, J.; Brouwers, J.; Clarysse, S.; Vertzoni, M.; Tack, J.; Annaert, P.; Augustijns, P. Drug supersaturation in simulated and human intestinal fluids representing different nutritional states. *J. Pharm. Sci.* **2010**, *99*, 4525–4534. [CrossRef] [PubMed]
29. Cahn, J.W. On spinodal decomposition. *Acta Metall.* **1961**, *9*, 795–801. [CrossRef]
30. Bonnett, P.E.; Carpenter, K.J.; Dawson, S.; Davey, R.J. Solution crystallisation via a submerged liquid-liquid phase boundary: Oiling out. *Chem. Commun.* **2003**, 698–699. [CrossRef]
31. Deneau, E.; Steele, G. An In-Line Study of Oiling Out and Crystallization. *Org. Process Res. Dev.* **2005**, *9*, 943–950. [CrossRef]
32. Rodríguez-Spong, B.; Acciacca, A.; Fleisher, D.; Rodríguez-Hornedo, N. PH-induced nanosegregation of ritonavir to lyotropic liquid crystal of higher solubility than crystalline polymorphs. *Mol. Pharm.* **2008**, *5*, 956–967. [CrossRef] [PubMed]
33. Indulkar, A.S.; Box, K.J.; Taylor, R.; Ruiz, R.; Taylor, L.S. pH-Dependent Liquid–Liquid Phase Separation of Highly Supersaturated Solutions of Weakly Basic Drugs. *Mol. Pharm.* **2015**, *12*, 2365–2377. [CrossRef] [PubMed]

9

In Vitro Methods to Study Colon Release: State of the Art and an Outlook on New Strategies for Better *In-Vitro* Biorelevant Release Media

Marie Wahlgren [1,*], Magdalena Axenstrand [1], Åsa Håkansson [1], Ali Marefati [1] and Betty Lomstein Pedersen [2]

1 Department of Food technology engineering and nutrition, Lund University, P.O. Box 124, 221 00 Lund, Sweden; magdalenaaxenstrand@gmail.com (M.A.); asa.hakansson@food.lth.se (A.H.); ali.marefati@food.lth.se (A.M.)

2 Ferring International PharmaScience Center (IPC), Kay Fiskers Plads 11, 2300 Copenhagen, Denmark; Betty.Pedersen@ferring.com

* Correspondence: marie.wahlgren@food.lth.se

Abstract: The primary focus of this review is a discussion regarding in vitro media for colon release, but we also give a brief overview of colon delivery and the colon microbiota as a baseline for this discussion. The large intestine is colonized by a vast number of bacteria, approximately 10^{12} per gram of intestinal content. The microbial community in the colon is complex and there is still much that is unknown about its composition and the activity of the microbiome. However, it is evident that this complex microbiota will affect the release from oral formulations targeting the colon. This includes the release of active drug substances, food supplements, and live microorganisms, such as probiotic bacteria and bacteria used for microbiota transplantations. Currently, there are no standardized colon release media, but researchers employ in vitro models representing the colon ranging from reasonable simple systems with adjusted pH with or without key enzymes to the use of fecal samples. In this review, we present the pros and cons for different existing in vitro models. Furthermore, we summarize the current knowledge of the colonic microbiota composition which is of importance to the fermentation capacity of carbohydrates and suggest a strategy to choose bacteria for a new more standardized in vitro dissolution medium for the colon.

Keywords: *in vitro* systems; colon delivery; colon microbiota

---

1. Introduction

Most drugs are adsorbed in the upper GI-tract. However, for a range of therapeutics, food supplements and probiotics delivery to the colon is important. This is especially true for a range of inflammatory diseases of the GI-tract such as Crohn's disease and Ulcerative colitis [1–6] but also for other diseases in the colon that would benefit from a local treatment including colon cancer [7,8], enteric nematodes [9] and enzyme replacement therapies [10]. Other areas of interest are colon delivery of proteins and peptides [11,12], probiotic bacteria [13,14] and microbiota replacement therapies [15]. In these cases, formulations are employed aiming at colon-targeted delivery and at the same time avoiding release in the upper GI-tract. Thus, these formulations can protect the active ingredient from degradation in the stomach and small intestine.

There are a range of colon delivery systems, but it is not within the scope of this article to do an in-depth review of these. Instead, we recommend some of the literature referred to in the next sections and the following general reviews [2,16]. The principle of these formulations will however define the demands on colon delivery in in vitro methods used as they are dependent on different triggers of release. The main release mechanisms described in the literature are based on a few different triggers.

Degradation by the colonic microbiota: One strategy is to use excipients that are degraded by the microorganisms in the colon. Two of the most common classes of excipients used are carbohydrates and azo compounds. The bacteria of colon produce a large repertoire of enzymes, among which some are able to digest complex carbohydrates that have escaped digestion in the small intestine. These include enzymes such as amylases, pectinases and β-D-galactosidases to mention a few. Such enzymes have the ability to hydrolyze polysaccharide-specific bonds. Polysaccharides that can be used as coatings for this purpose are resistant starches, guar gum, pectin, dextran, inulin, and chitosan [10,13,17–21]. These are all molecules that can only be degraded by the microorganisms in the colon. Another colon bacterial-induced release is azore-reductive bacterial activities [22]. For a more thorough overview of these systems, we recommend the review by Sinha and Kumria [23]. One drawback with this principle is that some patients especially with inflammatory disease have a different colonic microbiota that could affect these extracellular enzymes [2,24].

Time-controlled release: These are primarily based on slow eroding or dissolving polymer films or matrixes [25–27]. In such systems, the polymer or wax (primarily natural waxes have been used) responsible for the release should not be sensitive to pH, enzymes or other components of the lumen such as bile salts. These types of formulations will be partly affected by transport of water and components in the GI tract fluid into the formulation and thus, the kinetics of this transport are expected to be highly affected by the increased viscosity of the lumen [28] when water is adsorbed in the colon, as has also been seen for some formulations [29]. The effect flow-behavior in the intestinal lumen has also been seen to influence the uptake of nutrients from food and this has been extensively discussed in a review by Takahashi [30]. Furthermore, the rate of gastric emptying will also influence if the time delayed formulations will release in the colon. It is well known that the gastric emptying time will vary considerable for larger objects such as a tablet.

pH controlled release: These formulations are based on the difference in pH along the GI-tract and are based on film coating that dissolves at different pH [31,32]. In order to secure release in the colon, some employ two or more films with different properties [32]. In some cases, pH dependence and time dependence are combined [33–36]. The main drawback of these systems is the large intra-individual variation in pH along the GI-tract, especially for patients with GI-tract diseases. A recent expert opinion concluded that due to the variation of pH in the GI-tract, colon delivery formulations that is only dependent on pH difference has a major risk of both premature drug release and no release at all [37].

Pressure-controlled delivery: This is based on the fact that the high viscosity of the lumen combined with the smooth muscle contractions of the colon assert a mechanical pressure on the formulation that ruptures a film coating or a capsule [38,39]. Primarily for capsules, the film strength of the capsule can be designed in such way that it ruptures at these pressures [16]. The drawback is that the main colonic motor pattern, pan-colonic pressurizations, can be severally reduced for example in patients with chronic constipation [40]. Furthermore, the less frequent high-amplitude propagating sequences that might be especially important for these formulations are only present after meals and not in all individuals studied [41].

Nanoparticle drug delivery systems: Various types of advanced nanoparticle formulations for colon delivery have been investigated by numerous researchers. These can for example be based on poly(lactic-*co*-glycolic acid) (PLGA), lipids, chitosan or silica, and these nanoparticles could be targeting inflamed mucosa. More details can be found in the reviews by Zhang et al. [42], Hua et al. [43] and by Vass et al. [44]. These types of formulation have the potential to deliver better treatment to the patients but there is a need for more attention to the practical design of the final dosage forms that successfully deliver the nanoparticles to the colon.

All of these formulation principles have their pros and cons and few of them have been found to deliver drugs to the whole colon. Thus, there is still a need to develop new colon-targeting formulations. In both early and late formulation development phases, there is a need for suitable and biorelevant in vitro media for evaluation of the various formulation concepts. Furthermore, during the formulation development of chosen concepts there is a need to evaluate the release profiles from different formulation designs and manufacturing principles.

The recommended dissolution media in the European and US Pharmacopeias are focused on simulating the upper GI tract. There is no Pharmacopeia in vitro dissolution method for colon delivery as such and the release media employed by several researchers for the evaluation of colon release differs a lot. It is the purpose of this review to discuss the benefit and draw backs of different colon release-testing media and also to suggest novel release media based on microorganisms present in the colon. In discussing in vitro methods, we also have to look at the whole passage through the GI-tract. Thus, this review will briefly describe the GI-tract and some of the dissolution media used to resemble the upper parts of the GI-tract.

Also within food research there is an interest in understanding release and digestion, especially concerning functional foods which are developed with the aim of promoting health and preventing diseases such as obesity, cancer, diabetes, neurodegenerative diseases (Alzheimer and Parkinson), and others [45]. These systems are developed in a way that the bioactive ingredient is protected while controlling and targeting the release to the specific location in the human gastrointestinal tract where they act [45]. The bioactive ingredients include polyphenols, carotenoids, fatty acids, proteins, peptides, amino acids, vitamins, minerals, and even live probiotic bacteria [46]. The challenge of inclusion of these bioactive ingredients is that they are susceptible to the conditions dictated by processing, storage and digestion that may lead to a decline in bioaccessibility as well as bioavailability. As a result, and in order to see the fate of bioactive compounds in human gastrointestinal conditions, simulated in vitro and in vivo digestion models are frequently used. In this review, we will do a comparison between the methods used in pharmaceutical development with those used for food research.

Even though the dissolution media are the focus of this review, it is important to bear in mind that an in vitro release profile from an oral dosage form is determined by the choice of dissolution method which comprises the (1) dissolution medium (composition and volume), (2) physical apparatus design, and (3) apparatus settings, that determine the hydrodynamics during release from the dosage form.

The review will discuss the pros and cons of most existing dissolution medias used for colon release. However, the main focus will be on media containing microorganisms. These medias are complex but should be the most biorelevant ones as the microbiota is the component that primarily governs the environmental conditions in the colon. Using live microorganisms ensures that the media contains a range of enzymes, and that these enzymes are constantly renewed by the bacteria. This is especially important when the release mechanism is based on degradation by the colonic microbiota. One could also suspect that a complex live microbiota to some extent could adapt to the nutrients given for example if carbohydrate-based formulations are investigated. One of the advantages of using a complex media is that different formulations, for example formulations based on different carbohydrates, can be investigated.

2. The GI Tract

2.1. The Upper GI-Tract

Drugs that are administrated orally are exposed to a changing environment, and if a drug is intended to target the colon, it will be exposed both to the upper part of the GI tract and colon. Figure 1 illustrates the changing conditions encountered during passage through the GI-tract. One of the key uses is the changing pH in the GI tract. In the stomach the pH normally varies between 1 and 3.5. Higher gastric pH up to 4.6 has been observed in healthy human subjects by Koziolek et al. [47] and higher gastric pH can be expected in patients receiving gastric acid blocker therapy and in the elderly it can be elevated up to pH > 5 [48]. Traditionally, oral formulations that are designed to avoid gastric release are coated with a polymer that is insoluble at low pH but soluble at higher pH, the so-called enteric coatings.

The content of the stomach is released into the small intestine. The surface area of the small intestinal mucosa is large due to the presence of villi and microvilli's that increase the contact area between the lumen and the epithelial cell wall which promotes drug absorption [49]. The pH of the small intestine ranges between 5.5 and 7.5 [50,51]. The lumen of the intestine also contains numerous enzymes as well as bile salts. The enzymes include hydrolases and proteases such as trypsin, chymotrypsin and carboxypeptidases as well as lipases and amylases. Bile salt are reabsorbed in ileum and about 95% of the bile salts are recirculated [52]. The concentration of bile and enzymes show considerable individual variation and vary between the fasted or fed state. Compared to the colon, the upper GI-tract contains only a minor amount of bacteria, of around 10^3–10^4 CFU/mL [53,54], and thus, enzyme from bacteria play a minor role compared to the endogenous enzymes in the small intestine.

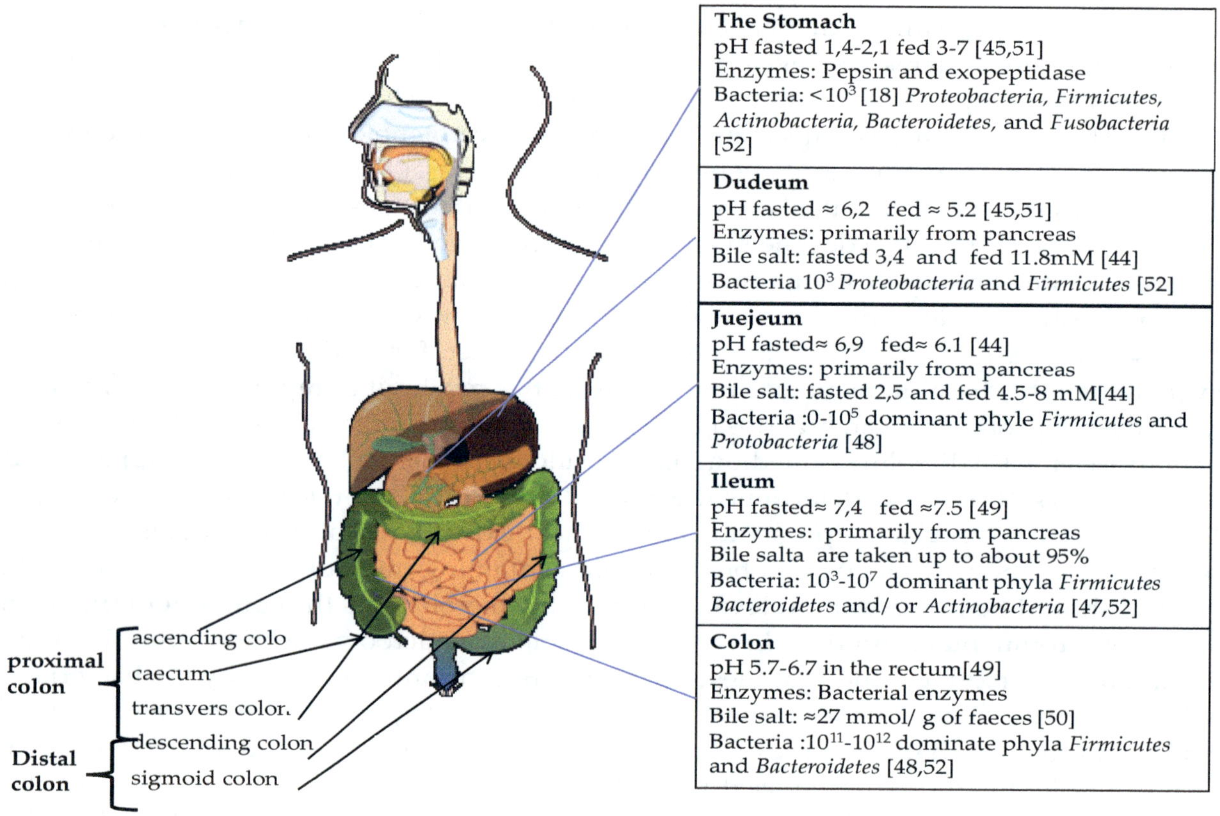

Figure 1. An overview of the conditions in the GI-tract with a focus on the composition of the liquid content. Data from References [18,50,51,53–58]. The picture of the GI-tract is by Mariana Ruiz, Jmarchn from Wikimedia commons. (https://commons.wikimedia.org/wiki/File:Digestive_system_without_labels.svg)

2.2. The Physiology of Colon

The main function of the colon is uptake of water and different ions from the colonic content, and it serves as a storage and compaction space for feces The microorganisms that reside in the colon have important consequences for human health, being active fermenters of undigested polysaccharides, and the community composition and activities are known to be strongly influenced by the dietary carbohydrate content [59–61]. The addition of probiotic bacteria has for example been seen to affect such diverse disorders as stress [62], colonic carcinogenesis and hepatic injuries [63] and obesity management [64,65]. Another emerging topic is fecal transplantation focusing on not one microorganism but the whole microbiota from healthy donors [66].

The colon makes up the final 1.5 m of the GI tract and can be further divided into smaller parts such as the caecum, ascending, transverse and descending colon, see Figure 1. The pH of colon varies between 5.7 and 6.7 along the large intestine. It is lowest in the ascending colon and then it increases. It should also be noted that for patients with diseases such as Crohn's disease and Ulcerative colitis, the pH can often be reduced compared to the pH in healthy subjects [2].

Colon is a strictly anaerobic environment and its microbiota is a dense and complex community comprised by mainly obligate anaerobe bacteria. Compared to the stomach and small intestine, the colon harbors a much larger population of bacteria with up to 10^{11} bacteria per gram of intestinal content. The microbiota of the colon is different in different regions. Close to the epithelial barrier, there is a nearly bacterial free zone of mucus and then the microorganisms are spatially organized with different compositions of bacteria closer to the mucin than those in contact with lumen. The microbiota of the mucosa also varies along the colon [67,68]. These microorganisms produce a large panel of enzymes that are active in the breakdown of dietary fibers that escape digestion in the small intestine. Tasse et al. [69] used coupled functional screens and sequence-based metagenomics to identify highly prevalent genes encoding enzymes that are involved in the catabolism of dietary fibers by the human gut microbiome and found that they produce a range of carbohydrate digestive enzymes such as beta-glucanase, hemicellulase, galactanase, amylase, or pectinase [69]. The bacteria of the colon also metabolize the bile salts that has not been taken up in ileum. Thus, the bile salt composition is different in the colon compared to the small intestine, see Table 1. The pancreatic enzymes are also digested in the colon and amylase was for example found to decrease by 50% while protease decreased by 70% [70].

Table 1. Bile salt composition in the small intestines and colon. Data are from Ridlon et al. [52].

Bile Salt	Small Intestines	Colon
Cholic acid CA	35%	2%
Chenodeoxycholic acid CDCA	35%	2%
Deoxycholic acid (DCA)	25%	34%
Lithocholic acid LCA	1%	29%
Ursodeoxycholic acid UDCA	2%	2%
12-oxy-LCA		3%
Others	2%	28%

Compared to the upper GI-tract, most of the nutrients in lumen have already been adsorbed when reaching the colon [71]. However, the amount of free fatty acids is increased from around 6–8 mM in ileum to 32–29 mM in cecum. In a fed state, the nutrient content of cecum was around 6 mg/mL of protein and 10 mg/mL of soluble carbohydrates [71]. This can be compared to the content in jejunum where the protein content of 1 mg/mL in the fasted state and 5 mg/mL in the fed state has been determined using the Loc-in-Gut technique [72].

3. In Vitro Release Methods

A dissolution test is a key tool for determining the release profile during the development of an oral drug product and it is especially important for controlled release formulations. Although research on dissolution processes goes back to the 1890s, when the topic was mainly studied by physical chemists, it took many years before its applicability and importance in pharmaceuticals was implemented. Until the 1950s, it was believed that the bioavailability of drugs was only dependent on disintegration of the tablet [73]. However, in 1957, Nelson related theophylline blood concentration to dissolution rate [74]. His work was followed by several other studies investigating the correlation between dissolution and bioavailability. During this time, it was discovered that the formulation of the drug could affect the pharmacological effect. In the 1970s, large differences were discovered between different formulations and brands of the drug digoxin [75],which further supported the theory that the release from formulation influences bioequivalence. Cases of drug toxicity and reduced drug effects as a result of alternation of an excipient were observed [76]. Incidents like these led to the realization of the importance of dissolution studies for the purpose of quality control and the introduction of dissolution requirements in pharmacopeias of dissolution data for tablets and capsules. Additionally, standard dissolution methods were introduced in the Unites States Pharmacopeia, National Formulary [73] and also in other Pharmacopeias such as those for Europe and Japan. The physical designs of the most frequently employed standard pharmaceutical apparatus are described in the Pharmacopoeias. These are the Basket (USP 1) and Paddle (USP 2) apparatus, the reciprocating cylinder apparatus (USP 3) and flow through apparatus (USP 4). The Pharmacopoeias also recommend the range of settings that determine the hydrodynamics during the dissolution test. More biorelevant apparatus have been suggested by several researchers and some of these were reviewed together with the standard dissolution equipment by Kostewicz et al. [77]. Another relevant apparatus is the Dynamic Colon Model that is designed to mimic the architecture, physical pressures and motility patterns in the proximal colon [78].

One key use of in vitro release testing is to try to use it for prediction of *in vivo* uptake, the so called in vitro–in vivo correlation (IVIVC). There are three different levels of IVIVC [79,80]. In Level A correlations, all data collected (both dissolution and blood plasma concentration) is used to create a point-to-point relationship. It is considered to be the highest level of correlation and is usually, but not always, a linear relationship. This direct relationship between in vivo and in vitro data can be used to predict in vivo performance. In Level B, all the obtained data is used just as in Level A correlations, however, a point-to-point relationship is not created, instead the mean in vitro dissolution time is related to the mean in vivo dissolution time or mean in vivo residence time. A Level C correlation is a single point correlation where only one point from the in vitro dissolution profile is related to an in vivo parameter such as maximum blood plasma concentration, Cmax. No prediction of the in vivo blood concentration profile can be made using this type of correlation. Developing a meaningful IVIVC is, however, always challenging since there are many factors to consider, such as transit time and composition of the gastric and intestinal content including pH, bile salts and enzymes that affects the release and uptake of a drug [81].

When conducting in vitro studies, the choice of dissolution media is important. There are several strategies on how to choose the media going from very simple solutions, in some cases even just water, to very complex ones that are more biologically relevant [80]. It is important to point out that the purpose of a dissolution method is not to simulate the exact conditions in vivo, which of course is impossible. It is, however, important that the dissolution method resembles the characteristics of the in vivo situation that determines the release profile. This does not mean that the method should not be as realistic as possible, but the goal is to be able to compare a system over time and between different laboratories. Without a reproducible way to do this, the test loses its meaning. Thus, there is often a tradeoff between highly realistic and complex media and the reproducibility. In designing a dissolution method, the purpose of the method often sets the degree of complexity. For dissolution methods that are going to be used in quality control, reproducibility and capability is in focus since it is more important to detect production variability than the biological relevance of the method. For research and development purpose as well as for establishing an IVIVC, the biorelevance of the dissolution media is of high importance.

In the case of oral formulations, it is the GI tract that has to be simulated during the dissolution studies. Due to the variation in pH along the GI tract, the pH may be adjusted during the in vitro experiment to simulate the transit through the GI tract. This is important for understanding the interaction of the formulation with pH, the dissolution of acids and bases and to understand the survival of probiotics [14]. In the case of probiotics, the aim is to modulate the microbiota to give health benefits to the consumer. In most cases, probiotics are given as a cost supplement but with growing evidence of the effects on several diseases, the interest to use live bacteria also as a pharmaceutical product is increasing. The demands on such a pharmaceutical product will be different from most current probiotics and for oral products survival through the stomach and upper GI tract will be crucial for the probiotics to work properly. As pointed out by Quigley, there is a need for both better formulations and quality controls when it comes to many of these products [82]. For further reading on probiotics, we recommend some of the following recent reviews on the topic [82–86].

Both the stomach and small intestine can be simulated using the pharmacopoeia dissolution media. These media range from simple solutions with low complexity to solutions containing surfactants or enzymes which complexity wise can be categorized as medium to high, respectively (see Table 2). For the sake of this review, the media in Table 2 have been categorized with regards to a representation of either the fasted or fed state. Furthermore, it is worth noting that the USP <1092> [79] is suggesting the option that dissolution media may simulate the gastric and intestinal fluids more closely with regards to both the ionic strength and molarity of the buffers employed.

For conducting dissolution tests of controlled release formulations, these are normally conducted in series. The European Pharmacopoeia recommends pH steps and timings for dissolution tests involving steps with increasing pH [87]. These steps start in acidic milieu (pH 1.0–1.5) representing the stomach and may end at the highest pH levels (pH 7.2–7.5) representing the lower parts of the small intestines. Typically, the formulation is left in gastric conditions for the approximated transit time through the stomach, usually 1 or 2 h [87,88]. This is followed by an adjustment of the solution to the conditions for simulated small intestinal juice. Normally, it is only the upper parts of the GI-tract that are studied during the release tests but for colon delivery also the release in simulated colon conditions has to be studied. These testing conditions do not include a step simulating the colonic fluid.

Table 2. Dissolution media in Pharmacopoeias and Guidelines resembling the upper GI tract.

GI Site Represented	Suggested Prandial State	Media	Complexity	References
Stomach	Fasted	pH 1.0–1.5	Low	[87,89–91]
		pH < 4.0 + Surfactant(s)	Medium	[79,87]
		pH < 4.0 + Enzymes (pepsin)	High	[87,89]
	Fed	Stomach pH + Physiological Surfactant(s)	Medium	[79]
No specific site	Fasted	pH 4.5	Low	[79,87,90,92]
	Fed	pH > 4.0 and < 6.8 + Enzymes (Papain)	High	[89]
Small intestines	Fasted	pH 5.5, 5.8, 6.5, 6.8 *, 7.2, 7.5	Low	[87,89,90]
		Intestinal pH + Physiological Surfactant(s)	Medium	[79]
	Fed	Intestinal pH + Physiological Surfactant(s)	Medium	[79]
		pH ≥ 6.8 + Enzymes (Pancreatic powder)	High	[87,89]

* pH 6.8 is the most frequently employed pH resembling the small intestines.

Important changes induced by food ingestion include an increase in pH, and stimulation of secretion of bile salts and pancreatic enzymes. For this reason, simulations of fasted and fed conditions have been developed by several pharmaceutical researcher and in-depth reviews covering both simulated gastric and intestinal dissolution media have been made by Reppas et al. [93] and Bergström et al. [50]. For example, Vertzoni et al. suggested a fasted state simulated gastric fluid (FaSSGF) which besides hydrochloric acid contains pepsin as well as low amounts of bile salt and lecithin [94]. Simulation of the fed state in the stomach has been achieved by using milk for example. In a study from 2013, Christophersen and colleagues used milk together with bile salt and lipase to simulate a fed condition in the stomach and duodenum [95]. Worth noting is that the fed state is more complicated to simulate since the environment in the stomach changes over time as the food is digested and emptied into the small intestine [96]. For the simulation of the small intestinal fluids, the pioneering work by Prof. Dressman has led to standardized dissolution medias for fasted and fed state in the small intestines. These fasted states simulated intestinal fluids (FaSSIF) and fed state simulated intestinal fluids (FeSSIF) are extensively discussed in the review by Markopoulos et al. [97]. Biorelevant dissolution media are categorized by Markopoulos et al. in four levels. At level 0 media, only the difference in physiological pH along the GI tract is taken in to consideration while for level

I, the distinction between fasted and fed is done based on both pH and buffer capacity of the media. At level II, the difference in bile components, lipids and their digestion products, and the osmolality are also considered, and in the most complex versions of level III, considerations such as changes in viscosity and digestive enzymes are included [97]. Another important aspect to consider when constructing biorelevant dissolution tests is that gastric emptying occurs less frequently when food is ingested which is why the gastric simulation step should be longer when simulating a fed state compared to a fasted state [50].

Interestingly, there are actually two different traditions in developing complex release media for simulating the GI tract, one based on pharmaceutical research and one based on food research. The perspective of these two traditions varies of course as the food research primarily focuses on the digestion of food components while pharmaceutical research focuses on the release of the active compound. For example, food research might include the chewing of the food, a part that is seldom relevant for pharmaceuticals. This means that also the enzymes from the mouth are included in such studies [98]. The in vitro models used in food research can be static [99] or dynamic [100,101] and batch or continuous [102]; however, regardless of the nature of the methods, all of them consist of simulated oral (mouth), gastric, and intestinal compartments and may or may not include the colon. Due to the complexity of these models, they are often adopted to the specific conditions of each system. In order to do so, the system is categorized to either protein-based, lipid-based or carbohydrate-based systems and the digestive conditions are chosen for the system being analyzed. In this way, if a protein-based delivery system is being evaluated, the main focus would be the gastric and intestinal steps where the corresponding proteases exist (i.e. pepsin in the stomach, trypsin and chymotrypsin in the small intestine). In a similar way, when lipid-based delivery systems are being evaluated, gastric and intestinal lipases are included; however, the focus is more on the intestinal lipolysis. Finally, if a carbohydrate-based delivery system is being analyzed, the oral and intestinal amylases are to be included. In some cases for simplification of the in vitro evaluation, whatever passes the oral, gastric and intestinal steps is considered to be delivered to the colon [103,104].

Many of the in vitro methods that are used for food research are more complex than the traditional pharmaceutical models. In the early 1990s, Molly et al. [105] developed a comprehensive dynamic model called "the simulator of the human intestinal microbial ecosystem" (SHIME). Through a multi-chamber system controlled by a computer, simulation of the conditions in the stomach, duodenum, jejunum, ileum, caecum, proximal, transverse, and distal colon, this model enabled scientist to control the concentrations of enzymes, bile, pH, temperature, feed composition, transit time, and anaerobic environment in each reactor.

Another model developed by Minekus, Marteau and Havenaar [101] was comprised of two separate models. TIM-1 simulates the conditions of the stomach, duodenum, jejunum, and ileum while TIM-2 simulates the large intestine controlled by a computer. An advantage of this model to SHIME was the possibility of controlled peristaltic movements and water absorption. It was later in that decade when Macfarlane, Macfarlane and Gibson [102] developed the three-stage continuous system which simulates the proximal, transverse and distal colon (differing slightly in pH and volume) containing fecal microbiota of healthy individuals and the system was then, in the late 1990s, validated against sudden death victims. The results of these types of evaluations have shown that the majority of carbohydrate breakdown and short-chain fatty acid production occurred in the proximal part of the colon while amino acid metabolism occurred in the transverse and distal colon [102]. Although these methods were developed for food and probiotic applications, they have since also been used in pharmaceutical research [106,107].

In addition to those models, the Dynamic Gastric Model (DGM) developed in the former Institute of Food Research in Norwich, UK as well as the Human Gastric Simulator (HGS) developed at UC-Davis, can be mentioned [108]. Similarly, simulated intestinal models were developed to investigate mass transfer from the luminal side [109]. Despite their potentials, these models have limitations due to limited accessibility worldwide and therefore, a consensus static digestion method was developed within the COST (European Cooperation in Science and Technology) Action, the so called InfoGest method [99,110]. The InfoGest method consists of a simulated upper GI (mouth to small intestines) method. Although this method is very good in providing details on the type and activity of the enzymes, ratios of digestive fluids, pH, ionic strength, and time, it is still very complicated, laborious and time-consuming.

Finally, one of the more advanced in vitro systems developed has been in the area of understanding how different components can affect the human gut microbiome. This in vitro microbiome modulation is performed in a three-stage culture system GIS2 simulator and the effect of the components on the microbiota is analyzed by determining the microbiological fingerprint using qPCR analysis [111].

Colon Release

Most oral pharmaceutical formulation dissolution tests covering the stomach and small intestine are sufficient. However, for drugs that are intended to target the colon, an additional step simulating the large intestine needs to be added. This has proven to be challenging as the colon is a very complex environment and is therefore difficult to mimic. There is a severe lack of simple and relevant ways to perform dissolution tests for formulations that target the colon, and the methods available today have significant drawbacks.

Current methods available for simulating the large intestine include dissolution in buffers of relevant pH, the use of mixtures of enzymes that are known to be produced by bacteria in the colon, caecum content from animals (primarily rats), human fecal slurries, and fermentation of selected bacteria. Below, we give a short description of these methods, for a more thorough review on the first four methods, we recommend the review by Yang [112].

Release in buffers: This is the simplest and most reproducible system to use but its biological relevance is low. The system can be used for formulations based on pH triggered and time-dependent release. These buffers might be able to represent the key mechanism of release in vivo but the pH levels chosen are typically representing a mean in vivo pH and not the range of pH actually found in vivo. With regards to some formulations, the viscosity of the release media could also be of importance and as discussed in the introduction, the viscosity changes in the colonic lumen and could affect the transport of molecules and release from formulations. However, one has to be aware that many excipients are also degraded by the enzymes of the microbiota and to obtain relevant results, buffers can only be used when one is sure that no such degradation occurs. This being said, there are still several cases when pH control is the only method used [32–34]. Usually this is done in systems where no enzymatic break down would be expected but unfortunately also in cases where such break downs are an obvious risk.

Use of enzymes present in the colon: The use of an enzyme or mixtures of enzymes that are known to be produced by bacteria in the colon has the clear benefit of being considerably easy to handle, comparably inexpensive and has high reproducibility. The drawback is of course that even a mixture of enzymes is a very large simplification compared to the large range of bacterial enzymes in the colon. However, by choosing a high concentration of one enzyme, good correlation with fecal dissolution systems can sometimes be achieved as shown by Siew et al. [113]. In Table 3, we list some example of the enzymes that have been used in colon-simulating release media. The problem is still that different methods for colon delivery will be susceptible to different enzymes, and thus, the possibility to compare for example different carbohydrates for colon delivery is not straight forward using enzymatic release media. Instead, media such as feces and rat caecum, have been used.

Table 3. Examples of colon bacterial enzymes used in simulated colon media for dissolution.

Type of Formulation Components	Enzyme	Refences
Azo-structures, polymers and conjugates	Azoreductase	[114,115]
Guar gum	Galactomannanase, α-galactosidase	[116,117]
Chitosane	β-glucosidase	[118,119]
Pectin	Pectinase	[120,121]
Starch	Amylase	[113]
Dextrane	Dextranase	[122]
Inuline	Inulase	[122]

Use of rat caecum content: To incubate the drug in a slurry of rat caecum content is one of the more common methods employed when the investigator prefer a more biologically relevant media. The benefits are that caecum can be treated in such a way that the anaerobic condition is maintained, and by adhering to a strict protocol of animal feeding, a rather high degree of reproducibility should be able to be obtained. Furthermore, the rats can be given a special diet to increase the bacterial species that are sensitive to the system investigated [123]. The drawback is primarily that the method involves the sacrifice of animals and results obtained from experiments on animals may not be directly applicable to humans due to microbiota compositional differences [124]. The microbiota in rodents might differ from humans, for example, lactobacilli is a major group in mice [125] but in humans lactobacilli are regularly present but in a smaller proportion [126].

Another interesting thing to note is that different research teams have been using quite different protocols for these experiments which means that it can be difficult to compare the results. Several groups have based their method on the work done by Prasad et al. [127], who used a USP bath with 4% of rat caecum in phosphate buffer pH 6.8, and to keep the system semi-anaerobic, the solution was bubbled through with CO_2. There are slight variations to this method, for example, by using different pHs, 6.5 [128]–7.5 [129], using nitrogen in some steps of the method instead of CO_2 [128], using variations in caecum content, 2%–10% [129,130], and varying the type of USP setup [128] or using sealed bottles [131]. In systems based on azo-structures, the intact or sonicated caecum (to release intracellular enzymes) have been mixed with co-factors such as benzyl viologen, NADP, glucose-6-phosphate dehydrogenase, and glucose-6-phosphate [122,132,133]. Caecum content from other animal species has also been used and for example guinea pig caecum was more similar to human fecal slurry in its breakage of azo-bonds than rat caecum [134].

Using fecal slurries from animals or humans: This has either been done using the same principle as for rat caecum, dispersing the sample in buffer and following the release in this solution during anaerobic conditions [135,136], or by using the fecal slurry to include a more complex fermentation step [4,100,137]. The main advantage of using fecal samples is that animals do not have to be sacrificed and it is possible to use human samples. One additional benefit is that it is possible to use fecal samples also from patients [138]. Using human feces makes it more relevant but the fact that it is fecal samples and not samples from the earlier parts of the colon is a problem. Primarily, these samples will not be harvested in anaerobic conditions, and thus, especially in the case of fermentation, there is a high risk that the anaerobic bacteria dominating in the colon are not viable in feces. The other problems are that the microbiota in the lower part of the colon is not the same as in the earlier parts of the colon and by using human samples there will be a large variation between samples from different individuals. Culturing the samples of feces or caecum for that matter before the addition of the formulation increases the activity of the system and can increase the rate of degradation as seen for example in the breakage of azo-bonds [134]. However, many of the studies are based on simply dispersing the feces (around 10%) in buffers with varying pH and incubating with the formulation as the only additional source of nutrient under anaerobic conditions [135,136,139,140]. Interesting to note, is that in most cases the pH employed is around 7.5. That is a pH closer to that of feces and not to the lower pH of the upper colon where most of the fermentation will take place in vivo. There are also, as discussed previously, several complex systems using coupled fermentation reactors to simulate the changing properties of the whole GI-tract or colon. This includes systems such as SHIME®, EnteroMix, Lacroix model and TIM-2, for a thorough review of these systems, please see Venema et al. [141]. When using a fermentation medium, the composition of the fermentation medium used for this purpose may be a simple but optimized and still complete medium, containing all principal components of a full-fermentation medium. However, it could also be of a more complex nature, mimicking a certain dietary habit, for example the prevailing Western-style diet [142,143].

Using selected bacteria: One of the earliest examples of using selected bacteria was the work by Karroute et al. [138], who used bifidobacteria, *Bacteroides* and *E. coli* to study release from pellets coated with Nutriose. In a study from 2015, Singh and colleagues used a probiotic mixture to simulate the large intestine when testing drug release from Sulfasalazine spheroids coated with different polysaccharides [144]. This system was compared to fecal slurries of humans, rats and goats, and the release profiles of carbohydrate-based formulations were rather similar, especially to the rat caecum content medium, even though the release in the probiotic release media was slightly slower [145]. The composition of the probiotic release media is presented in Table 4. In a similar study by Kotla et al. [146], a probiotic culture was once again used to mimic the colonic environment to examine drug release from 5-fluorouracil granules coated with polysaccharides. The species used are listed in Table 4. While no specific concentrations for each species were given by Kotal et al, the cultured media contained a total amount of 9.8×10^{10} CFU (colony forming units). In this study, the drug release profiles obtained from the tests with probiotic mixture, rat caecum content and human fecal slurries were to some extent comparable. In general, the probiotic mixture resulted in a slightly faster release than the other two media [146]. Unfortunately, the choice of bacteria was not thoroughly discussed in these articles although the authors suggested that these bacteria can simulate the conditions in the colon. The problem is, however, that although the colon contains some probiotic bacterial species as part of the microbiota composition, these are not the dominating species. In order to give suggestions for a more relevant media to simulate the colon, we present an overview of the literature that has investigated the microbiota of human colon. This has been done, especially with focus on carbohydrate degradation in the human large intestine. Based on this we suggest some key species that could be used for such systems.

Table 4. Species selected for the bacterial mixture, as well as the amounts of different bacteria used to create a dissolution media simulating the colon by Singh et al. [144] and Kotla et al. [146].

Singh, et.al., 2015 [140]		Kotla et al., 2016 [142]
Composition	**Bacterial Count/Amount (CFU)**	**Composition**
Lactobacillus acidophilus	0.75×10^{12}	Lactobacillus acidophilus
Lactobacillus rhamnosus	0.75×10^{12}	Lactobacillus rhamnosus
Bifidobacterium longum	0.75×10^{12}	Bifidobacterium longum
Bifidobacterium bifidum	0.50×10^{12}	Bifidobacterium infantis
Saccharomyces boulardii	0.10×10^{12}	Lactobacillus plantarum
		Lactobacillus casei
		Bifidobacterium breve
		Streptococcus thermophilus
		Saccharomyces boulardii

4. The Gut Microbiota

There are not many relevant studies on the human microbiota, i.e. human studies including identification and quantification of colonic bacteria on a species-specific level and based on a significant number of individuals. This suggests that although this particular microbial community has been studied extensively, it is still not very well understood. It appears that the general consensus is that the bacteria of the large intestine belong mainly to the phyla *Firmicutes* and *Bacteroidetes*. While several studies have indicated that species belonging to the *Clostridium* clusters IV and XIVa as well as to the *Bacteroidetes* phylum dominate the colonic flora, there is often a lack of examples of which bacteria dominate in the colon on a species-specific level. According to a study performed by Tap and colleagues where 16s rRNA sequencing was used to characterize the microbiota of colon, 79.4% and 16.9% of the sequences belonged to *Firmicutes* and *Bacteroidetes*, respectively [147]. This is further supported by the work of Yang et al., who by searching the Ribosomal Database Project identified bacteria that belonged to 13 phyla [148]; see Figure 2 for the most frequent phyla. However, it is not completely evident which species are dominant or most commonly occurring in humans. A reason for this is that there is a clear inter-individual diversity of the colonic microbiota among humans as a result of, for example, differences in dietary intake, age and presence of diseases, and the studies usually include only a few subjects [61]. It is therefore difficult to tell how representative the results are. As for differences in dietary intake, it has, for example, been observed that *Prevotella* spp. and other *Bacteroidetes* are more common in a group of rural African children while *Firmicutes* are more prevalent in Italian children. These variations were ascribed to differences in starch and fiber intake [60].

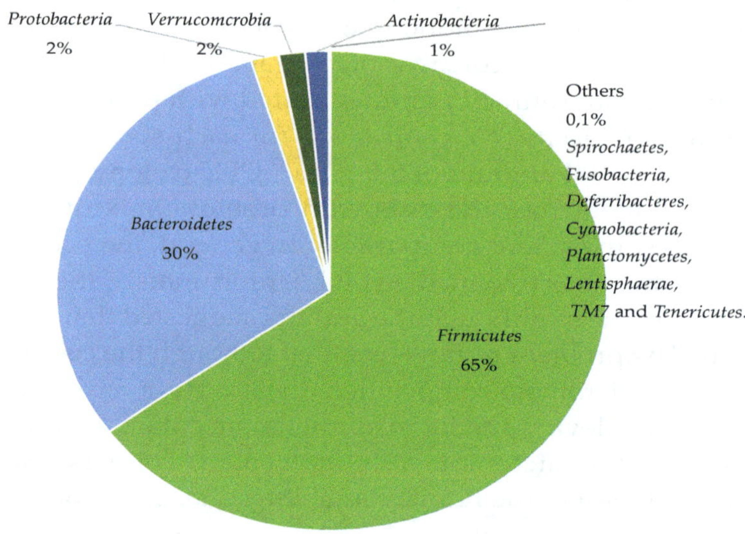

Figure 2. The phyla composition of the human gut from Yang et al. [148].

The above-mentioned study performed by Tap et al. [147], aimed at finding an intestinal microbiota phylogenetic core (a part of the microbiota that was common for more than 50% of the patients) among 17 healthy, both male and female, individuals. It was found that 2.1% of the detected operational taxonomic units (OTUs) were present in more than 50% of the individuals. Using quantitative PCR, they found that *Clostridium leptum* cluster IV, *Clostridium coccoides* cluster XIV and *Bacteroides/Prevotella* were the most dominating groups. The OTUs could be connected to species such as *Faecalibacterium prausnitzii* (present in 16 of 17 individuals), *Bacteroides vulgatus*, *Roseburia intestinalis*, *Ruminococcus bromii*, *Eubacterium rectale*, *Coprobacillus* sp. and *Bifidobacterium lognum*. It was found that the abundance of a certain OTU did not necessarily always relate to the frequency of observation. After applying a statistical model, it could be concluded that the 10 most frequent OTUs were related to *F. prausnitzii*, *Anaerostipes caccae*, *Clostridium spiroforme*, and *Bacteroides uniformis* among others [147]. Another study based on 16s rRNA stable isotope probing displayed a strong prevalence of sequences related to *Prevotella* spp. (*Bacteroidetes*), *Ruminococcus obeum* (*Clostridium* cluster XIVa), *R. bromii* (*Clostridium* cluster IV), *E. rectale* (*Clostridium* cluster XIVa), and *Bifidobacterium adolescentis* (*Actinobacteria*) [149]. Results also suggested that *R. bromii* might act as a primary starch degrader while the remaining species further degrade metabolites generated by *R. bromii*. This type of cross-feeding is not uncommon; on the contrary, it appears to be a central property of some anaerobic microbial communities [61].

In 1999, Suau and colleagues investigated the human bacterial colonic community by analyzing feces for adult males using cloned 16s rRNA sequences [126]. They found that 95% of the clones belonged to the *Bacteroides* group and to the species *Clostridium coccoides* and *Clostridium leptum*.

The majority of recovered sequences did not belong to known cultivated microorganisms; however, sequences were found that correspond to bacteria such as *B. thetaiotaomicron*, *F. prausnitzii*, *B. uniformis*, *B. vulgatus*, *Eubacterium eligens*, *E. rectale*, and *R. bromii*. [126]. In yet another study, using 16S rRNA gene sequencing, Wang and colleagues detected and quantitated 12 bacterial species in human and animal fecal samples [150]. They found that *F. prausnitzii*, *Peptostreptococcus productus*, and *Clostridium clostridiiforme* had high PCR titers in all fecal samples. Additionally, high PCR titers were detected for *B. thetaiotaomicron*, *B. vulgatus*, and *Eubacterium limosum* in human adult fecal samples. The authors stated that their results are consistent with previous studies, however, some differences were detected when compared to cultured-based methods, and the findings were explained by some species being non-culturable, making enumeration using such methods dependent on how easily bacteria can be cultivated. In contrast, PCR can detect both unculturable and dead bacteria. Additionally, their PCR method detected the bacteria in situ while detection occurs after enrichment when using culture-based methods. Moore and Holdeman [151] used anaerobic tube culture techniques to evaluate the microbial composition in human feces from 20 healthy Japanese–Hawaiian males. They observed 113 different microorganisms using this method which accounted for 94% of all viable cells, and the microorganisms included *B. fragilis ss. vulgatus*, *F. prausnitzii*, *B. adolescentis*, *Eubacterium aerofaciens*, *P. productus*, *rectale*, and *R. bromii* among others. In another clinical trial, Wang et al. [152] found that sequences related to *Bacteroidetes* and *Clostridium* cluster XIV and IV dominated the clone libraries created from mucosal biopsies from the distal ileum, ascending colon and rectum. However, no examples of predominant species of the ascending colon were mentioned.

In the studies mentioned above, fecal samples were used for the characterization attempts. This is due to the fact that such samples are easy to collect, and it is believed that they represent the colonic microbiota well. However, it should be kept in mind that certain microorganisms may not be well-represented by fecal samples since they might be part of the colonic mucosal microflora. In a study by Hold and colleagues [153], 16s rRNA gene sequencing was performed on colonic tissue samples instead of fecal samples. The colonic tissue was taken from elderly people, DNA was extracted, and 16s rDNA was used for PCR amplification before it was cloned into vector plasmids. In this study, 46% of the clones that were analyzed belonged to the *Clostridium* cluster XIVa. Most sequences did not show the closest resemblance to current species-type strains, however, 16 of 51 sequences were loosely related to *Eubacterium ramulus*, *E. rectale*, *Roseburia cecicola* and *Eubacterium halii*; 14.5% of the sequences belonged to the *Clostridium* cluster IV where 6 out of 16 sequences belonged to *Ruminococcus* spp and 4 out of 16 showed the closest resemblance to *F. prausnitzii*. Sequences belonging to the genus *Bacteroides* constituted 26% of the analyzed clones with most of the sequences being closely related to *B. vulgatus* and *B. uniformis*. Additionally, sequence similarity to *Prevotella enoeca* was found in one of the three samples [153].

5. Can a Novel Media Based on the Microbiota be Developed?

A media based on chosen microorganisms instead of fecal samples would have several benefits. Primarily, the reproducibility of such a media would be considerably higher and if the bacteria are grown anaerobically the media would also to some extent be more relevant for the colon. However, the choice of bacteria, in regard to the variability of the microbiota, is not straight forward. The media should also have a relevant pH and the addition of other components such as human enzymes and bile salts could be considered. However, as the bile salts to a large extent are reabsorbed before the colon and the fact that the dominating enzymes are those produced by the bacteria, it could be possible to simplify the system by excluding these endogenous components. If a simulated colon dissolution media should be developed, there are several standards that should be fulfilled. Primarily, the bacteria chosen should be relevant for the colon but also relevant for the components in the formulation. Thus, bacteria that are known to produce extracellular enzymes that break down carbohydrates should be considered. There are also practical concerns such as the number of bacterial species used should not make the system too complex and the bacteria chosen should be compatible with each other.

Furthermore, the media chosen for growth of the bacteria should be as simple as possible and relevant for the colon but at the same time assure good growth of all bacteria chosen. Below we describe five possible bacterial candidates and the rationale for choosing these candidates for a novel colon dissolution media, primarily for evaluating carbohydrate-based formulations.

Faecalibacterium prausnitzii ATCC 27768. The species *F. prausnitzii* belongs to the phylum *Firmicutes*, which, as mentioned before, is one of the phyla dominating the colonic microbiota. In a study performed by Hold et al. where fecal samples from 10 healthy individuals consuming a Western diet were collected, it was shown that *prausnitzii* made up between 1.4 and 5.9% of the total microbiota [154]. *F. prausnitzii* is one of the most important producers of the short chain fatty acid butyrate and therefore the species has an influence on human health [155]. In a study comparing fecal samples from 20 patients diagnosed with colorectal cancer, with 17 healthy individuals it was shown that the amounts of *F. prausnitzii* and *E. rectale* in patients with colorectal cancer were almost four times lower. According to a study performed by Lopez–Siles and colleagues, in an attempt to determine what substrate promotes the growth of *F. prausnitzii*, no growth was observed when using arabinogalactan and little or no growth on soluble starch. No fermentation was observed on Xylan, only a few of the used strains were able to grow well on inulin, and while most strains grew well on apple pectin, the same was not observed with citrus pectin. Additionally, most strains were able to grow on the host-derived substrate *N*-acetylglucosamine and D-glucosamine and D-glucuronic acid could be used by some strains [156]. This indicates that *F. prausnitzii* can switch between non-host substrates and host substrates which gives it a competitive advantage when dietary intake is reduced [61]. The fact that *F. prausnitzii* was able to compete for apple pectin as a substrate with two species found in human feces that have been reported to utilize pectin, namely *Bacteroides thetaiotaomicron* and *E. eligens* [157], suggests that *F. prausnitzii* might play a significant role in pectin fermentation in the colon of humans [156]. There are also studies available that indicate that *F. prausnitzii* can utilize prebiotics such as galactooligosaccharides for growth [158]. Additionally, in a study performed by Ramirez-Farias and colleagues, consumption of inulin-oligofructose increased the levels of *F. prausnitzii*. However, more research on the effect of inulin on growth of this species is necessary since no effect on counts of *F. prausnitzii* was observed as a result of higher inulin intake in yet another study [159].

Ruminococcus bromii ATCC 27255 *R. bromii* is an anaerobic, Gram-positive bacterial species that belongs to the *Firmicutes*. It has been reported to be a starch-degrading species. In a study performed by Ze et al. [160]. the ability of *R. bromii* to use different starches was compared to that of three other amylolytic species present in the human large intestine, namely *E. rectale*, *B. thetaiotaomicron* and *B. adolescentis*. It was noted that the starch utilization varied between the species depending on the type of starch and its pretreatment. Overall, *R. bromii* and *B. adolescentis* appeared to be more active than the other two species and they were notably more active in degrading raw or boiled resistant starches. Additionally, when all four species were grown together, it was observed that the starch utilization was higher compared to when the combinations with the other three species without *R. bromii* were co-cultivated. From the results, it was concluded that *R. bromii* was the most potent resistant starch degrader in the experiment. In the same study, the ability of the species to utilize starch metabolites was investigated. While not being able to utilize glucose, *R. bromii* could make use of breakdown products such as fructose and pullulan. It was also observed that some breakdown products created by *R. bromii* could be used by the three remaining species, indicating that there is a possibility of cross-feeding between the species used in this study [160]. There are also articles available that report an increase in *R. bromii* in individuals on diets with a higher amount of resistant starch. In a study from 2011, where fecal samples from obese men on different diets were compared, an increase in the number of *R. bromii* and *E. rectale* was observed when subjects were given a diet rich in resistant starch. It also appeared that a resistant starch-enriched diet stimulated an increase in species related to *R. bromii* and *E. rectale* [59]. A similar increase in *R. bromii*-related species was observed in a study using healthy individuals on diets supplemented with resistant starch. Additionally, despite the fact that an increase in SCFAs was noted in fecal samples when the subjects were on the resistant starch diet, this observation could not be connected to the abundance of *R. bromii* [161].

Eubacterium rectale ATCC 33656. As previously mentioned, *E. rectale* is a *Firmicutes* species belonging to the *Clostridia* cluster XIVa, that has been reported to be abundant in the human colon. Studies have shown that the species has an ability to degrade resistant starch and that its abundance in feces increases on a resistant starch-enriched diet [59]. Additionally, in a study from 2007, it was observed that the number of bacterial groups consisting of relatives of *E. rectale* and *Roseburia* spp. decreased significantly when subjects were on a diet low in carbohydrates. It was also noted that the concentration of SCFAs, and specifically butyrate, decreased in the feces in the same manner leading to the theory that these play an important role in butyrate production in the colon [162]. An *E. rectale* strain used in a study by Scott and colleagues, also proved to be able to grow on short chain fructooligosaccharides, xylooligosaccharides and amylopectin potato starch but failed to grow well on long chain inulin. The production of SCFA was also assessed in culture supernatants after 24 h of growth and showed butyrate, formate and lactate as the main fermentation products of *E. rectale* [163].

Bacteroides uniformis belongs to the *Bacteroidetes* phylum and allegedly has the ability to ferment a variety of polysaccharides. In a recent study from 2017, a strain of *B. uniformis* was isolated from infant stools, sequenced and grown on different carbon sources. Additionally, the genome expression patterns resulting from growth on these substrates were examined. The carbon sources used in the experiment were glucose, inulin, gum arabic (consisting of a complex mixture of branched polymers of galactose, rhamnose, arabinose, and glucuronic acid), pectin, wheat bran extract (mostly composed of a mixture of low weight xylo- and arabinoxylo-oligosaccharides) and mucin. It was observed that *B. uniformis* was able to grow on all these substrates. However, it was noted that the more complex polysaccharides such as those present in gum arabic, inulin and pectin were fermented less efficiently than the simpler oligosaccharides. It was concluded that this observation could be related to the origin of the bacterial strain, which in this case, came from infant stool. The analysis of the genome of *B. uniformis* showed that the species possesses a large panel of genes coding for so-called CAZymes (carbohydrate-active enzymes) compared to other *Bacteroides* species such as *B. thetaiotaomicron* and *Bacteroides cellulosyliticus*. Its ability to degrade mucin suggests that it might be able to grow on host-derived substrates and colonize the mucosa of the colon. Additionally, it was observed that production of the neurotransmitter GABA (gamma-amino butyric acid) increased significantly when *B. uniformis* was grown on mucin and pectin compared to growth on glucose. Lastly, pectin, gum arabic, and especially mucin, upregulated the expression of genes involved in butyrate production [164].

Prevotella copri CCUG 58058T. Even though *Prevotella* is mentioned as a family of bacteria that is common in the large intestine, it was difficult to find an example of a specific dominating species. Therefore, a random species known to exist in the large intestine was chosen, namely *Prevotella copri*. The species is a Gram-negative bacterium that belongs to the phylum *Bacteroidetes*. Scher and colleagues found that it is present in the stool of both healthy individuals and patients with rheumatoid arthritis, however, the species appeared to be overexpressed in the latter case. Since the prevalence of *P. copri* was similar in healthy individuals and in treated patients with reduced disease activity, they speculated that *P. copri* benefits from inflammatory conditions [165]. The fermentation of carbohydrates by *P. copri* in the large intestine does not seem to have been thoroughly explored. However, in a study from 2015, the gut microbiota was compared between healthy individuals who responded to the consumption of barley kernel-based bread, to those healthy individuals who did not respond or responded the least. Kovatcheva–Datchary and colleagues discovered an increased *Prevotella/Bacteroides* ratio in the responders compared to the non-responder. It was found that *P. copri* was the most abundant out of the *Prevotellaceae* species in the responders and this was also associated with an increased potential in fermentation of complex polysaccharides [166].

6. Conclusions

In this review, we have presented the most commonly used methods to study colon release. Although colon delivery has been studied extensively and there exists several different methods for in vitro studies of colon release and digestion of food, we think there is still a need for new in vitro methods. Primarily, there is a need for methods that include microorganisms but that are more reproducible and to some extent experimentally simpler than the current praxis of using fecal samples or caecum content.

Acknowledgments: This article was done with financial support from Vinnova-Swedish Governmental Agency for Innovation Systems within the NextBioForm Competence Centre.

References

1. Kotla, N.G.; Rana, S.; Sivaraman, G.; Sunnapu, O.; Vemula, P.K.; Pandit, A.; Rochev, Y. Bioresponsive drug delivery systems in intestinal inflammation: State-of-the-art and future perspectives. *Adv. Drug Deliv. Rev.* **2018**. [CrossRef] [PubMed]
2. Sharma, S.; Sinha, V.R. Current pharmaceutical strategies for efficient site specific delivery in inflamed distal intestinal mucosa. *J. Control. Release* **2018**, *272*, 97–106. [CrossRef] [PubMed]
3. Tuleu, C.; Basit, A.; Waddington, W.; Ell, P.; Newton, J. Colonic delivery of 4-aminosalicylic acid using amylose-ethylcellulose-coated hydroxypropylmethylcellulose capsules. *Aliment. Pharmacol. Ther.* **2002**, *16*, 1771–1779. [CrossRef] [PubMed]
4. Milojevic, S.; Newton, J.M.; Cummings, J.H.; Gibson, G.R.; Botham, R.L.; Ring, S.G.; Stockham, M.; Allwood, M.C. Amylose as a coating for drug delivery to the colon: Preparation and in vitro evaluation using 5-aminosalicylic acid pellets. *J. Control. Release* **1996**, *38*, 75–84. [CrossRef]
5. Leopold, C.S.; Eikeler, D. Eudragit E as coating material for the pH-controlled drug release in the topical treatment of inflammatory bowel disease (IBD). *J. Drug Target.* **1998**, *6*, 85–94. [CrossRef]
6. Wang, Q.S.; Wang, G.F.; Zhou, J.; Gao, L.N.; Cui, Y.L. Colon targeted oral drug delivery system based on alginate-chitosan microspheres loaded with icariin in the treatment of ulcerative colitis. *Int. J. Pharm.* **2016**, *515*, 176–185. [CrossRef]
7. Andishmand, H.; Hamishehkar, H.; Babazadeh, A.; Taghvimi, A.; Mohammadifar, M.A.; Tabibiazar, M. A Colon Targeted Delivery System for Resveratrol Enriching in pH Responsive-Model. *Pharm. Sci.* **2017**, *23*, 42–49. [CrossRef]
8. Gulbake, A.; Jain, A.; Jain, A.; Jain, A.; Jain, S.K. Insight to drug delivery aspects for colorectal cancer. *World J. Gastroenterol.* **2016**, *22*, 582–599. [CrossRef]
9. Krishnaiah, Y.S.R.; Veer Raju, P.; Dinesh Kumar, B.; Bhaskar, P.; Satyanarayana, V. Development of colon targeted drug delivery systems for mebendazole. *J. Control. Release* **2001**, *77*, 87–95. [CrossRef]
10. Blemur, L.; Le, T.C.; Marcocci, L.; Pietrangeli, P.; Mateescu, M.A. Carboxymethyl starch/alginate microspheres containing diamine oxidase for intestinal targeting. *Biotechnol. Appl. Biochem.* **2016**, *63*, 344–353. [CrossRef]
11. Del Curto, M.; Maroni, A.; Foppoli, A.; Zema, L.; Gazzaniga, A.; Sangalli, M. Preparation and evaluation of an oral delivery system for time-dependent colon release of insulin and selected protease inhibitor and absorption enhancer compounds. *J. Pharm. Sci.* **2009**, *98*, 4661–4669. [CrossRef] [PubMed]
12. Jiang, B.; Yu, H.; Zhang, Y.; Feng, H.; Hoag, S.W. A Multiparticulate Delivery System for Potential Colonic Targeting Using Bovine Serum Albumin as a Model Protein: Theme: Formulation and Manufacturing of Solid Dosage Forms Guest Editors: Tony Zhou and Tonglei Li. *Pharm. Res.* **2017**, *34*, 2663–2674. [CrossRef] [PubMed]
13. Calinescu, C.; Mateescu, M. Carboxymethyl high amylose starch: Chitosan self-stabilized matrix for probiotic colon delivery. *Eur. J. Pharm. Biopharm.* **2008**, *70*, 582–589. [CrossRef] [PubMed]
14. Dodoo, C.C.; Wang, J.; Basit, A.W.; Stapleton, P.; Gaisford, S. Targeted delivery of probiotics to enhance gastrointestinal stability and intestinal colonisation. *Int. J. Pharm.* **2017**, *530*, 224–229. [CrossRef] [PubMed]
15. Khanna, S. Microbiota Replacement Therapies: Innovation in Gastrointestinal Care. *Clin. Pharmacol. Ther.* **2018**, *103*, 102–111. [CrossRef] [PubMed]

16. Philip, A.K.; Philip, B. Colon targeted drug delivery systems: A review on primary and novel approaches. *Oman Med. J.* **2010**, *25*, 79–87. [CrossRef] [PubMed]
17. Chourasia, M.K.; Jain, S.K. Polysaccharides for colon targeted drug delivery. *Drug Deliv.* **2004**, *11*, 129–148. [CrossRef] [PubMed]
18. Vandamme, T.F.; Lenourry, A.; Charreau, C.; Chaumeil, J.-C. The use of polysaccharides to target drugs to colon. *Carbohydr. Polym.* **2002**, *48*, 219–231. [CrossRef]
19. Basit, A.; Short, M.; McConnell, E. Microbiota-triggered colonic delivery: Robustness of the polysaccharide approach. *J. Drug Target.* **2009**, *17*, 64–71. [CrossRef]
20. Freire, C.; Podczeck, F.; Veiga, F.; Sousa, J. Starch-based coatings for colon-specific delivery. Part II: Physicochemical properties and in vitro drug release from high amylose maize starch films. *Eur. J. Pharm. Biopharm.* **2009**, *72*, 587–594. [CrossRef]
21. Chen, J.; Li, X.; Chen, L.; Xie, F. Starch film-coated microparticles for oral colon-specific drug delivery. *Carbohydr. Polym.* **2018**, *191*, 242–254. [CrossRef] [PubMed]
22. Hou, L.; Shi, Y.; Jiang, G.; Liu, W.; Han, H.; Feng, Q.; Ren, J.; Yuan, Y.; Wang, Y.; Shi, J.; et al. Smart nanocomposite hydrogels based on azo crosslinked graphene oxide for oral colon-specific drug delivery. *Nanotechnology* **2016**, *27*, 315105. [CrossRef] [PubMed]
23. Sinha, V.R.; Kumria, R. Polysaccharides in colon-specific drug delivery. *Int. J. Pharm.* **2001**, *224*, 19–38. [CrossRef]
24. Forbes, J.D.; Chen, C.Y.; Knox, N.C.; Marrie, R.A.; El-Gabalawy, H.; de Kievit, T.; Alfa, M.; Bernstein, C.N.; Van Domselaar, G. A comparative study of the gut microbiota in immune-mediated inflammatory diseases-does a common dysbiosis exist? *Microbiome* **2018**, *6*, 221. [CrossRef] [PubMed]
25. Maroni, A.; Zema, L.; Cerea, M.; Foppoli, A.; Palugan, L.; Gazzaniga, A. Erodible drug delivery systems for time-controlled release into the gastrointestinal tract. *J. Drug Deliv. Sci. Technol.* **2016**, *32*, 229–235. [CrossRef]
26. Sangalli, M.E.; Maroni, A.; Zema, L.; Busetti, C.; Giordano, F.; Gazzaniga, A. In vitro and in vivo evaluation of an oral system for time and/or site-specific drug delivery. *J. Control. Release* **2001**, *73*, 103–110. [CrossRef]
27. Hu, M.Y.; Peppercorn, M.A. MMX mesalamine: A novel high-dose, once-daily 5-aminosalicylate formulation for the treatment of ulcerative colitis. *Expert Opin. Pharmacother.* **2008**, *9*, 1049–1058. [CrossRef] [PubMed]
28. Lentle, R.G.; Janssen, P.W.M. Physical characteristics of digesta and their influence on flow and mixing in the mammalian intestine: A review. *J. Comp. Physiol. B* **2008**, *178*, 673–690. [CrossRef]
29. Shameem, M.; Katori, N.; Aoyagi, N.; Kojima, S. Oral Solid Controlled Release Dosage Forms: Role of GI-Mechanical Destructive Forces and Colonic Release in Drug Absorption Under Fasted and Fed Conditions in Humans. *Pharm. Res.* **1995**, *12*, 1049–1054. [CrossRef]
30. Takahashi, T. Flow Behavior of Digesta and the Absorption of Nutrients in the Gastrointestine. *J. Nutr. Sci. Vitaminol.* **2011**, *57*, 265–273. [CrossRef]
31. McConnell, E.; Short, M.; Basit, A. An in vivo comparison of intestinal pH and bacteria as physiological trigger. *J. Control. Release* **2008**, *130*, 154–160. [CrossRef]
32. Li, J.; Yang, L.; Ferguson, S.M.; Hudson, T.J.; Watanabe, S.; Katsuma, M.; Fix, J.A. In vitro evaluation of dissolution behavior for a colon-specific drug delivery system (CODES™) in multi-pH media using United States Pharmacopeia apparatus II and III. *AAPS PharmSciTech* **2002**, *3*, 59. [CrossRef] [PubMed]
33. Akhgari, A.; Heshmati, Z.; Afrasiabi Garekani, H.; Sadeghi, F.; Sabbagh, A.; Sharif Makhmalzadeh, B.; Nokhodchi, A. Indomethacin electrospun nanofibers for colonic drug delivery: In vitro dissolution studies. *Colloids Surf. B* **2017**, *152*, 29–35. [CrossRef] [PubMed]
34. Handali, S.; Moghimipour, E.; Rezaei, M.; Kouchak, M.; Ramezani, Z.; Dorkoosh, F.A. In vitro and in vivo evaluation of coated capsules for colonic delivery. *J. Drug Deliv. Sci. Technol.* **2018**, *47*, 492–498. [CrossRef]
35. Oshi, M.A.; Naeem, M.; Bae, J.; Kim, J.; Lee, J.; Hasan, N.; Kim, W.; Im, E.; Jung, Y.; Yoo, J.-W. Colon-targeted dexamethasone microcrystals with pH-sensitive chitosan/alginate/Eudragit S multilayers for the treatment of inflammatory bowel disease. *Carbohydr. Polym.* **2018**, *198*, 434–442. [CrossRef]
36. Linares, V.; Casas, M.; Caraballo, I. Printfills: 3D printed systems combining fused deposition modeling and injection volume filling. Application to colon-specific drug delivery. *Eur. J. Pharm. Biopharm.* **2019**, *134*, 138–143. [CrossRef] [PubMed]
37. Maroni, A.; Moutaharrik, S.; Zema, L.; Gazzaniga, A. Enteric coatings for colonic drug delivery: State of the art. *Expert Opin. Drug Deliv.* **2017**, *14*, 1027–1029. [CrossRef] [PubMed]

38. Hu, Z.; Kimura, G.; Mawatari, S.-S.; Shimokawa, T.; Yoshikawa, Y.; Takada, K. New preparation method of intestinal pressure-controlled colon delivery capsules by coating machine and evaluation in beagle dogs. *J. Control. Release* **1998**, *56*, 293–302. [CrossRef]
39. Ishibashi, T.; Pitcairn, G.R.; Yoshino, H.; Mizobe, M.; Wilding, I.R. Scintigraphic Evaluation of a New Capsule-Type Colon Specific Drug Delivery System in Healthy Volunteers. *J. Pharm. Sci.* **1998**, *87*, 531–535. [CrossRef] [PubMed]
40. Corsetti, M.; Pagliaro, G.; Demedts, I.; Deloose, E.; Gevers, A.; Scheerens, C.; Rommel, N.; Tack, J. Pan-Colonic Pressurizations Associated With Relaxation of the Anal Sphincter in Health and Disease: A New Colonic Motor Pattern Identified Using High-Resolution Manometry. *Am. J. Gastroenterol.* **2017**, *112*, 479–489. [CrossRef] [PubMed]
41. Dinning, P.G.; Wiklendt, L.; Maslen, L.; Gibbins, I.; Patton, V.; Arkwright, J.W.; Lubowski, D.Z.; O'Grady, G.; Bampton, P.A.; Brookes, S.J.; et al. Quantification of in vivo colonic motor patterns in healthy humans before and after a meal revealed by high-resolution fiber-optic manometry. *Neurogastroenterol. Motil.* **2014**, *26*, 1443–1457. [CrossRef] [PubMed]
42. Zhang, S.; Langer, R.; Traverso, G. Nanoparticulate drug delivery systems targeting inflammation for treatment of inflammatory bowel disease. *Nano Today* **2017**, *16*, 82–96. [CrossRef]
43. Hua, S.; Marks, E.; Schneider, J.J.; Keely, S. Advances in oral nano-delivery systems for colon targeted drug delivery in inflammatory bowel disease: Selective targeting to diseased versus healthy tissue. *Nanomed. Nanotechnol. Biol. Med.* **2015**, *11*, 1117–1132. [CrossRef] [PubMed]
44. Vass, P.; Démuth, B.; Hirsch, E.; Nagy, B.; Andersen, S.K.; Vigh, T.; Verreck, G.; Csontos, I.; Nagy, Z.K.; Marosi, G. Drying technology strategies for colon-targeted oral delivery of biopharmaceuticals. *J. Control. Release* **2019**, *296*, 162–178. [CrossRef] [PubMed]
45. Benshitrit, R.C.; Levi, C.S.; Tal, S.L.; Shimoni, E.; Lesmes, U. Development of oral food-grade delivery systems: Current knowledge and future challenges. *Food Funct.* **2012**, *3*, 10–21. [CrossRef]
46. Sagalowicz, L.; Leser, M.E. Delivery systems for liquid food products. *Curr. Opin. Colloid Interf. Sci.* **2010**, *15*, 61–72. [CrossRef]
47. Koziolek, M.; Grimm, M.; Becker, D.; Iordanov, V.; Zou, H.; Shimizu, J.; Wanke, C.; Garbacz, G.; Weitschies, W. Investigation of pH and Temperature Profiles in the GI Tract of Fasted Human Subjects Using the Intellicap((R)) System. *J. Pharm. Sci.* **2015**, *104*, 2855–2863. [CrossRef]
48. Russell, T.L.; Berardi, R.R.; Barnett, J.L.; Dermentzoglou, L.C.; Jarvenpaa, K.M.; Schmaltz, S.P.; Dressman, J.B. Upper Gastrointestinal pH in Seventy-Nine Healthy, Elderly, North American Men and Women. *Pharm. Res.* **1993**, *10*, 187–196. [CrossRef]
49. Helander, H.F.; Fändriks, L. Surface area of the digestive tract—Revisited. *Scand. J. Gastroenterol.* **2014**, *49*, 681–689. [CrossRef]
50. Bergstrom, C.A.; Holm, R.; Jorgensen, S.A.; Andersson, S.B.; Artursson, P.; Beato, S.; Borde, A.; Box, K.; Brewster, M.; Dressman, J.; et al. Early pharmaceutical profiling to predict oral drug absorption: Current status and unmet needs. *Eur. J. Pharm. Sci.* **2014**, *57*, 173–199. [CrossRef]
51. Pentafragka, C.; Symillides, M.; McAllister, M.; Dressman, J.; Vertzoni, M.; Reppas, C. The impact of food intake on the luminal environment and performance of oral drug products with a view to in vitro and in silico simulations: A PEARRL review. *J. Pharm. Pharmacol.* **2018**. [CrossRef] [PubMed]
52. Ridlon, J.M.; Kang, D.J.; Hylemon, P.B. Bile salt biotransformations by human intestinal bacteria. *J. Lipid Res.* **2006**, *47*, 241–259. [CrossRef] [PubMed]
53. Villmones, H.C.; Haug, E.S.; Ulvestad, E.; Grude, N.; Stenstad, T.; Halland, A.; Kommedal, O. Species Level Description of the Human Ileal Bacterial Microbiota. *Sci. Rep.* **2018**, *8*, 4736. [CrossRef] [PubMed]
54. Sundin, O.H.; Mendoza-Ladd, A.; Zeng, M.; Diaz-Arevalo, D.; Morales, E.; Fagan, B.M.; Ordonez, J.; Velez, P.; Antony, N.; McCallum, R.W. The human jejunum has an endogenous microbiota that differs from those in the oral cavity and colon. *BMC Microbiol.* **2017**, *17*, 160. [CrossRef] [PubMed]
55. Fallingborg, J. Intraluminal pH of the human gastrointestinal tract. *Dan. Med. Bull.* **1999**, *46*, 183–196. [PubMed]
56. Mudd, D.G.; Mckelvey, S.T.D.; Norwood, W.; Elmore, D.T.; Roy, A.D. Faecal bile acid concentrations of patients with carcinomaor increased risk of carcinoma in the large bowel. *Gut* **1980**, *21*, 587–590. [CrossRef] [PubMed]

57. Dressman, J.B.; Berardi, R.R.; Dermentzoglou, L.C.; Russell, T.L.; Schmaltz, S.P.; Barnett, J.L.; Jarvenpaa, K.M. Upper Gastrointestinal (GI) pH in Young, Healthy Men and Women. *Pharm. Res.* **1990**, *7*, 756–761. [CrossRef] [PubMed]
58. Hakansson, A.; Molin, G. Gut Microbiota and Inflammation. *Nutrients* **2011**, *3*, 637–682. [CrossRef]
59. Walker, A.W.; Ince, J.; Duncan, S.H.; Webster, L.M.; Holtrop, G.; Ze, X.; Brown, D.; Stares, M.D.; Scott, P.; Bergerat, A.; et al. Dominant and diet-responsive groups of bacteria within the human colonic microbiota. *ISME J.* **2011**, *5*, 220–230. [CrossRef]
60. De Filippo, C.; Cavalieri, D.; Di Paola, M.; Ramazzotti, M.; Poullet, J.B.; Massart, S.; Collini, S.; Pieraccini, G.; Lionetti, P. Impact of diet in shaping gut microbiota revealed by a comparative study in children from Europe and rural Africa. *Proc. Nat. Acad. Sci. USA* **2010**, *107*, 14691–14696. [CrossRef]
61. Flint, H.J.; Scott, K.P.; Duncan, S.H.; Louis, P.; Forano, E. Microbial degradation of complex carbohydrates in the gut. *Gut Microbes* **2012**, *3*. [CrossRef] [PubMed]
62. Andersson, H.; Tullberg, C.; Ahrné, S.; Hamberg, K.; Lazou Ahrén, I.; Molin, G.; Sonesson, M.; Håkansson, Å. Oral Administration of Lactobacillus plantarum 299v Reduces Cortisol Levels in Human Saliva during Examination Induced Stress: A Randomized, Double-Blind Controlled Trial. *Int. J. Microbiol.* **2016**, *2016*. [CrossRef] [PubMed]
63. Håkansson, Å.; Bränning, C.; Molin, G.; Adawi, D.; Hagslätt, M.L.; Jeppsson, B.; Nyman, M.; Ahrné, S. Blueberry husks and probiotics attenuate colorectal inflammation and oncogenesis, and liver injuries in rats exposed to cycling DSS-treatment. *PLoS ONE* **2012**, *7*. [CrossRef] [PubMed]
64. Ejtahed, H.S.; Angoorani, P.; Soroush, A.R.; Atlasi, R.; Hasani-Ranjbar, S.; Mortazavian, A.M.; Larijani, B. Probiotics supplementation for the obesity management; A systematic review of animal studies and clinical trials. *J. Funct. Foods* **2019**, *52*, 228–242. [CrossRef]
65. Karlsson, C.L.J.; Molin, G.; Fåk, F.; Johansson Hagslätt, M.L.; Jakesevic, M.; Håkansson, Å.; Jeppsson, B.; Weström, B.; Ahrné, S. Effects on weight gain and gut microbiota in rats given bacterial supplements and a high-energy-dense diet from fetal life through to 6 months of age. *Br. J. Nutr.* **2011**, *106*, 887–895. [CrossRef] [PubMed]
66. Filip, M.; Tzaneva, V.; Dumitrascu, D.L. Fecal transplantation: Digestive and extradigestive clinical applications. *Clujul Med.* **2018**, *91*, 259–265. [CrossRef] [PubMed]
67. Zhang, Z.; Geng, J.; Tang, X.; Fan, H.; Xu, J.; Wen, X.; Ma, Z.S.; Shi, P. Spatial heterogeneity and co-occurrence patterns of human mucosal-associated intestinal microbiota. *ISME J.* **2014**, *8*, 881–893. [CrossRef]
68. Aguirre de Carcer, D.; Cuiv, P.O.; Wang, T.; Kang, S.; Worthley, D.; Whitehall, V.; Gordon, I.; McSweeney, C.; Leggett, B.; Morrison, M. Numerical ecology validates a biogeographical distribution and gender-based effect on mucosa-associated bacteria along the human colon. *ISME J.* **2011**, *5*, 801–809. [CrossRef]
69. Tasse, L.; Bercovici, J.; Pizzut-Serin, S.; Robe, P.; Tap, J.; Klopp, C.; Cantarel, B.L.; Coutinho, P.M.; Henrissat, B.; Leclerc, M.; et al. Functional metagenomics to mine the human gut microbiome for dietary fiber catabolic enzymes. *Genome Res.* **2010**, *20*, 1605–1612. [CrossRef]
70. Macfarlane, G.T.; Cummings, J.H.; Macfarlane, S.; Gibson, G.R. Influence of retention time on degradation of pancreatic enzymes by human colonic bacteria grown in a 3-stage continuous culture system. *J. Appl. Bacteriol.* **1989**, *67*, 521–527. [CrossRef]
71. Reppas, C.; Karatza, E.; Goumas, C.; Markopoulos, C.; Vertzoni, M. Characterization of Contents of Distal Ileum and Cecum to Which Drugs/Drug Products are Exposed During Bioavailability/Bioequivalence Studies in Healthy Adults. *Pharm. Res.* **2015**, *32*, 3338–3349. [CrossRef] [PubMed]
72. Persson, E.M.; Gustafsson, A.S.; Carlsson, A.S.; Nilsson, R.G.; Knutson, L.; Forsell, P.; Hanisch, G.; Lennernas, H.; Abrahamsson, B. The effects of food on the dissolution of poorly soluble drugs in human and in model small intestinal fluids. *Pharm. Res.* **2005**, *22*, 2141–2151. [CrossRef] [PubMed]
73. Dokoumetzidis, A.; Macheras, P. A century of dissolution research: From Noyes and Whitney to the biopharmaceutics classification system. *Int. J. Pharm.* **2006**, *321*, 1–11. [CrossRef] [PubMed]
74. Nelson, E. Solution rate of theophylline salts and effects from oral administration. *J. Am. Pharm. Assoc.* **1957**, *46*, 607–614. [CrossRef]
75. Lindenbaum, J.; Mellow, M.H.; Blackstone, M.O.; Butler, V.P., Jr. Variation in biologic availability of digoxin from four preparations. *N. Engl. J. Med.* **1971**, *285*, 1344–1347. [CrossRef] [PubMed]
76. Tyrer, J.H.; Eadie, M.J.; Sutherland, J.M.; Hooper, W.D. Outbreak of anticonvulsant intoxication in an Australian city. *Br. Med. J.* **1970**, *4*, 271–273. [CrossRef] [PubMed]

77. Kostewicz, E.S.; Abrahamsson, B.; Brewster, M.; Brouwers, J.; Butler, J.; Carlert, S.; Dickinson, P.A.; Dressman, J.; Holm, R.; Klein, S.; et al. In vitro models for the prediction of in vivo performance of oral dosage forms. *Eur. J. Pharm. Sci.* **2014**, *57*, 342–366. [CrossRef]
78. Stamatopoulos, K.; Batchelor, H.K.; Simmons, M.J.H. Dissolution profile of theophylline modified release tablets, using a biorelevant Dynamic Colon Model (DCM). *Eur. J. Pharm. Biopharm.* **2016**, *108*, 9–17. [CrossRef] [PubMed]
79. <1092> The Dissolution Procedure: Development and Validation. In *The United States Pharmacopeia (USP)*; The United States Pharmacopeial Convention North Bethesda: Rockville, MD, USA, 2018.
80. González-García, I.; Mangas-Sanjuán, V.; Merino-Sanjuán, M.; Bermejo, M. In vitro–in vivo correlations: General concepts, methodologies and regulatory applications. *Drug Dev. Ind. Pharm.* **2015**, *41*, 1935–1947. [CrossRef]
81. Lu, Y.; Kim, S.; Park, K. In vitro-in vivo correlation: Perspectives on model development. *Int. J. Pharm.* **2011**, *418*, 142–148. [CrossRef] [PubMed]
82. Quigley, E.M.M. Prebiotics and Probiotics in Digestive Health. *Clin. Gastroenterol. Hepatol.* **2019**, *17*, 333–344. [CrossRef] [PubMed]
83. Lee, E.S.; Song, E.J.; Nam, Y.D.; Lee, S.Y. Probiotics in human health and disease: From nutribiotics to pharmabiotics. *J. Microbiol.* **2018**, *56*, 773–782. [CrossRef] [PubMed]
84. Ooi, S.L.; Correa, D.; Pak, S.C. Probiotics, prebiotics, and low FODMAP diet for irritable bowel syndrome—What is the current evidence? *Complement. Ther. Med.* **2019**, *43*, 73–80. [CrossRef]
85. Kothari, D.; Patel, S.; Kim, S.K. Probiotic supplements might not be universally-effective and safe: A review. *Biomed. Pharmacother.* **2019**, *111*, 537–547. [CrossRef] [PubMed]
86. Astó, E.; Méndez, I.; Audivert, S.; Farran-Codina, A.; Espadaler, J. The Efficacy of Probiotics, Prebiotic Inulin-Type Fructans, and Synbiotics in Human Ulcerative Colitis: A Systematic Review and Meta-Analysis. *Nutrients* **2019**, *11*. [CrossRef] [PubMed]
87. Recommendations on dissolution testing. In *European Pharmacopoeia 9.0*; EDQM-Council of Europe: Strasbourg, France, 2016.
88. Dissolution test for solid dosage forms. In *European Pharmacopoeia 9.0*; EDQM-Council of Europe: Strasbourg, France, 2016.
89. <711> Dissolution. In *The United States Pharmacopeia (USP)*; The United States Pharmacopeial Convention North Bethesda: Rockville, MD, USA, 2018.
90. SUPAC. Guidance for Industry Immediate Release Solid Oral Dosage Forms Scale-Up and Postapproval Changes: Chemistry, Manufacturing, and Controls, In Vitro Dissolution Testing, and In Vivo Bioequivalence Documentation. 1995. Available online: https://www.fda.gov/downloads/Drugs/Guidances/UCM456594.pdf (accessed on 2 February 2019).
91. Dissolution Testing and Acceptance Criteria for Immediate-Release Solid Oral Dosage Form Drug Products Containing High Solubility Drug Substances Guidance for Industry. 2018. Available online: https://www.fda.gov/downloads/Drugs/Guidances/UCM456594.pdf (accessed on 2 February 2019).
92. Guideline on the Investigation of Bioequivalence. 2010. Available online: https://www.ema.europa.eu/documents/scientific-guideline/guideline-investigation-bioequivalence-rev1_en.pdf (accessed on 2 February 2019).
93. Reppas, C.; Vertzoni, M. Biorelevant in-vitro performance testing of orally administered dosage forms. *J. Pharm. Pharmacol.* **2012**, *64*, 919–930. [CrossRef] [PubMed]
94. Vertzoni, M.; Dressman, J.; Butler, J.; Hempenstall, J.; Reppas, C. Simulation of fasting gastric conditions and its importance for the in vivo dissolution of lipophilic compounds. *Eur. J. Pharm. Biopharm.* **2005**, *60*, 413–417. [CrossRef] [PubMed]
95. Christophersen, P.C.; Christiansen, M.L.; Holm, R.; Kristensen, J.; Jacobsen, J.; Abrahamsson, B.; Mullertz, A. Fed and fasted state gastro-intestinal in vitro lipolysis: In vitro in vivo relations of a conventional tablet, a SNEDDS and a solidified SNEDDS. *Eur. J. Pharm. Sci.* **2014**, *57*, 232–239. [CrossRef]
96. Jantratid, E.; Janssen, N.; Reppas, C.; Dressman, J.B. Dissolution media simulating conditions in the proximal human gastrointestinal tract: An update. *Pharm. Res.* **2008**, *25*, 1663–1676. [CrossRef]
97. Markopoulos, C.; Andreas, C.J.; Vertzoni, M.; Dressman, J.; Reppas, C. In-vitro simulation of luminal conditions for evaluation of performance of oral drug products: Choosing the appropriate test media. *Eur. J. Pharm. Biopharm.* **2015**, *93*, 173–182. [CrossRef]

98. Granfeldt, Y.; Bjorck, I.; Drews, A.; Tovar, J. An in vitro procedure based on chewing to predict metabolic response to. *Eur. J. Clin. Nutr.* **1992**, *46*, 649–660.
99. Egger, L.; Ménard, O.; Delgado-Andrade, C.; Alvito, P.; Assunção, R.; Balance, S.; Barberá, R.; Brodkorb, A.; Cattenoz, T.; Clemente, A.; et al. The harmonized INFOGEST in vitro digestion method: From knowledge to action. *Food Res. Int.* **2016**, *88*, 217–225. [CrossRef]
100. Molly, K.; De Smet, I.; Nollet, L.; Vande Woestyne, M.; Verstraete, W. Effect of Lactobacilli on the Ecology of the Gastrointestinal Microbiota Cultured in the SHIME Reactor. *Microb. Ecol. Health Dis.* **1996**, *2*, 79–89. [CrossRef]
101. Minekus, M.; Marteau, P.; Havenaar, R. Multicompartmental dynamic computer-controlled model simulating the stomach and small intestine. *Altern. Lab. Anim. ATLA* **1995**.
102. Macfarlane, G.T.; Macfarlane, S.; Gibson, G.R. Validation of a Three-Stage Compound Continuous Culture System for Investigating the Effect of Retention Time on the Ecology and Metabolism of Bacteria in the Human Colon. *Microb. Ecol.* **1998**, *35*, 180–187. [CrossRef] [PubMed]
103. Marefati, A.; Bertrand, M.; Sjöö, M.; Dejmek, P.; Rayner, M. Storage and digestion stability of encapsulated curcumin in emulsions based on starch granule Pickering stabilization. *Food Hydrocolloids* **2017**, *63*, 309–320. [CrossRef]
104. Tikekar, R.V.; Pan, Y.; Nitin, N. Fate of curcumin encapsulated in silica nanoparticle stabilized Pickering emulsion during storage and simulated digestion. *Food Res. Int.* **2013**, *51*, 370–377. [CrossRef]
105. Molly, K.; Vande Woestyne, M.; Verstraete, W. Development of a 5-step multi-chamber reactor as a simulation of the human intestinal microbial ecosystem. *Appl. Microbiol. Biotechnol.* **1993**, *39*, 254–258. [CrossRef] [PubMed]
106. Verwei, M.; Minekus, M.; Zeijdner, E.; Schilderink, R.; Havenaar, R. Evaluation of two dynamic in vitro models simulating fasted and fed state conditions in the upper gastrointestinal tract (TIM-1 and tiny-TIM) for investigating the bioaccessibility of pharmaceutical compounds from oral dosage forms. *Int. J. Pharm.* **2016**, *498*, 178–186. [CrossRef] [PubMed]
107. Claeys, B.; Vervaeck, A.; Hillewaere, X.K.; Possemiers, S.; Hansen, L.; De Beer, T.; Remon, J.P.; Vervaet, C. Thermoplastic polyurethanes for the manufacturing of highly dosed oral sustained release matrices via hot melt extrusion and injection molding. *Eur. J. Pharm. Biopharm.* **2015**, *90*, 44–52. [CrossRef] [PubMed]
108. Kong, F.; Singh, R.P. A human gastric simulator (HGS) to study food digestion in human stomach. *J. Food Sci.* **2010**, *75*, E627–E635. [CrossRef]
109. Tharakan, A.; Norton, I.; Fryer, P.; Bakalis, S. Mass transfer and nutrient absorption in a simulated model of small intestine. *J. Food Sci.* **2010**, *75*, E339–E346. [CrossRef] [PubMed]
110. Minekus, M.; Alminger, M.; Alvito, P.; Ballance, S.; Bohn, T.; Bourlieu, C.; Carriere, F.; Boutrou, R.; Corredig, M.; Dupont, D. A standardised static in vitro digestion method suitable for food—An international consensus. *Food Funct.* **2014**, *5*, 1113–1124. [CrossRef] [PubMed]
111. Vamanu, E.; Gatea, F.; Sarbu, I. In Vitro Ecological Response of the Human Gut Microbiome to Bioactive Extracts from Edible Wild Mushrooms. *Molecules* **2018**, *23*. [CrossRef] [PubMed]
112. Yang, L. Biorelevant dissolution testing of colon-specific delivery systems activated by colonic microflora. *J. Control. Release* **2008**, *125*, 77–86. [CrossRef] [PubMed]
113. Siew, L.F.; Man, S.M.; Newton, J.M.; Basit, A.W. Amylose formulations for drug delivery to the colon: A comparison of two fermentation models to assess colonic targeting performance in vitro. *Int. J. Pharm.* **2004**, *273*, 129–134. [CrossRef]
114. Yadav, S.; Deka, S.R.; Tiwari, K.; Sharma, A.K.; Kumar, P. Multi-Stimuli Responsive Self-Assembled Nanostructures Useful for Colon Drug Delivery. *IEEE Trans. NanoBiosci.* **2017**, *16*, 764–772. [CrossRef]
115. Rao, J.; Khan, A. Enzyme sensitive synthetic polymer micelles based on the azobenzene motif. *J. Am. Chem. Soc.* **2013**, *135*, 14056–14059. [CrossRef] [PubMed]
116. Gliko-Kabir, I.; Yagen, B.; Baluom, M.; Rubinstein, A. Phosphated crosslinked guar for colon-specific drug delivery: II. In vitro and in vivo evaluation in the rat. *J. Control. Release* **2000**, *63*, 129–134. [CrossRef]
117. Tuğcu-Demiröz, F.; Acartürk, F.; Takka, S.; Konuş-Boyunağa, Ö. In-vitro and in-vivo evaluation of mesalazine-guar gum matrix tablets for colonic drug delivery. *J. Drug Target.* **2004**, *12*, 105–112. [CrossRef]
118. Yamada, K.; Iwao, Y.; Bani-Jaber, A.; Noguchi, S.; Itai, S. Preparation and Evaluation of Newly Developed Chitosan Salt Coating Dispersions for Colon Delivery without Requiring Overcoating. *Chem. Pharm. Bull.* **2015**, *63*, 799–806. [CrossRef] [PubMed]

119. Jyoti, K.; Bhatia, R.K.; Martis, E.A.F.; Coutinho, E.C.; Jain, U.K.; Chandra, R.; Madan, J. Soluble curcumin amalgamated chitosan microspheres augmented drug delivery and cytotoxicity in colon cancer cells: In vitro and in vivo study. *Colloids Surf. B* **2016**, *148*, 674–683. [CrossRef] [PubMed]
120. Andishmand, H.; Tabibiazar, M.; Mohammadifar, M.A.; Hamishehkar, H. Pectin-zinc-chitosan-polyethylene glycol colloidal nano-suspension as a food grade carrier for colon targeted delivery of resveratrol. *Int. J. Biol. Macromol.* **2017**, *97*, 16–22. [CrossRef] [PubMed]
121. Gunter, E.A.; Popeyko, O.V. Calcium pectinate gel beads obtained from callus cultures pectins as promising systems for colon-targeted drug delivery. *Carbohydr. Polym.* **2016**, *147*, 490–499. [CrossRef] [PubMed]
122. Stubbe, B.; Maris, B.; Van den Mooter, G.; De Smedt, S.C.; Demeester, J. The in vitro evaluation of 'azo containing polysaccharide gels' for colon delivery. *J. Control. Release* **2001**, *75*, 103–114. [CrossRef]
123. Krishnaiah, Y.S.R.; Bhaskar Reddy, P.R.; Satyanarayana, V.; Karthikeyan, R.S. Studies on the development of oral colon targeted drug delivery systems for metronidazole in the treatment of amoebiasis. *Int. J. Pharm.* **2002**, *236*, 43–55. [CrossRef]
124. Imaoka, A.; Setoyama, H.; Takagi, A.; Matsumoto, S.; Umesaki, Y. Improvement of human faecal flora-associated mouse model for evaluation of the functional foods. *J. Appl. Microbiol.* **2004**, *96*, 656–663. [CrossRef]
125. Savage, D.C.; Dubos, R.; Schaedler, R.W. The gastrointestinal epithelium and its autochthonous bacterial flora. *J. Exp. Med.* **1968**, *127*, 67–76. [CrossRef]
126. Suau, A.; Bonnet, R.; Sutren, M.; Godon, J.J.; Gibson, G.R.; Collins, M.D.; Doré, J. Direct analysis of genes encoding 16S rRNA from complex communities reveals many novel molecular species within the human gut. *Appl. Environ. Microbiol.* **1999**, *65*, 4799–4807. [PubMed]
127. Rama Prasad, Y.V.; Krishnaiah, Y.S.R.; Satyanarayana, V. In vitro evaluation of guar gum as a carrier for colon-specific drug delivery. *J. Control. Release* **1998**, *51*, 281–287. [CrossRef]
128. Kumar Dev, R.; Bali, V.; Pathak, K. Novel microbially triggered colon specific delivery system of 5-Fluorouracil: Statistical optimization, in vitro, in vivo, cytotoxic and stability assessment. *Int. J. Pharm.* **2011**, *411*, 142–151. [CrossRef]
129. Vaidya, A.; Jain, A.; Khare, P.; Agrawal, R.K.; Jain, S.K. Metronidazole Loaded Pectin Microspheres for Colon Targeting. *J. Pharm. Sci.* **2009**, *98*, 4229–4236. [CrossRef] [PubMed]
130. Sirisha, V.N.l.; Eswariah, M.C.; Rao, A.S. A Novel Approach of Locust Bean Gum Microspheres for Colonic Delivery of Mesalamine. *Int. J. Appl. Pharm.* **2018**, *10*. [CrossRef]
131. Das, A.; Wadhwa, S.; Srivastava, A.K. Cross-Linked Guar Gum Hydrogel Discs for Colon-Specific. Delivery of Ibuprofen: Formulation and In Vitro Evaluation. *Drug Deliv.* **2006**, *13*, 139–142. [CrossRef] [PubMed]
132. Kalala, W.; Kinget, R.; Van den Mooter, G.; Samyn, C. Colonic drug-targeting: In vitro release of ibuprofen from capsules coated with poly(ether-ester) azopolymers. *Int. J. Pharm.* **1996**, *139*, 187–195. [CrossRef]
133. Van den Mooter, G.; Samyn, C.; Kinget, R. The Relation Between Swelling Properties and Enzymatic Degradation of Azo Polymers Designed for Colon-Specific Drug Delivery. *Pharm. Res.* **1994**, *11*, 1737–1741. [CrossRef]
134. Kopečková, P.; Rathi, R.; Takada, S.; Říhová, B.; Berenson, M.M.; Kopeček, J. Bioadhesive N-(2-hydroxypropyl) methacrylamide copolymers for colon-specific drug delivery. *J. Control. Release* **1994**, *28*, 211–222. [CrossRef]
135. McConnell, E.L.; Tutas, J.; Mohamed, M.A.M.; Banning, D.; Basit, A.W. Colonic drug delivery using amylose films: The role of aqueous ethylcellulose dispersions in controlling drug release. *Cellulose* **2006**, *14*, 25–34. [CrossRef]
136. Siew, L.F.; Basit, A.W.; Newton, J.M. The potential of organic-based amylose-ethylcellulose film coatings as oral colon-specific drug delivery systems. *AAPS PharmSciTech* **2000**, *1*, 53–61. [CrossRef]
137. Macfarlane, S.; Quigley, M.E.; Hopkins, M.J.; Newton, D.F.; Macfarlane, G.T. Polysaccharide degradation by human intestinal bacteria during growth under multi-substrate limiting conditions in a three-stage continuous culture system. *FEMS Microbiol. Ecol.* **1998**, *26*, 231–243. [CrossRef]
138. Karrout, Y.; Neut, C.; Wils, D.; Siepmann, F.; Deremaux, L.; Flament, M.P.; Dubreuil, L.; Desreumaux, P.; Siepmann, J. Novel polymeric film coatings for colon targeting: Drug release from coated pellets. *Eur. J. Pharm. Sci.* **2009**, *37*, 427–433. [CrossRef] [PubMed]
139. Simonsen, L.; Hovgaard, L.; Mortensen, P.B.; Brøndsted, H. Dextran hydrogels for colon-specific drug delivery. V. Degradation in human intestinal incubation models. *Eur. J. Pharm. Sci.* **1995**, *3*, 329–337. [CrossRef]

140. Wilson, P.J.; Basit, A.W. Exploiting gastrointestinal bacteria to target drugs to the colon: An in vitro study using amylose coated tablets. *Int. J. Pharm.* **2005**, *300*, 89–94. [CrossRef]
141. Venema, K.; van den Abbeele, P. Experimental models of the gut microbiome. *Best Pract. Res. Clin. Gastroenterol.* **2013**, *27*, 115–126. [CrossRef] [PubMed]
142. Fooks, L.J.; Gibson, G.R. Mixed culture fermentation studies on the effects of synbiotics on the human intestinal pathogens Campylobacter jejuni and Escherichia coli. *Anaerobe* **2003**, *9*, 231–242. [CrossRef]
143. O'Donnell, M.M.; Rea, M.C.; Shanahan, F.; Ross, R.P. The Use of a Mini-Bioreactor Fermentation System as a Reproducible, High-Throughput ex vivo Batch Model of the Distal Colon. *Front. Microbiol.* **2018**, *9*. [CrossRef] [PubMed]
144. Singh, S.K.; Yadav, A.K.; Prudhviraj, G.; Gulati, M.; Kaur, P.; Vaidya, Y. A novel dissolution method for evaluation of polysaccharide based colon specific delivery systems: A suitable alternative to animal sacrifice. *Eur. J. Pharm. Sci.* **2015**, *73*, 72–80. [CrossRef] [PubMed]
145. Yadav, A.K.; Sadora, M.; Singh, S.K.; Gulati, M.; Maharshi, P.; Sharma, A.; Kumar, B.; Rathee, H.; Ghai, D.; Malik, A.H.; et al. Novel biorelevant dissolution medium as a prognostic tool for polysaccharide-based colon-targeted drug delivery system. *J. Adv. Pharm. Technol. Res.* **2017**, *8*, 150–155. [CrossRef] [PubMed]
146. Kotla, N.G.; Singh, S.; Maddiboyina, B.; Sunnapu, O.; Webster, T.J. A novel dissolution media for testing drug release from a nanostructured polysaccharide-based colon specific drug delivery system: An approach to alternative colon media. *Int. J. Nanomed.* **2016**, *11*, 1089–1095. [CrossRef]
147. Tap, J.; Mondot, S.; Levenez, F.; Pelletier, E.; Caron, C.; Furet, J.P.; Ugarte, E.; Muñoz-Tamayo, R.; Paslier, D.L.E.; Nalin, R.; et al. Towards the human intestinal microbiota phylogenetic core. *Environ. Microbiol.* **2009**, *11*, 2574–2584. [CrossRef]
148. Yang, X.; Xie, L.; Li, Y.; Wei, C. More than 9,000,000 unique genes in human gut bacterial community: Estimating gene numbers inside a human body. *PLoS ONE* **2009**, *4*, e6074. [CrossRef] [PubMed]
149. Kovatcheva-Datchary, P.; Egert, M.; Maathuis, A.; Rajilić-Stojanović, M.; De Graaf, A.A.; Smidt, H.; De Vos, W.M.; Venema, K. Linking phylogenetic identities of bacteria to starch fermentation in an in vitro model of the large intestine by RNA-based stable isotope probing. *Environ. Microbiol.* **2009**, *11*, 914–926. [CrossRef] [PubMed]
150. Wang, R.F.; Cao, W.W.; Cerniglia, C.E. PCR detection and quantitation of predominant anaerobic bacteria in human and animal fecal samples. *Appl. Environ. microbiol.* **1996**, *62*, 1242–1247. [PubMed]
151. Moore, W.E.C.; Holdeman, L.V. Human fecal flora: The normal flora of 20 Japanese Hawaiians. *J. Appl. Microbiol.* **1974**, *27*, 961–979.
152. Wang, M.; Ahrné, S.; Jeppsson, B.; Molin, G. Comparison of bacterial diversity along the human intestinal tract by direct cloning and sequencing of 16S rRNA genes. *FEMS Microbiol. Ecol.* **2005**, *54*, 219–231. [CrossRef] [PubMed]
153. Hold, G.L.; Pryde, S.E.; Russell, V.J.; Furrie, E.; Flint, H.J. Assessment of microbial diversity in human colonic samples by 16S rDNA sequence analysis. *FEMS Microbiol. Ecol.* **2002**, *39*, 33–39. [CrossRef] [PubMed]
154. Hold, G.L.; Schwiertz, A.; Aminov, R.I.; Blaut, M.; Flint, H.J. Oligonucleotide probes that detect quantitatively significant groups of butyrate-producing bacteria in human feces. *Appl. Environ. Microbiol.* **2003**, *69*, 4320–4324. [CrossRef]
155. Louis, P.; Flint, H.J. Diversity, metabolism and microbial ecology of butyrate-producing bacteria from the human large intestine. *FEMS Microbiol. Lett.* **2009**, *294*, 1–8. [CrossRef]
156. Lopez-Siles, M.; Khan, T.M.; Duncan, S.H.; Harmsen, H.J.M.; Garcia-Gil, L.J.; Flint, H.J. Cultured representatives of two major phylogroups of human colonic Faecalibacterium prausnitzii can utilize pectin, uronic acids, and host-derived substrates for growth. *Appl. Environ. Microbiol.* **2012**, *78*, 420–428. [CrossRef] [PubMed]
157. Salyers, A.A.; Vercellotti, J.R.; West, S.E.H.; Wilkins, T.D. Fermentation of mucin and plant polysaccharides by strains of Bacteroides from the human colon. *Appl. Environ. Microbiol.* **1977**, *33*, 319–322.
158. Davis, L.M.G.; Martínez, I.; Walter, J.; Goin, C.; Hutkins, R.W. Barcoded pyrosequencing reveals that consumption of galactooligosaccharides results in a highly specific bifidogenic response in humans. *PLoS ONE* **2011**, *6*. [CrossRef] [PubMed]
159. Kleessen, B.; Schwarz, S.; Boehm, A.; Fuhrmann, H.; Richter, A.; Henle, T.; Krueger, M. Jerusalem artichoke and chicory inulin in bakery products affect faecal microbiota of healthy volunteers. *Br. J. Nutr.* **2007**, *98*, 540–549. [CrossRef] [PubMed]

160. Ze, X.; Duncan, S.H.; Louis, P.; Flint, H.J. Ruminococcus bromii is a keystone species for the degradation of resistant starch in the human colon. *ISME J.* **2012**, *6*, 1535–1543. [CrossRef] [PubMed]
161. Abell, G.C.J.; Cooke, C.M.; Bennett, C.N.; Conlon, M.A.; McOrist, A.L. Phylotypes related to Ruminococcus bromii are abundant in the large bowel of humans and increase in response to a diet high in resistant starch. *FEMS Microbiol. Ecol.* **2008**, *66*, 505–515. [CrossRef] [PubMed]
162. Duncan, S.H.; Belenguer, A.; Holtrop, G.; Johnstone, A.M.; Flint, H.J.; Lobley, G.E. Reduced dietary intake of carbohydrates by obese subjects results in decreased concentrations of butyrate and butyrate-producing bacteria in feces. *Appl. Environ. Microbiol.* **2007**, *73*, 1073–1078. [CrossRef] [PubMed]
163. Scott, K.P.; Martin, J.C.; Duncan, S.H.; Flint, H.J. Prebiotic stimulation of human colonic butyrate-producing bacteria and bifidobacteria, in vitro. *FEMS Microbiol. Ecol.* **2014**, *87*, 30–40. [CrossRef]
164. Benítez-Páez, A.; Gómez del Pulgar, E.M.; Sanz, Y. The glycolytic versatility of Bacteroides uniformis CECT 7771 and Its genome response to oligo and polysaccharides. *Front. Cell. Infect. Microbiol.* **2017**, *7*. [CrossRef]
165. Scher, J.U.; Sczesnak, A.; Longman, R.S.; Segata, N.; Ubeda, C.; Bielski, C.; Rostron, T.; Cerundolo, V.; Pamer, E.G.; Abramson, S.B.; et al. Expansion of intestinal Prevotella copri correlates with enhanced susceptibility to arthritis. *eLife* **2013**, *2013*. [CrossRef]
166. Kovatcheva-Datchary, P.; Nilsson, A.; Akrami, R.; Lee, Y.S.; De Vadder, F.; Arora, T.; Hallen, A.; Martens, E.; Björck, I.; Bäckhed, F. Dietary Fiber-Induced Improvement in Glucose Metabolism Is Associated with Increased Abundance of Prevotella. *Cell Metab.* **2015**, *22*, 971–982. [CrossRef]

10

In Vitro–In Vivo Correlations Based on In Vitro Dissolution of Parent Drug Diltiazem and Pharmacokinetics of its Metabolite

Constantin Mircioiu [1], Valentina Anuta [2], Ion Mircioiu [3], Adrian Nicolescu [4] and Nikoletta Fotaki [5,*]

1 Department of Applied Mathematics and Biostatistics, Faculty of Pharmacy, "Carol Davila" University of Medicine and Pharmacy, 020956 Bucharest, Romania
2 Department of Physical and Colloidal Chemistry, Faculty of Pharmacy, "Carol Davila" University of Medicine and Pharmacy, 020956 Bucharest, Romania
3 Department of Biopharmacy and Pharmacokinetics, Titu Maiorescu University, 004051 Bucharest, Romania
4 Department of Medicine, Queen's University, Kingston, ON K7L 3N6, Canada
5 Department of Pharmacy and Pharmacology, University of Bath, Claverton Down, Bath BA2 7AY, UK
* Correspondence: n.fotaki@bath.ac.uk

Abstract: In this study a novel type of in vitro–in vivo correlation (IVIVC) is proposed: The correlation of the in vitro parent drug dissolution data with the in vivo pharmacokinetic data of drug's metabolite after the oral administration of the parent drug. The pharmacokinetic data for the parent drug diltiazem (DTZ) and its desacetyl diltiazem metabolite (DTZM) were obtained from an in vivo study performed in 19 healthy volunteers. The pharmacokinetics of the parent drug and its metabolite followed a pseudomono-compartmental model and deconvolution of the DTZ or DTZM plasma concentration profiles was performed with a Wagner–Nelson-type equation. The calculated in vivo absorption fractions were correlated with the in vitro DTZ dissolution data obtained with USP 2 apparatus. A linear IVIVC was obtained for both DTZ and DTZM, with a better correlation observed for the case of the metabolite. This type of correlation of the in vitro data of the parent compound with the in vivo data of the metabolite could be useful for the development of drugs with active metabolites and prodrugs.

Keywords: in vitro–in vivo correlation (IVIVC); diltiazem; mathematical modeling; metabolites; dissolution

1. Introduction

One of the goals of in vitro–in vivo correlations (IVIVCs) is the estimation of the in vivo release of an active substance from orally administered pharmaceutical formulations based on in vitro dissolution data. For extended release formulations, reasonable linear correlations have been obtained from a number of IVIVC studies [1–5]. In other cases, linear correlations were not satisfactory [6–9], or the data could not be correlated [2,10,11]. Although in the case of extended release formulations linear relationships are frequently obtained, both the United States Pharmacopoeia (USP) and the Food and Drug Administration (FDA) state that non-linear models are also acceptable to describe IVIVCs [12–14]. Non-linear models have been proposed by Polli et al. and Dunne et al. [15–17]. Model-independent methods are commonly used for the development of IVIVCs, but model-dependent methods are also applied [15–20]. For example, Dunne et al. started from survival curve methods considering the time at which a drug enters the solution (in vitro or in vivo) as a random variable and correlated the in vitro and in vivo parameters postulating different relations between distribution functions or their probability densities [16,17]. The distribution functions were obtained by cumulative dissolution and the probability densities were determined by the rate at which the drug is released from the pharmaceutical formulation. These non-linear models were considered as scientifically sound IVIVCs that contrast with the "empirical" non-linear functions such as the sigmoid, Weibull, Higuchi, or Hixson–Crowell methods [21]. All these models remain essentially empirical, and the more complex the model is the more unstable is the fitting algorithm and the risk of non-uniqueness of the solutions [22,23].

Diltiazem (DTZ), a benzothiazepine calcium channel blocker, has been widely used in the treatment of stable, variant, and unstable angina pectoris, systemic hypertension, and supraventricular tachycardias [24,25]. It is subjected to extensive and highly variable hepatic first-pass metabolism by CYP3A4, and only 2%–4% of the unchanged drug is excreted in the urine. The pharmacokinetics of DTZ in healthy volunteers indicated a biphasic elimination with a distribution half-life of 0.3 ± 0.2 h, an elimination half-life of 3.1 ± 1 h and an apparent volume of distribution of 5.3 ± 1.7 L/kg after intravenous (i.v.) administration of 15 mg, and an elimination half-life of 3.2 ± 1.3 h after oral administration of 60 mg [26]. The absolute bioavailability of DTZ ranged from 24% to 74% (mean 42% ± 18%), and the inter-individual variability may be explained by the highly variable first-pass effect [24]. Non-linearity and a slight increase of the half-life were observed when the dose was increased. Notably, in young healthy volunteers DTZ did not show linear kinetics between single and multiple doses [27].

DTZ has several metabolites in humans: Desacetyl DTZ (DTZM), N-monodesmethyl DTZ, desacetyl N-monodesmethyl DTZ, and desacetyl DTZ N-oxide, with average maximum plasma concentrations of 10%, 15%, 26%, and 13%, respectively, of the mean maximum DTZ concentration [28]. Therefore, the analysis of the pharmacokinetics of DTZ and its metabolites, as well as the development of IVIVCs can be useful in improving the general administration schedule, the personalization of therapy and the development of DTZ formulations for oral administration.

The aim of this study was to develop IVIVCs for orally administered DTZ formulations. Apart from the traditional IVIVC approach in which the in vitro drug dissolution is correlated with its in vivo absorption calculated by deconvolution, a novel method was developed. The in vitro dissolution of DTZ was correlated to the in vivo absorption estimated by a deconvolution method that uses the pharmacokinetic data of the active metabolite (DTZM). This approach could be valuable for the development of IVIVCs for drugs with significant plasma levels of metabolites.

2. Materials and Methods

2.1. Chemicals and Reagents

Diltiazem hydrochloride (batch 4) and haloperidol (batch 1) reference standards were purchased from the European Directorate for the Quality of Medicines (EDQM, Strasbourg, France), while desacetyl diltiazem hydrochloride (batch JOC143) was obtained from the United States Pharmacopeia (USP, Rockville, MD, USA). Cardiazem® 60 mg tablets (Hoechst Marion Roussel, batch number 1099841) were used for the in vitro and in vivo studies.

HPLC gradient grade acetonitrile and methanol were purchased from Merck KGaA (Darmstadt, Germany), whereas HPLC grade methyl tert-butyl ether was acquired from Sigma-Aldrich (Taufkirchen, Germany). All other reagents were of analytical grade and used without further purification. Ultrapure water (resistivity 18.2 MΩ·cm at 25 °C, Total Organic Carbon (TOC) < 5 ppb) was obtained from a Milli-Q (Millipore, Milford, MA, USA) water purification system. Blank human plasma was obtained from the Army Centre of Transfusion Hematology (Bucharest, Romania).

2.2. In Vitro Dissolution Studies

Dissolution studies of Cardiazem® 60 mg tablets were performed using a USP 2 dissolution apparatus (DT 800 Erweka GmbH, Heusenstamm, Germany) at 75 rpm. The dissolution medium (ultrapure water, 900 mL) was deaerated and maintained at 37 ± 0.5 °C. Aliquots of 5 ± 0.1 mL were withdrawn at 10, 15, 20, 30, 60, 120, and 180 min, and immediately replaced with an equal volume of fresh medium maintained at the same temperature. The samples were filtered through a 0.45 μm Teflon® filter, and the drug concentrations were determined by measuring the absorbance of each sample at 237 nm on a V-530 UV-VIS spectrophotometer (JASCO Ltd., Tokio, Japan). Diltiazem concentrations were calculated from linear calibration curves. Dissolution data for each compound are reported as mean values of 12 replicates, and the coefficient of variation (CV%; [mean value/standard deviation] × 100%) was calculated.

2.3. Clinical Study

In vivo data were obtained in a pharmacokinetic study after administration of two 60 mg Cardiazem® tablets to 19 healthy volunteers in a single-dose study under fasting conditions.

The study was carried out in accordance with the basic principles defined in the Helsinki Declaration of 1964 as revised in 2013, as well as with the International Conference on Harmonization (ICH) Good Clinical Practice regulations. The study was conducted at the National Institute for Aeronautical and Space Medicine «Gen. Dr. Av. Victor Atanasiu» within the Central Clinical Emergency Military Hospital in Bucharest (Romania).

The study protocol (protocol code: DILTZARE155/2002) was approved by the Institutional Ethics Committee of Biopharmacy & Pharmacol Res S.A. (approval number 32, 4 July 2007), as well as by the Romanian National Agency for Medicines and Medical Devices (approval number 337, 24 July 2007).

The study subjects ($n = 19$) were of Caucasian race, aged between 19 and 30 years (24.3 ± 3.34) and with a body mass index between 19 and 27 (22.43 ± 1.87). All subjects were healthy according to their medical and social history, physical examination, and laboratory tests. The subjects had no history of drug or alcohol abuse, hypersensitivity to the investigational products, and did not take any medication for two weeks before dosing. Alcohol, tobacco, as well as caffeine containing beverages were forbidden for 48 h before as well as during the study. All subjects gave written informed consent prior to study enrolment and were allowed to terminate their participation in the trial at any time, without restrictions. Standard meals were provided to the subjects at four and nine hours after drug administration.

Venous blood samples (5 mL) were collected into heparinized tubes through a catheter inserted in the antecubital vein before (time 0) and at 0.5, 1, 1.5, 2, 2.5, 3, 3.5, 4, 5, 6, 7, 8, 10, 12, and 24 h after drug administration. Blood samples were centrifuged at 5 °C for six minutes at approx. 3000 rpm. Plasma was separated in two equal aliquots (1.2–1.3 mL), transferred to labeled 1.5 mL polypropylene tubes and immediately frozen and stored at a < −20 °C until analysis.

2.4. Sample Treatment

Plasma samples (500 μL) were transferred to 10 mL disposable polypropylene tubes, to which 100 μL internal standard (IS) solution (containing 10 μg/mL haloperidol in methanol), 200 μL 0.2 M dipotassium phosphate buffer pH = 9 and 3 mL methyl *tert*-butyl ether were added. The tubes were vortex-mixed for 10 min and then centrifuged for 10 min at 4000 rpm. Of the organic layer 2.5 mL were removed and extracted with 200 μL 0.025 M phosphoric acid solution. After shaking for 10 min and centrifugation for 10 min at 4000 rpm, 25 μL of the acidic aqueous phase were analyzed by HPLC.

2.5. Preparation of Standard Solutions and Quality Control Samples

The stock solutions of DTZ and DTZM were prepared by dissolving an appropriate amount of each reference standard in methanol to yield concentrations of 100 μg/mL and 50 μg/mL, respectively, and serially diluted with the same solvent. 10 μL of the diluted solutions of each analyte were spiked into 80 μL of blank plasma, in order to obtain the calibration standard solutions with final concentrations of 2.5, 5, 10, 25, 50, 100, 250, and 500 ng/mL for DTZ and 1.25, 2.5, 5, 12.5, 25, 50 125, and 250 ng/mL for DTZM.

Quality control (QC) samples were prepared similarly, in order to obtain concentrations at the lower limit of quantification (LLOQ; 2.5 ng/mL for DTZ and 1.25 ng/mL for DTZM), and at low (QC_{low}

= 7.5 ng/mL DTZ and 3.75 ng/mL DTZM), medium (QC_{med} = 150 ng/mL DTZ and 75 ng/mL DTZM), and high (QC_{high} = 300 ng/mL DTZ and 150 ng/mL DTZM) concentration levels.

All stock and standard solutions were protected from light and stored at −20 °C until use.

2.6. Chromatographic Analysis

Chromatographic analyses were performed on a Waters liquid chromatographic system (Milford, MA 01757, USA) consisting of a quaternary gradient system (600E Multisolvent Delivery System), in line degasser (Waters model AF), UV tunable absorbance detector (Waters model 486), and auto sampler (Waters model 717 plus). Empower Pro software (Waters, Milford, MA 01757, USA) was used to control the system, acquire and process data. The UV detector was set at 235 nm. The chromatographic separation was achieved on an Ascentis 5C18, 5-μm 150 × 2.1 mm column (Supelco, Bellefonte, PA 16823, USA) at a constant temperature (35 °C). The mobile phase consisted of an isocratic mixture of 0.025 M potassium di-hydrogen phosphate buffer containing 0.2% triethylamine adjusted to pH 2.2 and acetonitrile in a 72:28 (*v/v*) ratio, and delivered at 0.35 mL/min flow rate. Of each sample 25 μL were injected into the chromatographic column.

Method validation was performed in accordance with the bioanalytical method validation guidelines of the FDA, including selectivity, linearity, limits of quantification, accuracy, precision, recovery, dilution effects, and stability [29]. Assay specificity was evaluated in relation to interferences from the endogenous matrix components of drug free plasma samples of six different origins. The calibration curves of both DTZ and DTZM were constructed by plotting DTZ or DTZM to IS peak area ratios versus concentration (ng/mL), using data obtained from triplicate analysis of the calibration standard solution (in the range 2.5–500 ng/mL for DTZ and 1.25–250 ng/mL for DTZM). The lower limit of quantification (LLOQ) was set as the lowest concentration on the calibration curve. Within-run and between runs precision and accuracy were estimated by analyzing five replicates of the LLOQ and the QC samples in a single analytical run and on five consecutive days, respectively. The acceptance criteria for precision and accuracy were: Relative Standard Deviation (RSD)% ≤15% and bias within ±15% for the QC samples and RSD% ≤20% and bias within ±20% for the LLOQ samples. The absolute recovery of DTZ and DTZM was determined using five replicates of the three concentration level QC samples. Bench-top, extract, stock solution, freeze-and-thaw, long-term, and post-preparative stability studies were also performed to evaluate the stability of both DTZ and DTZM.

2.7. Treatment of In Vivo Data

Estimation of pharmacokinetic parameters of the in vivo parameters by non-compartmental analysis was performed using subroutines of the KINETICA 4.2 software (Innaphase Corp, Philadelphia, PA 19102, USA). The maximum concentration (C_{max}) and the corresponding peak times (T_{max}) were determined from the individual drug plasma concentration-time profiles. The elimination rate constant (k_e) was obtained from the least-square fitted terminal log-linear portion of the plasma concentration–time profile. The elimination half-life ($t_{1/2}$) was calculated as $0.693/k_e$. The area under the curve to the last measurable concentration (AUC_{0-t}) was calculated by the trapezoidal rule method. The area under the curve extrapolated to infinity ($AUC_{0-\infty}$) was calculated as $AUC_{0-t} + C_t/k_e$, where C_t is the last measurable concentration. Shapiro–Wilk statistic W-test (SW–W) was used to evaluate normality of data distribution, with a $p < 0.05$ set as threshold for statistical significance.

Compartmental analysis of the in vivo data was performed using TOPFIT 2.0 software (Thomae GmbH, Germany). Fitting performance was assessed based on the Akaike (AIC) and Schwarz (SC) criteria (both based on the sum of "errors" corrected by a "penalty" function proportional to the number of parameters model: $AIC = N \cdot lnSS + 2p$; $SC = N \cdot lnSS + p \cdot lnN$) [22], where N is the sample size (i.e., number of data points), p represents the number of model parameters and SS is the sum of squares error.

The significance of the differences in the fitting performance of two nested models, a more complicated one (with p parameters) and a simpler one (with q parameters, $q < p$), was evaluated by comparing the relative increase in the sum of squares $\left(\frac{SS_q - SS_p}{SS_p}\right)$ with the relative decrease in degrees of freedom $\left(\frac{df_q - df_p}{df_p}\right)$ going from the more complicated to the simpler model, based on the F ratio:

$$F = \frac{SS_q - SS_p}{SS_p} \frac{df_p}{df_q - df_p}$$

where the degrees of freedom *df* equals the difference between the sample size *N* and the number of parameters of each model ($df_p = N - p$ and $df_q = N - q$, respectively).

A model is considered more efficient if it is simple, has a minimum number of parameters, is "phenomenologically" justified and errors are comparable with experimental errors and physiological variability.

2.8. Model-Independent Estimation of In Vivo Absorption/Dissolution by the Deconvolution of In Vivo Pharmacokinetics

The fraction of drug absorbed was calculated using the Wagner–Nelson equation [30]:

$$FRA(t_i) = \frac{c_{pd}(t_i) + \int_0^{t_i} k_e c_{pd} dt}{\int_0^{\infty} k_e c_{pd} dt} = \frac{c_{pd}(t_i) + k_e AUC(PD)_{0-t_i}}{k_e AUC(PD)_{0-\infty}},$$

where, *FRA*(t_i), fraction of the drug absorbed at time t_i; $c_{pd}(t_i)$, plasma concentration of the parent drug at time t_i; k_e, elimination rate constant for the parent drug; $AUC(PD)_{0-t_i}$, area under the concentration–time curve of the parent drug from time 0 to time t_i; $AUC(PD)_{0-\infty}$, area under the concentration–time curve of the parent drug from time 0 to infinity.

In the case of metabolites, a Wagner–Nelson type equation was applied for the calculation of the apparent fraction of the metabolized drug (FRM):

$$FRM(t_i) = \frac{c_m(t_i) + \int_0^{t_i} k_e^m c_m dt}{\int_0^{\infty} k_e^m c_m dt} = \frac{c_m(t_i) + k_e^m [AUC - M]_{0-t_i}}{k_e^m [AUC - M]_{0-\infty}},$$

where, *FRM*(t_i), fraction of the metabolized drug at time t_i; $c_m(t_i)$, plasma concentration of the metabolite at time t_i; k_e^m, elimination rate constant of the metabolite.

The elimination rate constant was estimated by performing both a non-compartmental analysis (linear regression of the last points of the logarithmic data) and a one-compartmental modeling of the mean plasma levels.

If the absorption and metabolism can be assumed to be rapid, *FRM*(t_i) could be considered an estimation of *FRA*(t_i). Based on this assumption, an in vitro dissolution–in vivo metabolism correlation could be expected.

3. Results

3.1. In Vitro Dissolution of Diltiazem

The individual DTZ dissolution profiles in water are presented in Figure 1 and the mean % dissolved over time are shown in Table 1. A 80.92% DTZ dissolved is observed after 3 h. Since DTZ is lipophilic (logP 2.7) [31], its administration as a hydrochloride salt helps the rapid dissolution in the stomach. Its precipitation in the intestine is likely unavoidable (pKa = 8.06) and could account for its absorption variability. Based on the small variability of the in vitro dissolution profiles, as revealed by the low values of CV% (Table 1), the mean dissolution profile can be used for the development of IVIVCs.

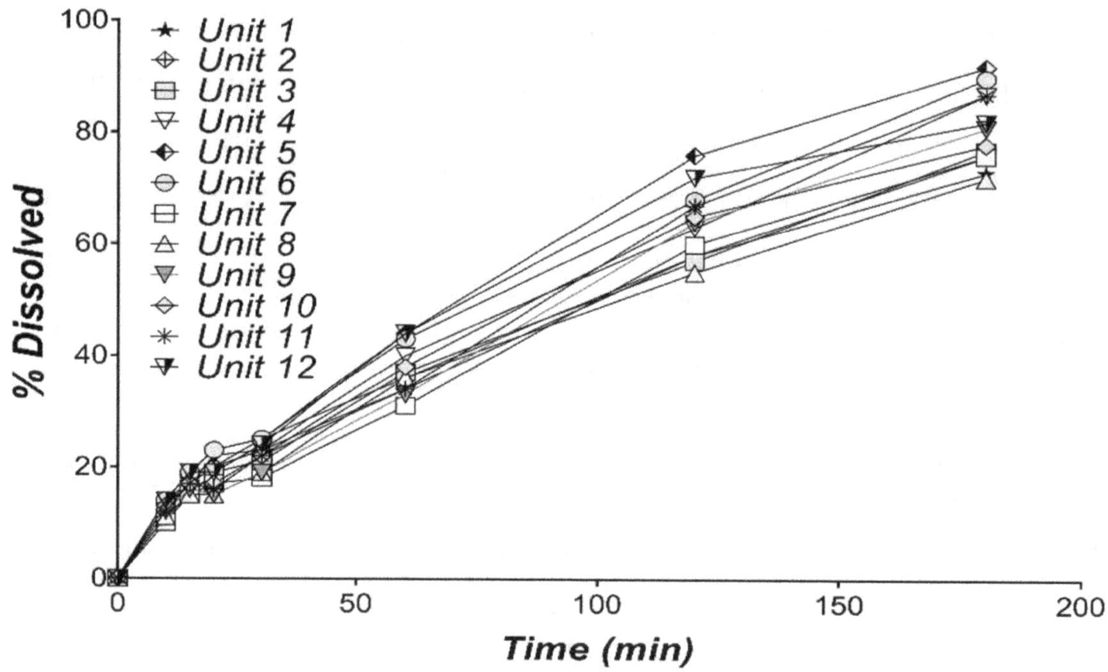

Figure 1. Individual in vitro dissolution profiles of DTZ from 60 mg Cardiazem® tablets in 900 mL water, using USP Apparatus 2, at 75 rpm (n = 12).

Table 1. In vitro dissolution of DTZ from 60 mg Cardiazem® tablets in 900 mL water, using USP Apparatus 2, at 75 rpm (n = 12).

Time (min)	Dissolved (%)	CV (%)
10	12.42	10.56
15	17.00	9.04
20	18.67	15.88
30	22.17	11.19
60	37.67	10.46
120	63.58	9.66
180	80.92	8.29

3.2. Chromatographic Method Validation

No interference between the endogenous matrix components and DTZ or DTZM was observed, indicating selectivity of the HPLC method in the plasma samples (Figure 2). Calibration curves were linear over the concentration range 2.5–500 ng/mL for DTZ (Y = 1.21e–003X + 2.03e–003; R^2 = 0.9997), and 1.25–250 ng/mL for DTZM (Y = 1.59e–003X + 2.33e–004; R^2 = 0.9997).

The LLOQ was 2.5 ng/mL for DTZ and 1.25 ng/mL for DTZM, suggesting a good sensitivity of the analytical method.

Both within-run and between runs accuracy and precision were within the accepted limits (Table 2) for the LLOQ and all the QC samples. The within-run precision (RSD%) ranged between 1.19% and 5.71%, whereas accuracy (% bias versus nominal concentration) ranged between 0.25% and 3.76%; the between run precision (RSD%) was between 3.53% and 8.03% whereas the % bias versus the nominal concentration was lower than 6% (Table 2).

The mean absolute recovery in plasma was 105.19% ± 4.81% for DTZ, 96.52 ± 5.59 for DTZM and 91.11 ± 3.32 for the IS, indicating lack of interference from the sample preparation method. Dilution effect was not observed either for DTZ or DTZM by means of a five-fold dilution with blank plasma.

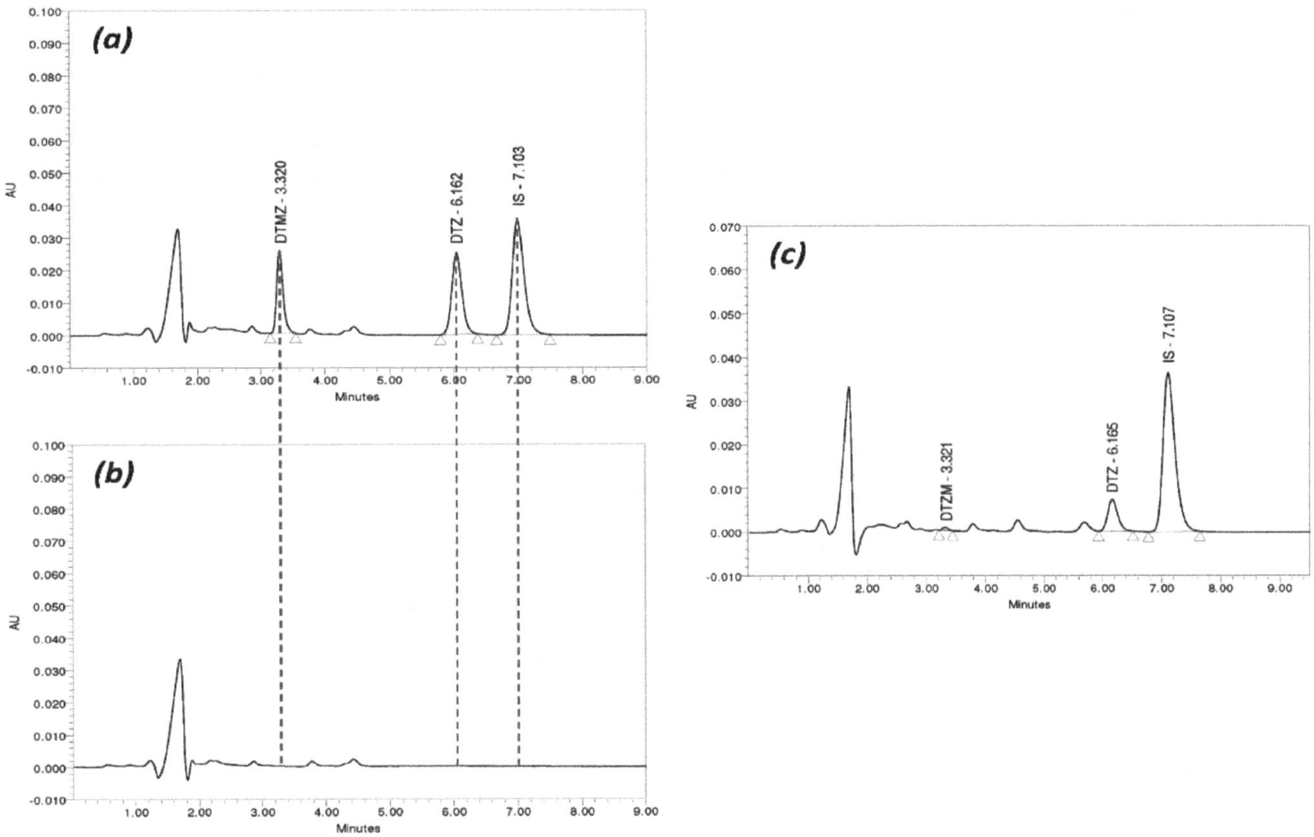

Figure 2. Typical HPLC chromatograms of DTZ and DTZM in plasma: (**a**) Chromatogram of a standard sample containing DTZ (500 ng/mL) and DTZM (250 ng/mL) and internal standard (IS); (**b**) chromatogram of blank plasma; (**c**) chromatogram of a plasma sample obtained from one on the study subjects two hours after drug administration (DTZ—154.4 ng/mL, DTZM—3.9 ng/mL).

Table 2. Accuracy and precision data for the determination of diltiazem (DTZ) and desacetyl DTZ (DTZM) in human plasma.

Sample Code	DTZ				DTZM			
	Nominal conc. (ng/mL)	Measured conc. (Mean ± SD, ng/mL)	RSD (%)	Bias (%)	Nominal conc. (ng/mL)	Measured conc. (Mean ± SD, ng/mL)	RSD (%)	Bias (%)
				Within-run				
LLOQ	2.5	2.49 ± 0.14	5.71	−0.56	1.25	1.26 ± 0.05	3.79	0.40
QC_{low}	7.5	7.48 ± 0.29	3.89	−0.25	3.75	3.72 ± 0.14	3.73	−0.85
QC_{med}	150	148.83 ± 2.76	1.85	−0.78	75	72.18 ± 1.65	2.29	−3.76
QC_{high}	300	310.46 ± 3.70	1.19	3.49	150	146.26 ± 2.47	1.69	−2.49
				Between runs				
LLOQ	2.5	2.63 ± 0.17	6.43	5.04	1.25	1.32 ± 0.07	5.32	5.60
QC_{low}	7.5	7.52 ± 0.31	4.15	0.24	3.75	3.74 ± 0.30	8.03	−0.30
QC_{med}	150	146.22 ± 6.68	4.57	−2.52	75	73.71 ± 3.42	4.64	−1.72
QC_{high}	300	298.91 ± 12.52	4.19	−0.36	150	149.37 ± 5.27	3.53	−0.42

Both DTZ and DTZM were stable in plasma for 5 h at room temperature, for 27 h during the chromatographic analysis (placed in autosampler) and for 97 days at −20 °C. There was no observed degradation of the samples under three cycles of freezing and thawing.

Typical HPLC chromatograms of DTZ and DTZM in plasma are presented in Figure 2.

3.3. *Pharmacokinetics of Diltiazem and Its Metabolite*

The individual and mean plasma level profiles of DTZ and DTZM after oral administration of 120 mg of DTZ (two 60 mg Cardiazem® tablets) were relatively homogenously distributed in the concentration–time space (Figure 3). The data could be interpreted as revealing three clusters, i.e., three volunteers with high, one with low plasma levels, and the remaining 15 volunteers having homogenously distributed profiles. The plasma concentrations of the metabolite DTZM were approximately 20 times lower than those of the parent drug.

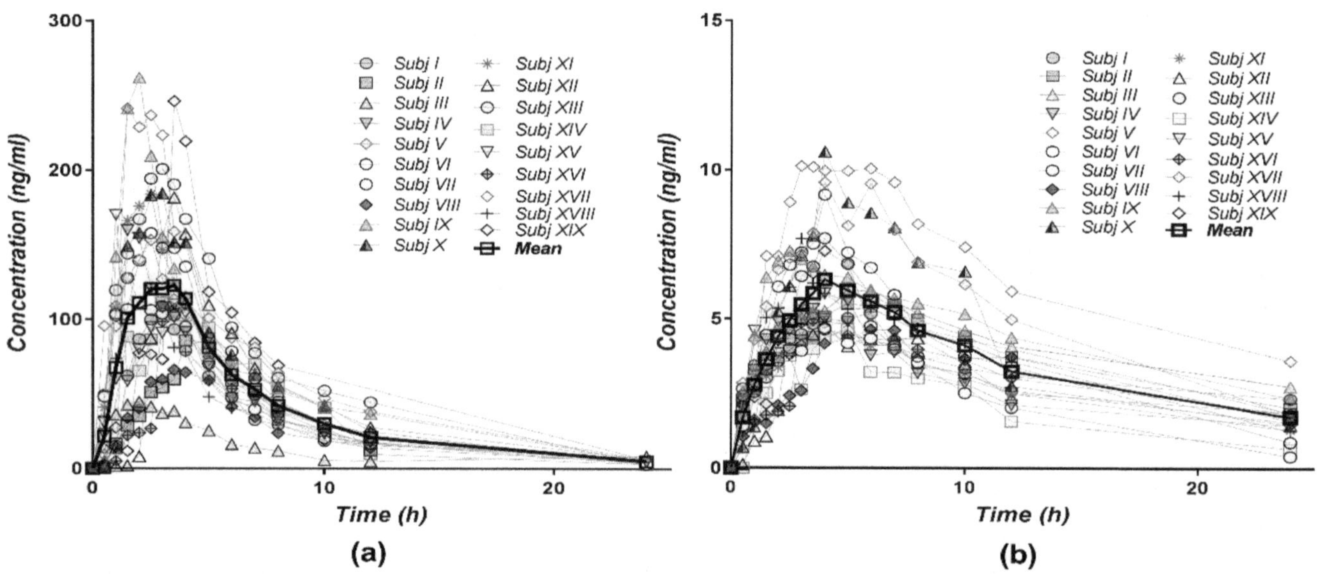

Figure 3. Individual and mean plasma concentration–time profiles for (**a**) DTZ and (**b**) DTZM after single dose oral administration of 120 mg diltiazem (2 × 60 mg Cardiazem® tablets) to 19 healthy subjects.

The distribution of the areas under curves of the plasma concentration profiles after the administration of 120 mg of DTZ in the 19 healthy volunteers was approximately normal (Figure 4).

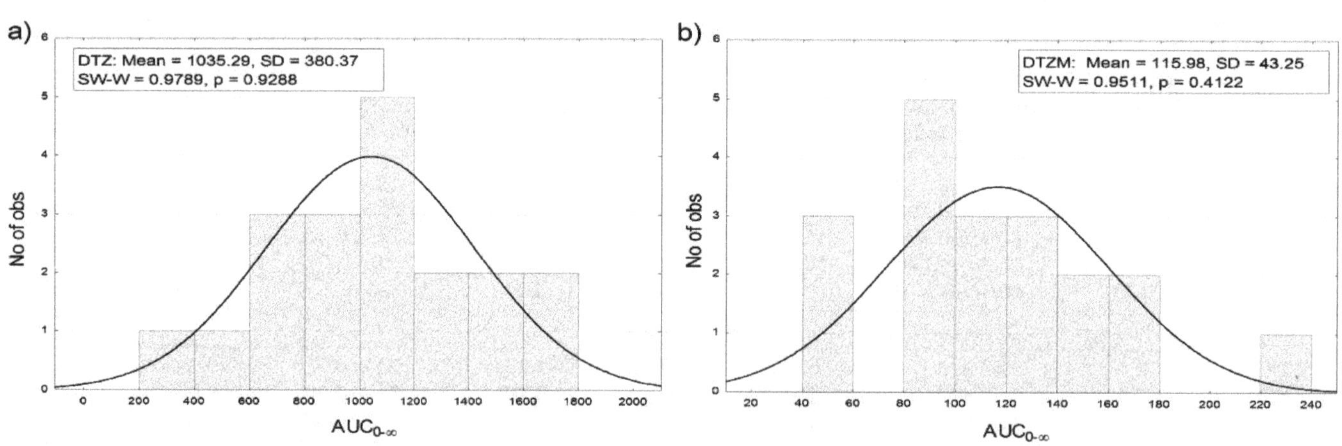

Figure 4. Frequency distribution of $AUC_{0-\infty}$ for (**a**) DTZ and (**b**) DTZM after the oral administration of 120 mg of DTZ in 19 healthy subjects (the observed significance level p of the Shapiro–Wilk statistic W (SW–W) indicates normality of the distribution ($p < 0.05$)).

The summary of the main pharmacokinetic parameters of DTZ and DTZM in the 19 healthy volunteers, estimated by non-compartmental analysis, is presented in Table 3.

Table 3. Summary pharmacokinetic parameters of DTZ and DTZM in healthy subjects estimated by non-compartmental analysis.

Parameter	DTZ		DTZM	
	Mean	SD	Mean	SD
C_{max} (ng/mL)	154	59.6	6.66	1.98
T_{max} (h)	2.66	0.898	4	1.12
k_e (1/h)	0.157	0.0237	0.074	0.0325
$t_{1/2}$ (h)	4.51	0.655	11.2	5.25

3.4. Compartmental Modeling of Diltiazem and Its Metabolite Pharmacokinetics

The pharmacokinetics of DTZ and DTZM were evaluated based on compartmental modeling. Based on work performed previously, it has been shown that the pharmacokinetics of the metabolites usually follow a pseudomono-compartmental model [32–34]. The pharmacokinetic modeling of DTZ and DTZM revealed that the mean plasma levels can be acceptably described by a one-compartment model after introducing a short lag-time (Figure 5). The use of the two compartmental model was just marginally better based on the Akaike and Schwarz criteria (Figure 6). Therefore, increase of the number of the parameters was not selected, as models with a high number of parameters are highly unstable, since small perturbations in the input data can lead to high differences in the solutions [23].

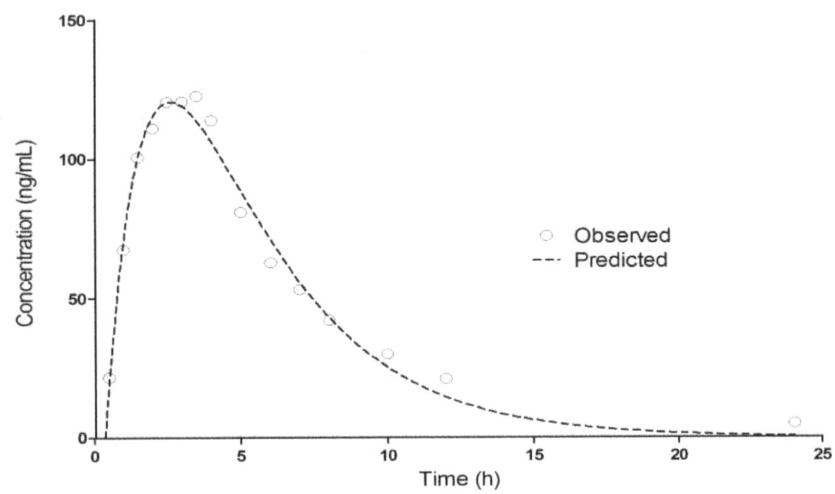

Figure 5. One-compartment pharmacokinetic modeling of DTZ mean plasma levels after oral administration of 120 mg DTZ (2 × 60 mg Cardiazem® tablets) in 19 healthy subjects.

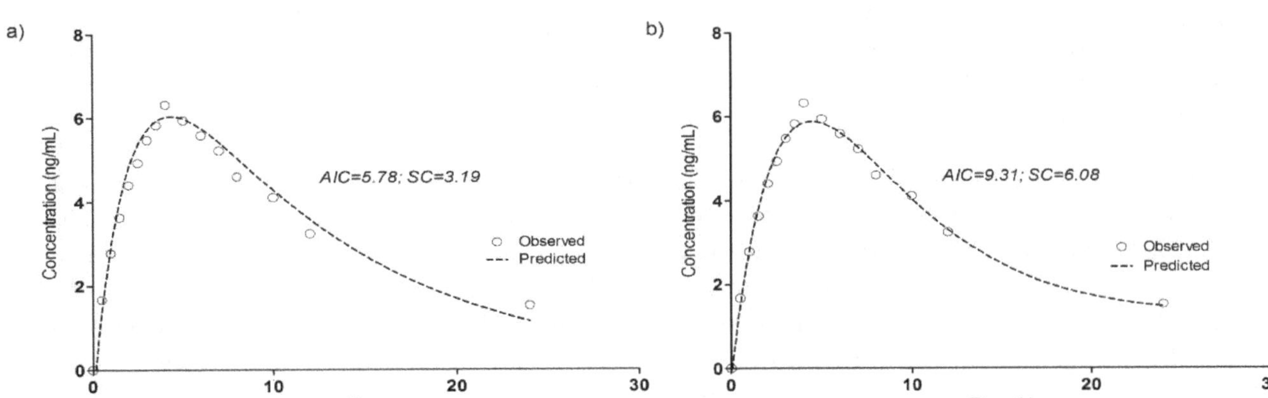

Figure 6. Pharmacokinetic modeling of DTZM mean plasma levels after oral administration of 120 mg DTZ (2 × 60 mg Cardiazem® tablets) in 19 healthy subjects. (**a**) One-compartment model; (**b**) two-compartment model.

The derived pharmacokinetic parameters from the one compartmental modeling of the mean plasma levels of DTZ and DTZM after the oral administration of 120 mg DTZ are summarized in Table 4.

Table 4. Pharmacokinetic parameters of DTZ and DTZM estimated by one-compartmental analysis of the mean concentration–time profiles after the oral administration of 120 mg of DTZ to 19 healthy subjects.

Parameter	DTZ	DTZM
k_e (1/h)	0.2861	0.0945
k_a (1/h)	0.0655	0.492
T_{lag} (h)	0.36	0.162
C_{max} (ng/mL)	120.5	6.04
T_{max} (h)	2.51	4.20
$AUC_{0-\infty}$ (ng/mL·h)	800.9	94.66
$t_{1/2}$ (h)	2.42	7.34

3.5. Model-Independent Estimation of In Vivo Absorption/Dissolution

The fractions of DTZ and DTZM absorbed over time as calculated by the Wagner–Nelson equations are presented in Figure 7. As the parent drug and metabolite follow a one-compartmental pharmacokinetic model (as presented in the previous section), this model independent deconvolution approach with the Wagner–Nelson method can be successfully applied to the in vivo DTZ and DTZM plasma concentration profiles.

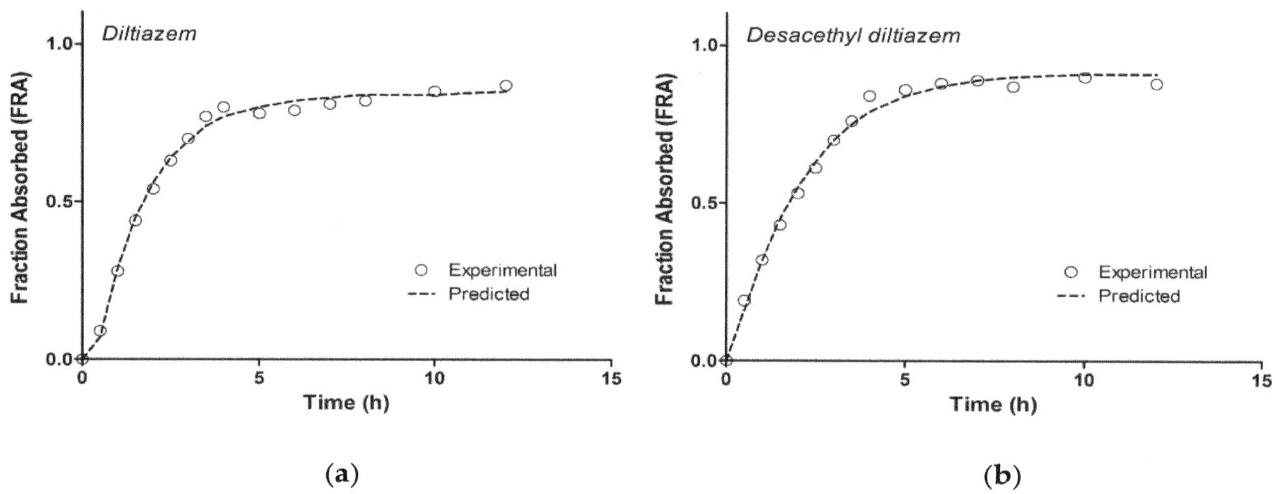

Figure 7. Fraction absorbed profiles calculated for (**a**) DTZ and (**b**) DTZM; observed: profiles calculated based on estimation of elimination rate constant with non-compartmental analysis, predicted: profiles calculated based on estimation of elimination rate constant with one-compartmental pharmacokinetic modeling.

The fraction absorbed profiles calculated based on estimation of elimination rate constant with both methods (non-compartmental analysis and one-compartmental pharmacokinetic modeling) were similar for DTZ and DTZM, revealing that the method used for the estimation of the elimination rate constant was robust. In the case of the DTZM, the elimination profile was simple and further metabolism was not observed. Furthermore, given the more polar character of DTZM compared to DTZ, its biliary excretion is less significant. Consequently, the variability of metabolite's elimination constant should be lower than that of the parent drug. This is an important argument for using the metabolite plasma levels rather than those of the parent drug for estimating the in vivo dissolution of the parent drug. The results obtained by following a Wagner–Nelson approach reflect the combination of the in vivo dissolution, absorption and metabolism of the parent drug. In this chain of processes, the slowest process determines the overall result.

3.6. Correlation of Apparent Absorbed/Metabolized Fraction with In Vitro Dissolution of Diltiazem

Since it is not possible to estimate separately the in vivo dissolution, gastric empting, absorption, and metabolism of the parent drug, a mechanistic approach is not realistic. Therefore, an empirical approach was followed. The "apparent fraction absorption" calculated from plasma levels of DTZ and DTZM was correlated with the in vitro dissolution of DTZ. A Level A correlation between in vitro dissolution and estimated in vivo dissolution starting from the parent drug and its metabolite plasma level was achieved (Figure 8). Both correlations were linear, with correlation coefficients greater than 0.98.

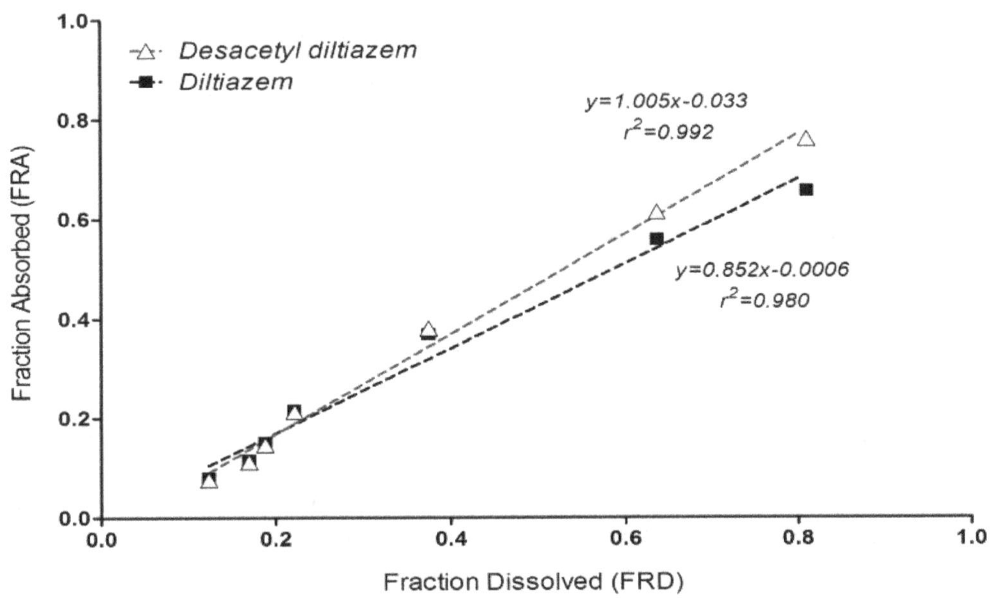

Figure 8. In vitro–in vivo correlation (IVIVC) model for DTZ (■) and DTZM (△).

The slope of the IVIVC model based on "metabolite pharmacokinetics—dissolution of parent drug" is close to 1, suggesting a superposition of the in vitro dissolution with the in vivo estimated absorption/dissolution from the pharmacokinetics of the metabolite.

4. Discussion

Considering the pharmacokinetics of drugs that undergo substantial metabolism, that would be classified as BDDCS (Biopharmaceutics Drug Disposition Classification System) Class 1 and 2 compounds [35], the following essential sequence should be considered: in vivo dissolution (correlated with the in vitro dissolution), absorption, and metabolism of the parent drug.

Since the rate and extent of absorption, and the metabolism are usually high, the slowest rate-determining step for the kinetics of entire process remains the release/dissolution of the parent drug from the pharmaceutical formulation. Consequently, the rate of metabolite appearance in the plasma is determined by the rate and extent of parent drug release and dissolution from the pharmaceutical formulation (Figure 9).

Since DTZ is lipophilic (logP 2.79) [31], the transfer rate constant from blood to peripheral compartments is higher than the reverse transport. The rate of return of DTZ to the blood would be small and could be neglected, and the transfer from the blood to the peripheral compartments can be integrated in a total elimination rate constant of the parent drug, k_e^{pd} (Figure 10).

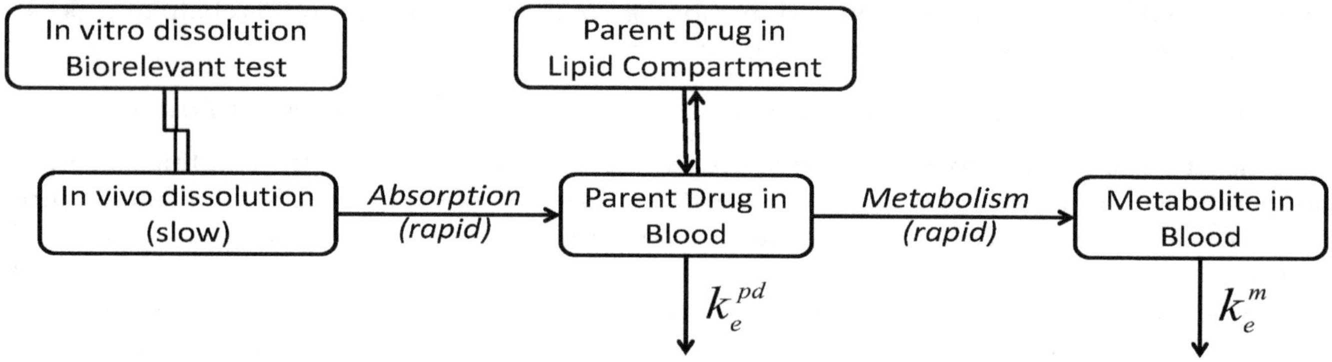

Figure 9. Schematic of processes involved in the pharmacokinetics of drugs that undergo substantial metabolism.

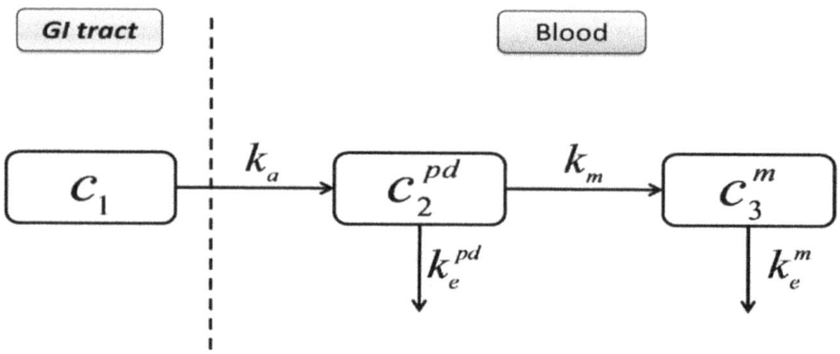

Figure 10. Simplified compartmental model describing the pharmacokinetics of DTZ and DTZM.

If the elimination of the metabolite is not rate limiting (that is when the slowest step is the elimination of the parent drug), the terminal half-life of the metabolite is the same or lower than the terminal half-life of the parent drug. This would be expected, as one of the "objectives" of metabolism is the transformation of drugs in more polar components, for an easier elimination. A one-compartment model can describe the pharmacokinetics of the metabolite, based on the following equation for extravascular administration: $c_m(T) = Ae^{-k_a T} + Be^{-k_e^m T}$. The apparent absorption rate constant k_a is a function of the in vivo dissolution, absorption, distribution, metabolism, and elimination of the parent drug, and k_e^m is the elimination rate constant for the metabolite. Consequently, it is expected that in vitro dissolution of parent drug - in vivo pharmacokinetics of metabolites correlations are possible for these drugs, and that these correlations account for the entire chain of in vivo processes, i.e., dissolution, absorption, metabolism of the parent drug, and direct appearance of the metabolite in the plasma.

The success of the correlation between the in vitro and in vivo dissolution would depend on the in vitro dissolution method. The good correlations between the in vitro dissolution of DTZ and the apparent absorption of DTZ, suggest that the rate determining process is the in vivo dissolution of the parent drug. In this study a successful prediction of DTZ pharmacokinetics after a single dose based on in vitro data only could be achieved.

5. Conclusions

Pharmacokinetic modeling of DTZ and DTZM mean plasma levels suggests a one-compartmental behavior. In the case of DTZ and, more generally, in the case of compounds subjected to extensive metabolism (BDDCS Class 1 and Class 2 compounds), the in vivo dissolution, absorption, metabolism of the parent drug, and the elimination of the metabolite would take place. Since the rate of absorption and the metabolism of BDDCS Class 1 and Class 2 compounds drugs are usually high, the rate of the appearance of the metabolites in the plasma is determined by the rate and extent of parent drug release from the pharmaceutical formulation. Under these conditions, a deconvolution method, similar to that of Wagner–Nelson method, can be applied to calculate the absorption and in vivo dissolution of a parent drug starting from the plasma levels of one of its metabolites. The correlation of the estimated in vivo dissolution curves with the in vitro dissolution curves proved to be linear, and in the case of the metabolite a very good superposition of the in vivo and in vitro dissolution kinetics was achieved. Upon further validation with more drugs, this type of correlations could be used for drugs with extensive metabolism, in which the plasma levels of the active metabolites that follow pseudomono-compartmental kinetics are higher than those of the parent drug.

Author Contributions: Conceptualization, C.M., V.A. and N.F.; methodology, V.A. and I.M.; software, V.A.; validation, V.A., N.F. and A.N.; formal analysis, I.M.; investigation, I.M.; resources, C.M.; data curation, A.N.; writing—original draft preparation, V.A.; writing—review and editing, N.F.; visualization, V.A.; supervision, C.M.; project administration, V.A.

References

1. Humbert, H.; Bosshardt, H.; Cabiac, M.-D.; Cabiac, M. In Vitro-in Vivo Correlation of a Modified-Release Oral Form of Ketotifen: In Vitro Dissolution Rate Specification. *J. Pharm. Sci.* **1994**, *83*, 131–136. [CrossRef] [PubMed]
2. Eddington, N.D.; Marroum, P.; Uppoor, R.; Hussain, A.; Augsburger, L. Development and Internal Validation of an In Vitro-in Vivo Correlation for a Hydrophilic Metoprolol Tartrate Extended Release Tablet Formulation. *Pharm. Res.* **1998**, *15*, 466–473. [CrossRef]
3. Mahayni, H.; Rekhi, G.; Uppoor, R.; Marroum, P.; Hussain, A.; Augsburger, L.; Eddington, N. Evaluation of "External" Predictability of an In Vitro–In Vivo Correlation for an Extended-Release Formulation Containing Metoprolol Tartrate. *J. Pharm. Sci.* **2000**, *89*, 1354–1361. [CrossRef]
4. Takka, S.; Rajbhandari, S.; Sakr, A. Effect of anionic polymers on the release of propranolol hydrochloride from matrix tablets. *Eur. J. Pharm. Biopharm.* **2001**, *52*, 75–82. [CrossRef]
5. Emami, J. In vitro-in vivo correlation: From theory to applications. *J. Pharm. Pharm. Sci.* **2006**, *9*, 169–189.
6. Lake, O.; Olling, M.; Barends, D. In vitro/in vivo correlations of dissolution data of carbamazepine immediate release tablets with pharmacokinetic data obtained in healthy volunteers. *Eur. J. Pharm. Biopharm.* **1999**, *48*, 13–19. [CrossRef]
7. Varshosaz, J.; Ghafghazi, T.; Raisi, A.; Falamarzian, M. Biopharmaceutical characterization of oral theophylline and aminophylline tablets. Quantitative correlation between dissolution and bioavailability studies. *Eur. J. Pharm. Biopharm.* **2000**, *50*, 301–306. [CrossRef]
8. Rao, B.S.; Seshasayana, A.; Saradhi, S.P.; Kumar, N.R.; Narayan, C.P.; Murthy, K.R. Correlation of 'in vitro' release and 'in vivo' absorption characteristics of rifampicin from ethylcellulose coated nonpareil beads. *Int. J. Pharm.* **2001**, *230*, 1–9.
9. Al-Behaisi, S.; Antal, I.; Morovján, G.; Szunyog, J.; Drabant, S.; Marton, S.; Klebovich, I. In vitro simulation of food effect on dissolution of deramciclane film-coated tablets and correlation with in vivo data in healthy volunteers. *Eur. J. Pharm. Sci.* **2002**, *15*, 157–162. [CrossRef]
10. Mircioiu, C.; Mircioiu, I.; Voicu, V.; Miron, D. Dissolution-Bioequivalence Non-Correlations. *Basic Clin. Pharmacol. Toxicol.* **2005**, *96*, 262–264. [CrossRef]
11. Meyer, M.C.; Straughn, A.B.; Mhatre, R.M.; Shah, V.P.; Williams, R.L.; Lesko, L.J. Lack of In Vivo/In Vitro Correlations for 50 mg and 250 mg Primidone Tablets. *Pharm. Res.* **1998**, *15*, 1085–1089. [CrossRef]
12. Food and Drug Administration-Center for Drug Evaluation and Research (CDER). Guidance for Industry: Extended Release Oral Dosage Forms: Development, Evaluation, and Application of In Vitro/In Vivo Correlations. Available online: https://www.fda.gov/media/70939/download (accessed on 19 February 2019).
13. Young, D. Significance of in Vitro in Vivo Correlation (ivivc). In *International Bioequivalence Standards: A New Era*; Amidon, G.L., Lesko, L.J., Midha, K.K., Shah, V.P., Hilfinger, J.M., Eds.; TSRL: Ann Arbor, MI, USA, 2006; pp. 41–48.
14. USP 34-NF 29. *The United States Pharmacopeia 32-the National Formulary 27*; United States Pharmacopeial Convention Inc.: Rockville, MD, USA, 2011.
15. Polli, J.E.; Crison, J.R.; Amidon, G.L. Novel approach to the analysis of in vitro-in vivo relationships. *J. Pharm. Sci.* **1996**, *85*, 753–760. [CrossRef]

16. Dunne, A.; O'Hara, T.; DeVane, J. A new approach to modelling the relationship between in vitro and in vivo drug dissolution/absorption. *Stat. Med.* **1999**, *18*, 1865–1876. [CrossRef]
17. Dunnex, A.; O'Hara, T.; DeVane, J.; Dunne, A. Level A in Vivo−in Vitro Correlation: Nonlinear Models and Statistical Methodology. *J. Pharm. Sci.* **1997**, *86*, 1245–1249. [CrossRef]
18. Sirisuth, N.; Augsburger, L.L.; Eddington, N.D. Development and validation of a non-linear IVIVC model for a diltiazem extended release formulation. *Biopharm. Drug Dispos.* **2002**, *23*, 1–8. [CrossRef]
19. Parojčić, J.; Ibric, S.; Djurić, Z.; Jovanović, M.; Corrigan, O.I. An investigation into the usefulness of generalized regression neural network analysis in the development of level A in vitro–in vivo correlation. *Eur. J. Pharm. Sci.* **2007**, *30*, 264–272. [CrossRef]
20. Corrigan, O.I.; Devlin, Y.; Butler, J. Influence of dissolution medium buffer composition on ketoprofen release from ER products and in vitro–in vivo correlation. *Int. J. Pharm.* **2003**, *254*, 147–154. [CrossRef]
21. Mendell-Harary, J.; Dowell, J.; Bigora, S.; Piscitelli, D.; Butler, J.; Farrell, C.; DeVane, J.G.; Young, D. Nonlinear in Vitro-in Vivo Correlations. In *Results and Problems in Cell Differentiation*; Springer Science and Business Media LLC: Berlin/Heidelberg, Germany, 1997; Volume 423, pp. 199–206.
22. Sandulovici, R.; Prasacu, I.; Mircioiu, C.; Voicu, V.A.; Medvedovici, A.; Anuta, V. Mathematical and phenomenological criteria in selection of pharmacokinetic model for m1 metabolite of pentoxyphylline. *FARMACIA* **2009**, *57*, 235–246.
23. Tvrdonova, M.; Dedik, L.; Mircioiu, C.; Miklovicova, D.; Ďurišová, M. Physiologically Motivated Time-Delay Model to Account for Mechanisms Underlying Enterohepatic Circulation of Piroxicam in Human Beings. *Basic Clin. Pharmacol. Toxicol.* **2009**, *104*, 35–42. [CrossRef]
24. Chaffman, M.; Brogden, R.N.; Speight, T.M.; Avery, G.S. A review of its pharmacological properties and therapeutic efficacy. *Drugs* **1985**, *29*, 387–454. [CrossRef]
25. Fagan, T.C. Diltiazem: Its place in the antihypertensive armamentarium. *J. Cardiovasc. Pharmacol.* **1991**, *18*, S26–S31. [CrossRef]
26. Hermann, P.; Rodger, S.D.; Remones, G.; Thenot, J.P.; London, D.R.; Morselli, P.L. Pharmacokinetics of diltiazem after intravenous and oral administration. *Eur. J. Clin. Pharmacol.* **1983**, *24*, 349–352. [CrossRef]
27. Caillé, G.; Boucher, S.; Spénard, J.; Lakhani, Z.; Russell, A.; Thiffault, J.; Grace, M.G. Diltiazem pharmacokinetics in elderly volunteers after single and multiple doses. *Eur. J. Drug Metab. Pharmacokinet.* **1991**, *16*, 75–80. [CrossRef]
28. Yeung, P.K.F.; Montague, T.J.; Tsui, B.; McGregor, C. High-Performance Liquid Chromatographic Assay of Diltiazem and Six of Its Metabolites in Plasma: Application to a Pharmacokinetic Study in Healthy Volunteers. *J. Pharm. Sci.* **1989**, *78*, 592–597. [CrossRef]
29. Food and Drug Administration-Center for Drug Evaluation and Research (CDER). Guidance for Industry: Bioanalytical Method Validation. Available online: https://www.fda.gov/regulatory-information/search-fda-guidance-documents/bioanalytical-method-validation-guidance-industry (accessed on 26 March 2019).
30. Wagner, J.G.; Nelson, E. Kinetic Analysis of Blood Levels and Urinary Excretion in the Absorptive Phase after Single Doses of Drug. *J. Pharm. Sci.* **1964**, *53*, 1392–1403. [CrossRef]
31. Kokate, A.; Li, X.; Williams, P.J.; Singh, P.; Jasti, B.R. In Silico Prediction of Drug Permeability Across Buccal Mucosa. *Pharm. Res.* **2009**, *26*, 1130–1139. [CrossRef]
32. Chrenova, J.; Durisova, M.; Mircioui, C.; Dedik, L.; Mircioiu, C. Effect of gastric emptying and entero-hepatic circulation on bioequivalence assessment of ranitidine. *Methods Find. Exp. Clin. Pharmacol.* **2010**, *32*, 413. [CrossRef]
33. Marchidanu, D.; Raducanu, N.; Miron, D.S.; Radulescu, F.S.; Anuta, V.; Mircioiu, I.; Prasacu, I. Comparative pharmacokinetics of rifampicin and 25-desacetyl rifampicin in healthy volunteers after single oral dose administration. *FARMACIA* **2013**, *61*, 398–410.
34. Mircioiu, C.; Ionica, G.; Danilceac, A.; Miron, D.; Mircioiu, I.; Radulescu, F.S. Pharmacokinetic and mathematical outliers for drugs with active metabolites. Note i. Model independent analyses for pentoxifylline. *FARMACIA* **2010**, *58*, 264–278.
35. Wu, C.Y.; Benet, L.Z. Predicting Drug disposition via application of BCS: Transport/absorption/elimination interplay and development of a biopharmaceutics. drug disposition classification SYSTEM. *Pharm. Res.* **2005**, *22*, 11–23. [CrossRef]

11

Gellan Gum/Laponite Beads for the Modified Release of Drugs: Experimental and Modeling Study of Gastrointestinal Release

Alessandra Adrover [1,*], Patrizia Paolicelli [2], Stefania Petralito [2], Laura Di Muzio [2], Jordan Trilli [2], Stefania Cesa [2], Ingunn Tho [3] and Maria Antonietta Casadei [2]

1 Dipartimento di Ingegneria Chimica, Materiali e Ambiente, Sapienza Universitá di Roma, Via Eudossiana 18, 00184 Rome, Italy
2 Dipartimento di Chimica e Tecnologie del Farmaco, Sapienza Universitá di Roma, Piazzale Aldo Moro 5, 00185 Rome, Italy; patrizia.paolicelli@uniroma1.it (P.P.); stefania.petralito@uniroma1.it (S.P.); laura.dimuzio@uniroma1.it (L.D.M.); jordan.trilli@uniroma1.it (J.T.); stefania.cesa@uniroma1.it (S.C.); mariaantonietta.casadei@uniroma1.it (M.A.C.)
3 Department of Pharmacy, University of Oslo, 0316 Oslo, Norway; ingunn.tho@farmasi.uio.no
* Correspondence: alessandra.adrover@uniroma1.it

Abstract: In this study, gellan gum (GG), a natural polysaccharide, was used to fabricate spherical porous beads suitable as sustained drug delivery systems for oral administration. GG was cross-linked with calcium ions to prepare polymeric beads. Rheological studies and preliminary experiments of beads preparation allowed to identify the GG and the $CaCl_2$ concentrations suitable for obtaining stable and spherical particles. GG beads were formed, through ionotropic gelation technique, with and without the presence of the synthetic clay laponite. The resultant beads were analyzed for dimensions (before and after freeze-drying), morphological aspects and ability to swell in different media miming biological fluids, namely SGF (Simulated Gastric Fluid, HCl 0.1 M) and SIF (Simulated Intestinal Fluid, phosphate buffer, 0.044 M, pH 7.4). The swelling degree was lower in SGF than in SIF and further reduced in the presence of laponite. The GG and GG-layered silicate composite beads were loaded with two model drugs having different molecular weight, namely theophylline and cyanocobalamin (vitamin B12) and subjected to in-vitro release studies in SGF and SIF. The presence of laponite in the bead formulation increased the drug entrapment efficiency and slowed-down the release kinetics of both drugs in the gastric environment. A moving-boundary swelling model with "diffuse" glassy-rubbery interface was proposed in order to describe the swelling behavior of porous freeze-dried beads. Consistently with the swelling model adopted, two moving-boundary drug release models were developed to interpret release data from highly porous beads of different drugs: drug molecules, e.g., theophylline, that exhibit a typical Fickian behavior of release curves and drugs, such as vitamin B12, whose release curves are affected by the physical/chemical interaction of the drug with the polymer/clay complex. Theoretical results support the experimental observations, thus confirming that laponite may be an effective additive for fabricating sustained drug delivery systems.

Keywords: beads; gellan gum; ionotropic gelation; laponite; modeling study; swelling; gastrointestinal drug release; polymer/clay composite

---

1. Introduction

Orally administered dosage forms are the most convenient formulations due to the easiness of employment, pre-determined and measured doses and overall non-invasive nature of administration, which increase the patient compliance. The successful oral formulation should deliver the required therapeutic dose to the specific site of action during the treatment period. However, the delivery of a drug by a simple conventional dosage form normally results in the immediate release of the active pharmaceutic ingredient and their use usually requires a high frequency of administration and uncontrolled absorption. These considerations have guided researchers to focus their efforts on improving oral delivery systems with the development of formulations providing more predictable release rates as well as an increased bioavailability. Sustained release formulations are extensively investigated in order to reduce the dosing frequency, thus resulting in increased patience compliance.

In the last decades, many biomaterials have been proposed as interesting materials in the design of modified oral drug delivery systems in order to accomplish therapeutic or convenience purposes not offered by conventional dosage forms.

Synthetic and natural polymers have been proposed for the development of oral extended-release dosage forms. However, naturally derived polymers offer many advantages over synthetic polymers related to their biocompatibility, biodegradability, non-toxicity and reasonable costs.

In particular, hydrophilic polymers, such as polysaccharides, are widely used as natural materials in sustained oral dosage forms and the interest in the application of these polymers for prolonging drug release has increased over the last decades [1]. The interest toward these polymers is related to their swelling and filmogen [2] capabilities as well as their pH-sensitive [3,4] or floating capability [5–8].

Natural gums, such as gellan gum (GG), an anionic, high molecular weight polysaccharide, has gained significant interest in the pharmaceutical field [9]. It consists of tetra-saccharide repeating units: α-L-rhamnose, β-D-glucuronic acid and β-D-glucose in the molar ratio 1:1:2.

GG has proven to be a versatile material in the formulation of polymeric hydrogels, including beads systems, due to its temperature sensitivity and ability to gel under mild conditions. In fact, it forms stable hydrogel networks in the presence of cationic cross-linkers [10,11], so that ionotropic gelation method can be employed for the synthesis of polymeric networks using divalent cations as cross-linking agents [12–14]. The contact of the polymer with cations results in the instantaneous formation of a gel matrix containing uniformly dispersed material throughout the crosslinked gellan gum matrix.

Polymeric beads are widely used for oral sustained release; after beads are ingested, the drug will slowly diffuse out from the polymer matrix, resulting in a prolonged release of the active agent. Nevertheless, some drawbacks, related to the higher porosity of the matrix or poor mechanical resistance of the polymeric network, could lead to a rapid and massive release in acidic dissolution medium [15]. Only a few polymers can be used in their pure form for the formulation of oral sustained release beads and therefore their combination with other biocompatible materials has been investigated in order to overcome these drawbacks. Clay minerals are one of the fillers that can be used, in combination with many biopolymers, to improve their drug delivery properties [16–19]. The ultimate goal is to bring together in the same material the best properties of the natural polymer and clay since each component plays a key role in improving the properties of the nanocomposite hydrogels.

In this scenario, clay hydrogel beads have been widely investigated in oral drug delivery applications, showing that mineral clays can be successfully used as functional additives in the development of bead-modified systems [20].

The most commonly used clay minerals belong to the smectite family. Among the smectite family, laponite $Na_{0.7}[(Si_8Mg_{5.5}Li_{0.3})O_{20}(OH)_4]_{0.7}$ is a synthetic clay composed of a layered structure (30–25 nm diameter, 1 nm thickness) that has been used to synthesize a wide range of nano-composite hydrogels [21–23]. Specifically, laponite (LAPO) nanoparticles can be uniformly dispersed within the polymeric matrix where they self-arrange and act as both filler and cross-linker during gel formation [24,25].

This study aims to verify the possibility of using laponite as an additive clay mineral to design new composite gellan gum beads with highly specific characteristics, such as appropriate swelling properties and release kinetics.

Rheological studies and preliminary experiments of bead preparation allowed selecting the gellan gum and crosslinker ($CaCl_2$) concentrations suitable for obtaining stable and spherical particles. Under optimized experimental conditions, laponite was uniformly dispersed in the polymeric solution allowing the formation of nano-composite GG beads with reduced mesh size. In order to investigate how the morphology, swelling and the release properties of the nano-composite hydrogels were affected by the laponite, beads were loaded with two model drugs having different molecular weights and release studies were performed in simulated gastric fluid (SGF) and in simulated intestinal one (SIF). Mathematical models for swelling and drug release from these highly porous beads were proposed. Reliable values of drug diffusion coefficients in different release media were obtained.

2. Materials and Methods

2.1. Chemicals

Theophylline, vitamin B12, methanol, acetic acid, hydrochloric acid and low acyl gellan gum (Gelzan^{TM}) were purchased from Sigma Aldrich Company (Darmstadt, Germany), and calcium chloride hydrate, potassium dihydrogen phosphate and sodium hydroxide from Carlo Erba Reagents S.r.l (Milan, Italy). We used bidistilled water from Carlo Erba Reagents S.r.l. for the HPLC analysis. For sample preparation and all the other analyses, we used demineralized water produced with a Pharma20 equipment, Culligan Italiana S.p.A (Bologna, Italy). Laponite XLG was a gift of Rockwood Additives Ltd. (Moosburg, Germany).

2.2. Rheological Measurements

Rheological experiments were performed with a Haake RheoStress 300 Rotational Rheometer (Dreieich, Germany) equipped with a Haake DC10 thermostat. Oscillatory experiments were performed at 25.0 ± 0.2 °C in the range 0.01–10 Hz on the hydrogels obtained from 1.0, 1.5 and 2.0% *w/w* GG solutions. Enough quantity of each sample was carefully poured to completely cover the 6 cm cone-plate geometry (angle of 1°). For each sample, the linear viscoelastic range was evaluated: a 1% maximum deformation was used.

2.3. Beads Preparation

Gellan gum (0.11, 0.165 or 0.22 g) was added to 11 mL of double distilled water and maintained under stirring for 5 h at 80 °C until a homogeneous solution was produced. This solution was cooled and kept at 40 °C. Then, 10 mL of this solution were carefully loaded into a syringe with a 21G needle, ensuring no air bubbles were present, and added to a solution of calcium chloride (50 mL, 0.3% and 0.6% *w/w*) drop wise. The beads were left cross-linking for 10 min (curing time), then filtered and washed four times with 10 mL of deionized water and freeze-dried. The curing time was optimized to have maximum entrapment efficiency of the model molecules used. In fact, while longer curing times increase the degree of crosslinking of the polymer, they also promote the effusion of the loaded molecule out of the beads, thus reducing the final drug loading.

Beads including laponite were produced starting from a solution (11 mL) of GG (1.5% *w/w*) and laponite (1.0% *w/w*) added drop wise to the solution of $CaCl_2$ (0.3% *w/w*), thus following the same procedure adopted for beads without laponite.

The diameter of fresh and freeze-dried beads was measured with a caliper along two orthogonal directions, taking the average of the measurements as the mean diameter of the beads, whereas the ratio between the two measurements was taken as the aspect ratio of the beads.

2.4. Determination of Swelling Degree

In order to quantify the swelling degree of the beads, 10 freeze-dried beads were weighed and placed into a tulle net and submerged into 25 mL of simulated gastric fluid (SGF, HCl 0.1 M) or simulated intestinal fluid (SIF, phosphate buffer 0.044 M, pH 7.4), maintained at 37.0 ± 0.5 °C. After

5 min, the beads were removed, lightly blotted on paper to remove the excess liquid and weighed. The beads were then submerged back into the medium and the process was repeated at established time intervals up to 24 h. The experiments were carried out in triplicate with each value representing the mean ± SD.

The swelling degree S was calculated using the following equation:

$$S = \frac{weight\ of\ swollen\ beads\ -\ weight\ of\ dry\ beads}{weight\ of\ dry\ beads}. \quad (1)$$

2.5. Preparation of Drug Loaded Beads

Gellan gum (0.165 g) was dissolved in 9 mL of distilled water using the method described in Section 2.3. Theophylline or vitamin B12 (0.0146 g) were solubilized in 2 mL of water and added to the cooled gellan gum solution, to make a final volume of 11 mL and a concentration of 1.5% *w/w* of GG. The solution was stirred at 100 rpm for 10 min to ensure the drug homogeneously dispersed. The beads were then formed using the method described in Section 2.3. Drug loaded beads including laponite were prepared from a starting solution (9 mL) of gellan gum (0.165 g) and laponite (0.11 g) and then following the same procedure adopted for drug loaded beads without laponite.

2.6. Drug Entrapment Efficiency

In order to determine the quantity of drug loaded into the beads, 15 mg of freeze-dried beads were stirred vigorously in SIF for 1 h, to destroy the beads and extract the drug. The solution was filtered and analyzed by HPLC. The apparatus consisted of a Perkin Elmer Series 200 LC pump, equipped with a 235 Diode Array Detector and a Total-Chrom data processor (Perkin Elmer, Waltham, MA, USA). HPLC analyses were carried out using a Merck Hibar LiChrocart (250–4.5 μm) RP-18 column under isocratic conditions (0.7 mL/min) using a mobile phase constituted by methanol and acetic acid (0.1 M) mixture in a proportion of 40:60 (*v:v*). Theophylline was monitored at $\lambda = 280$ nm and vitamin B12 at $\lambda = 360$ nm. Under these conditions, the retention time of theophylline was about 6 min, while that of vitamin B12 was about 4 min.

The drug entrapment efficiency was calculated using the following equation:

$$Drug\ entrapment\ efficiency\ (\%) = \frac{actual\ drug\ content\ of\ beads}{theoretical\ drug\ content\ of\ beads} \times 100. \quad (2)$$

All experiments were carried out in triplicate and each value reported representing the mean, ± SD.

2.7. In Vitro Release Studies

Release studies from drug loaded beads with different formulations were performed separately in SGF (HCl 0.1 M) and in SIF (phosphate buffer, pH 7.4) and sequentially in SGF and SIF to simulate the drug release in the entire gastrointestinal tract. A total of 15 mg of drug loaded beads were added to a known volume V_{res} of SIF or SGF, warmed to 37 °C in a water bath and stirred continuously at 200 rpm. At defined times, from 1 to 240 min, 1 mL of solution was withdrawn and replaced with 1 mL of fresh solution. Different volumes $V_{res} = 50, 75, 100, 150, 175$ mL were considered in order to investigate the influence of the release volume V_{res} on release curves. See Section 4.5.1 for a discussion on the role of V_{res}.

For gastrointestinal in-vitro release experiments, 15 mg of drug-loaded beads were added to 100 mL of SGF, warmed to 37 °C in a water bath and stirred continuously at 200 rpm. At defined times, from 1 to 120 min, 1 mL of solution was withdrawn and replaced with 1 mL of fresh SGF. After 120 min, the beads were drained to remove excess acid and transferred into 50 mL of SIF. Every 15 min, 1 mL of solution was withdrawn and replaced with the same volume of SIF until 240 min and then again after 24 h. By considering that, after the first 120 min, the beads had released from 60% to 95% of the initially loaded drug, depending on the bead formulation, we chose to carry out the subsequent release in SIF in a smaller release volume (half of that in SGF) to maintain the drug concentration in the release volume high enough to allow the subsequent HPLC analysis. Drug concentrations were determined by HPLC analysis as reported in the previous section.

After 24 h, the beads were collected from the media and destroyed to extract and quantify the drug still embedded into the beads. The release data were reported as drug concentration $C_{res}(t_w{}^i)$ [mg/mL] at withdrawal times $t_w{}^i$ [min] and as fraction of drug released up to time $t_w{}^i$ with respect to the total amount of drug loaded in the beads. The experiments were carried out in triplicate with each value reported representing the mean ± SD.

2.8. Statistics

Statistical tests were performed to evaluate the effect of laponite on gastrointestinal release rates of the two model molecules. Statistical analysis was performed with GraphPad Prism™ (Version 4.00) software (GraphPad Software, Inc., San Diego, CA, USA). The Student's t-test was applied to determine the statistical significance between two different experimental conditions. The values of $p < 0.05$ were considered significant.

3. Mathematical Modeling of Swelling and Drug release of Highly Porous Beads

3.1. Swelling Modeling

We adopted a radial one-dimensional model of swelling of spherical dry beads. A classical approach to swelling of glassy polymers requires the solution of a moving boundary model describing the solvent transport in the swollen gel and the time evolution of two fronts [26–28], the erosion front (rubbery-solvent interface at $r = S(t)$) and the swelling front (glassy-rubbery interface at $r = R(t)$), as shown in Figure 1.

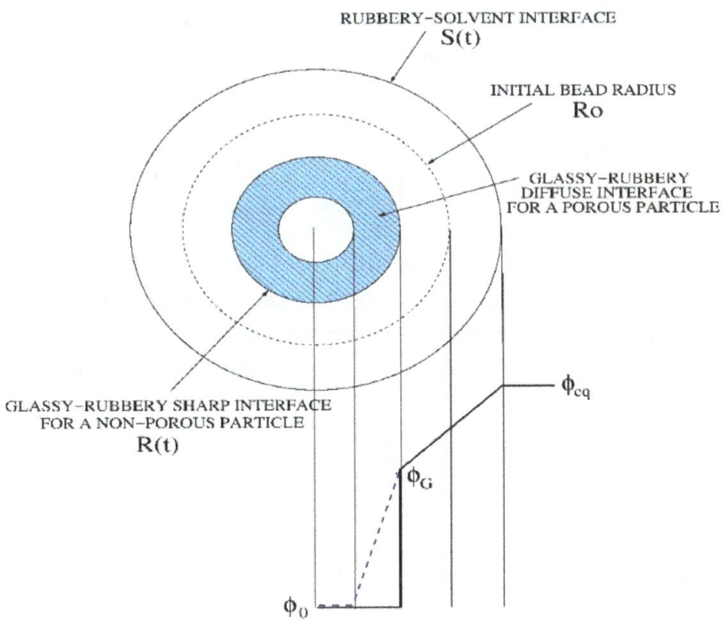

Figure 1. Schematic representation of moving fronts and solvent concentration profiles in a swelling process of a dry spherical bead. The two cases of a non-porous and a highly porous particle (blue dotted line) are shown.

The solvent balance equation, written in terms of the solvent volumetric fraction $\varphi(r,t)$ reads

$$\frac{\partial \varphi}{\partial t} = \frac{1}{r^2}\frac{\partial}{\partial r}\left(r^2 D_s(\varphi)\frac{\partial \varphi}{\partial r} - r^2 v_r^s(\varphi)\varphi\right) = \frac{1}{r^2}\frac{\partial}{\partial r}\left(r^2 D_s(\varphi)(1-\varphi)\frac{\partial \varphi}{\partial r}\right),\ R(t) < r < S(t), \quad (3)$$

where $v_r{}^s(\varphi)$ is the swelling velocity $v_r{}^s(\varphi) = D_s(\varphi)\partial\varphi/\partial r$ and $D_s(\varphi)$ is the solvent diffusion coefficient, that can be assumed constant or a function of the solvent volume fraction φ.

Equation (3) must be solved with the boundary conditions,

$$[\varphi]_{r=S(t)} = \varphi_{eq}, [\varphi]_{r=R(t)} = \varphi_G \; for \; R(t) > 0, \left[\frac{\partial\varphi}{\partial r}\right]_{r=0} = 0 \; for \; R(t) = 0, \quad (4)$$

and initial conditions $\varphi(r,0) = \varphi_0$ for $0 \le r \le R_0$, where R_0 is the initial radius of the dry particle, φ_{eq} is the volume fraction at equilibrium and φ_G is the threshold volume fraction to initiate swelling.

If we assume that the glassy phase for $r < R(t)$ is totally impermeable to the solvent (the solvent diffusivity is zero in the glassy phase) the two fronts, the glassy-rubbery at $r = R(t)$ and the rubbery-solvent at $r = S(t)$, evolve according to the Stefan boundary conditions,

$$(\varphi_G - \varphi_0)\frac{dR}{dt} = -D_s(\varphi_G)(1-\varphi_G)\left[\frac{\partial\varphi}{\partial r}\right]_{r=R(t)}, R(0) = R_0, \quad (5)$$

$$\frac{dS}{dt} = D_s(\varphi_{eq})\left[\frac{\partial\varphi}{\partial r}\right]_{r=S(t)}, \quad S(0) = R_0. \quad (6)$$

This model fits well with the case of a spherical initially non-porous particle for which the sharp glassy-rubbery interface progressively moves towards the center of the particle and spherical glassy inner core that progressively disappears. However, in the case of a porous particle, like the beads under investigation, we can imagine that the solvent can penetrate and diffuse inside the glassy core through the pore network and that the gelling transition occurs simultaneously both on the inside and on the external surface of the bead. Therefore, it is not possible to identify a net glassy-rubbery interface, but rather a "diffuse" interface as depicted in Figure 1. This phenomenon for porous-particles has been modeled by assuming a non-zero solvent diffusivity in the glassy phase, thus introducing a solvent concentration dependent diffusion coefficient as follows

$$D_s(\varphi) = D_s^{sg} f(\varphi), f(\varphi) = \left\{ \begin{array}{c} 1 \; for \; \varphi \ge \varphi_G \\ exp\left\{-\beta\frac{\varphi-\varphi_G}{\varphi_0-\varphi_G}\right\} \; for \; \varphi < \varphi_G \end{array} \right\}, \quad (7)$$

where $D_s{}^{sg}$ is the solvent diffusivity in the swollen gel, assumed constant for $\varphi > \varphi_G$, and β is a parameter controlling the decay of the diffusivity in the glassy core. The larger the porosity, the smaller β, the greater the ability of the solvent to penetrate in the glassy core.

The solvent transport equation and boundary conditions in highly porous particles read as

$$\frac{\partial\varphi}{\partial t} = \frac{1}{r^2}\frac{\partial}{\partial r}\left(r^2 D_s(\varphi)(1-\varphi)\frac{\partial\varphi}{\partial r}\right), 0 < r < S(t), \varphi(0 \le r \le R_0, t = 0) = \varphi_0, \quad (8)$$

$$[\varphi]_{r=S(t)} = \varphi_{eq}, \left[\frac{\partial\varphi}{\partial r}\right]_{r=0} = 0, \quad (9)$$

that are the same as Equations (3) and (4) with the basic difference that $\varphi(r,t)$ is now defined in the entire domain $0 \le r \le S(t)$ because the glassy-rubbery sharp interface $R(t)$ has been removed and solvent diffusion is allowed in the glassy region with diffusion coefficient given by Equation (7). The only moving boundary is the gel-solvent interface at $r = S(t)$, evolving in time according to Equation (6).

The "diffuse" interface swelling model introduces the only extra parameter β controlled by the bead porosity. Figure 2A,B shows the spatial behavior of the normalized solvent volume fraction $\varphi(r,t)/\varphi_{eq}$, for increasing times, as obtained from the numerical solution of the swelling model Equations (6)–(9), for two different values of β, namely $\beta = 2$ (Figure 2A) and $\beta = 8$ (Figure 2B).

Solvent concentration profiles for $\beta = 8$ show a very rapid decay of φ for $\varphi < \varphi_G$, thus exhibiting a very sharp interface, typical of a non-porous particle. On the contrary, for $\beta = 2$ (porous particle) concentration profiles exhibit a smoother behavior for $\varphi < \varphi_G$ because of solvent penetration in the glassy region.

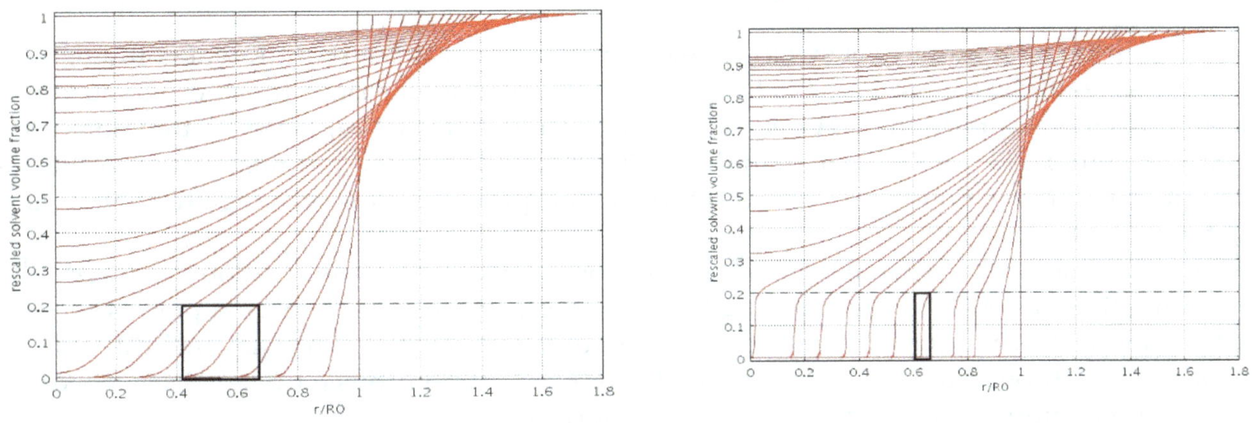

A **B**

Figure 2. Rescaled solvent volume fraction $\varphi(r,t)/\varphi_{eq}$, vs. dimensionless radius r/R_0 for increasing times during the swelling process. Dashed line indicates the value of φ_G/φ_{eq}, Black boxes highlight the thickness of the diffuse glassy-rubbery interface. (**A**) $\beta = 2$, porous particle; (**B**) $\beta = 8$, non-porous particle.

The estimate of model parameters D_s^{sg}, β and φ_{eq} can be obtained by comparing model predictions with experimental data for the temporal evolution and asymptotic value of the swelling degree $S(t)$

$$S(t) = \frac{weight\ of\ absorbed\ solvent}{weight\ of\ dry\ particle} = \frac{\rho_s \int_0^{S(t)} \varphi\ 4\pi r^2 dr}{\rho_b\ (4/3)\ \pi R_0^3} \tag{10}$$

where ρ_s and ρ_b are the solvent and the freeze-dried bead densities, respectively.

The estimate of model parameters is fully addressed in Section 4.3 in connection with the analysis of swelling data in both release media SGF and SIF.

3.2. Drug Release Modeling of No-Interacting Drugs

If we assume no physical/chemical interaction between the drug and the polymer or the clay-polymer complex, the transport model for the drug concentration $c_d(r,t)$, initially loaded in the glassy core, reads as

$$\frac{\partial c_d}{\partial t} = \frac{1}{r^2}\frac{\partial}{\partial r}\left(r^2 D_d(\varphi)\frac{\partial c_d}{\partial r} - r^2 v_r^s(\varphi) c_d\right), 0 < r < S(t), c_d(0 \leq r \leq R_0, t = 0) = c_d^0, \tag{11}$$

$$[c_d]_{r=S(t)} = C_{res}(t), \left[\frac{\partial c_d}{\partial r}\right]_{r=0} = 0, \tag{12}$$

where $v_r^s(\varphi)$ is the point wise swelling velocity and $D_d(\varphi) = D_d^{sg}(\varphi)f(\varphi)$ is the drug diffusivity, modeled exactly as the solvent diffusivity $D_s(\varphi)$. Indeed, D_d^{sg} is the drug diffusion coefficient in the swollen gel, assumed constant *for* $\varphi > \varphi_G$, and $f(\varphi)$ is the same function adopted to describe solvent penetration in the glassy core, Equation (7). Consistently with the solvent penetration model adopted, drug diffusion is allowed in the glassy core through the pore network, and the parameter β controlling diffusivity decay in the glassy core is assumed the same for the solvent and the drug.

The concentration $C_{res}(t)$, entering the boundary condition at the rubbery-solvent interface, represents the drug concentration in the reservoir in which the beads are immersed for release, with volume V_{res}, assumed perfectly mixed. $C_{res}(t)$ evolves in time according to the macroscopic balance equation accounting for drug release from swelling beads and withdrawals, modeled as an instantaneous depletion of drug concentration in the reservoir

$$V_{res}\frac{dC_{res}}{dt} = N_{beads}\left(-D_d^{sg}\left[\frac{\partial c_d}{\partial r}\right]_{r=S(t)} 4\pi S^2(t)\right) - \sum_{i=1}^{N_w^t} V_w C_{res}(t)\,\delta\left(t - t_w^i\right), \tag{13}$$

where N_{beads} is the total number of swelling/releasing beads, V_w is the withdrawal volume, $t_w{}^i$ is the time of the i-th withdrawal and $N_W{}^t$ is the number of withdrawals from time zero to current time t. The simplifying assumption of perfect sink condition is therefore replaced by the more accurate expression Equation (13) for $C_{res}(t)$ that, in the limit for $V_{res}/V_{beads} \rightarrow \infty$, permits to recover the perfect sink condition $C_{res}(t) = 0$. Equations (11)–(13) for drug transport must be solved together with Equations (6)–(9) for solvent diffusion.

Figure 3A,B shows the spatial behavior of the normalized drug concentration $(c_d - C_{res})/(c_d{}^0 - C_{res})$ for increasing times as obtained by choosing $\beta = 2$ (porous particle) and $\beta = 8$ (non-porous particle) for both $D_s(\varphi)$ and $D_d(\varphi)$. We observe that, for $\beta = 2$ (porous particle), the drug can smoothly diffuse out of the glassy core through the pore network while, for $\beta = 8$ (non-porous particle), drug concentration profiles exhibit a jump at the sharp glassy-rubber interface.

The estimate of the only model parameter $D_d{}^{sg}$ entering the drug release model is obtained by direct comparison of model predictions for $C_{res}(t)$ with experimental data for withdrawal drug concentrations $C_w{}^i = C_{res}(t_w{}^i)$ or by direct comparison of model predictions with experimental data of the integral release curve

$$\frac{M_t}{M_\infty} = \frac{V_{res}C_{res}(t) + \sum_{i=1}^{N_w^t} V_w C_{res}\left(t_w^i\right)}{V_{res}C_{res}(\infty) + \sum_{i=1}^{N_w} V_w C_{res}\left(t_w^i\right)}, \tag{14}$$

where $C_{res}(\infty)$ is the asymptotic concentration in the reservoir and N_W is the total number of withdrawals made during the entire release experiment.

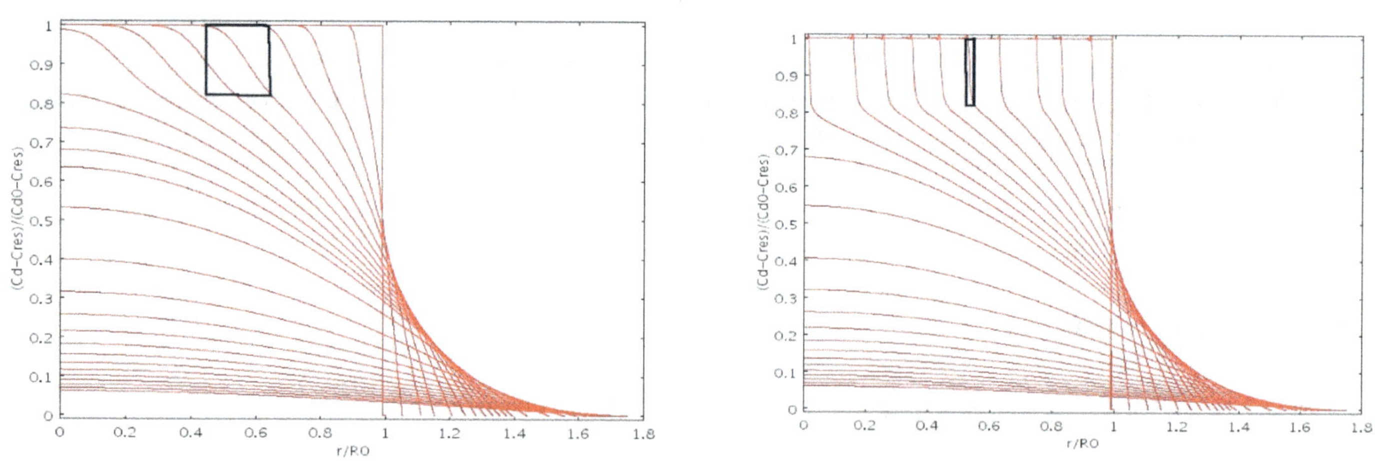

A **B**

Figure 3. Normalized drug concentration $(c_d - C_{res})/(c_d{}^0 - C_{res})$ vs. dimensionless radius r/R_0 for increasing times as obtained by adopting $\beta = 2$ ((**A**), highly porous particle) and $\beta = 8$ ((**B**), non-porous particle) for particle swelling and drug transport. Black boxes highlight the thickness of the diffuse glassy-rubbery interface.

3.3. *Drug Release Modeling of Interacting Drugs*

If we assume a physical/chemical interaction between the drug and the clay-polymer complex we need to introduce a two-phase model, analogous to that adopted by Singh et al. (1994) [29] and by Paolicelli et al. (2017) [30] modeling drug release from hydrogels via a diffusion transport equation coupled with a sorption/desorption mechanism. The "two-phases" model adopted in the present work introduces a fraction ε of drug molecules initially bounded to the clay-polymer complex by a physical bound and a "desorption" mechanism, occurring during solvent penetration, modeled as a linear transfer rate from the adsorbed "bounded" phase to the desorbed "free" (or gel-solvent) phase where the drug is free to diffuse with diffusion coefficient $D_d(\varphi)$, the same adopted in Section 3.2 for non-interacting drugs.

Let us then indicate with c_b and c_d the drug concentrations in the bounded and free (gel-solvent) phases, respectively. Drug concentration $c_b(r,t)$ evolves in space and time according to the transport equation for the clay-polymer complex during the swelling process

$$\frac{\partial c_b}{\partial t} = \frac{1}{r^2}\frac{\partial}{\partial r}\left(-r^2 v_r^s c_b\right) - k_{bg}(\varphi)c_b,\ 0 < r < S(t),\ c_b(r,t=0) = \epsilon c_d^0, \left[\frac{\partial c_b}{\partial r}\right]_{r=0} = 0, \quad (15)$$

but including a linear transfer rate from the bounded to the free phase $-r_{b\to g} = k_{bg}(\varphi)\, c_b$, induced by solvent penetration and modeled, according to the solvent diffusion model Equation (7), as $k_{bg}(\varphi) = k_{bg}{}^{sg} f(\varphi)$ where $k_{bg}{}^{sg}$ [1/s] is the transfer rate coefficient in the swollen gel, assumed constant for $\varphi > \varphi_G$. Correspondingly, the transport equation for drug molecules in the free (gel) phase $c_d(r,t)$ reads as

$$\begin{gathered}\frac{\partial c_d}{\partial t} = \frac{1}{r^2}\frac{\partial}{\partial r}\left(r^2 D_d(\varphi)\frac{\partial c_d}{\partial r} - r^2 v_r^s c_d\right) + k_{bg}(\varphi)c_b, 0 < \mathrm{r} < \mathrm{S}(t), \\ c_d(r,\ t=0) = (1-\epsilon)c_d^0,\end{gathered} \quad (16)$$

to be solved with the same boundary conditions Equation (12) adopted for the no-interaction model and with Equation (13) for the time evolution of the drug concentration in the reservoir $C_{res}(t)$.

The inverse of the transfer rate coefficient $1/k_{bg}{}^{sg}$ represents the characteristic time for the irreversible transfer of a drug molecule from the bounded to the free (gel) phase. This characteristic time $t_{bg} = 1/k_{bg}{}^{sg}$ can be compared to the characteristic drug diffusion time $t_D = R_0{}^2/D_d{}^{sg}$ by introducing the Thiele modulus $\Phi^2 = t_D/t_{bg} = k_{bg}{}^{sg}\, R_0{}^2/D_d{}^{sg}$ to identify the rate-controlling step.

The estimate of transport parameters, namely $D_d{}^{sg}$, and $k_{bg}{}^{sg}$ and is obtained by direct comparison of model predictions with experimental data for withdrawal drug concentrations $C_{res}(t_w{}^i)$ and for the integral release curves M_t/M_∞.

3.4. Numerical Issues

PDE equations and boundary conditions describing the one-dimensional swelling dynamics and drug release were numerically solved using finite elements method (FEM) in Comsol Multiphysics 3.5. The convection–diffusion package was coupled with ALE (Arbitrary Lagrangian Eulerian) moving mesh. Free displacement induced by boundary velocity conditions was set. Lagrangian quadratic elements were chosen. The linear solver adopted was UMFPACK, with relative tolerance 10^{-4} and absolute tolerance 10^{-7}. The number of finite elements is 10^4 with a non-uniform mesh. Smaller elements were located close to the boundary $r = S(t)$ in order to accurately compute concentration gradients controlling the velocity of the moving front.

4. Results and Discussion

4.1. Rheological Measurements

The concentration of gellan gum (GG) used for the preparation of the beads was carefully optimized on the basis of the rheological properties of its solutions. Specifically, GG solutions at 1.0, 1.5 and 2.0% *w/w* were prepared at 80 °C and, after complete solubilization, cooled to 40 °C. The flow curves obtained at this temperature for the three solutions of GG are reported in Figure 4A. The viscosity of the system increases by increasing the polymer concentration and the dependence of the viscosity on the shear rate is characteristic of a pseudo-plastic macromolecular system.

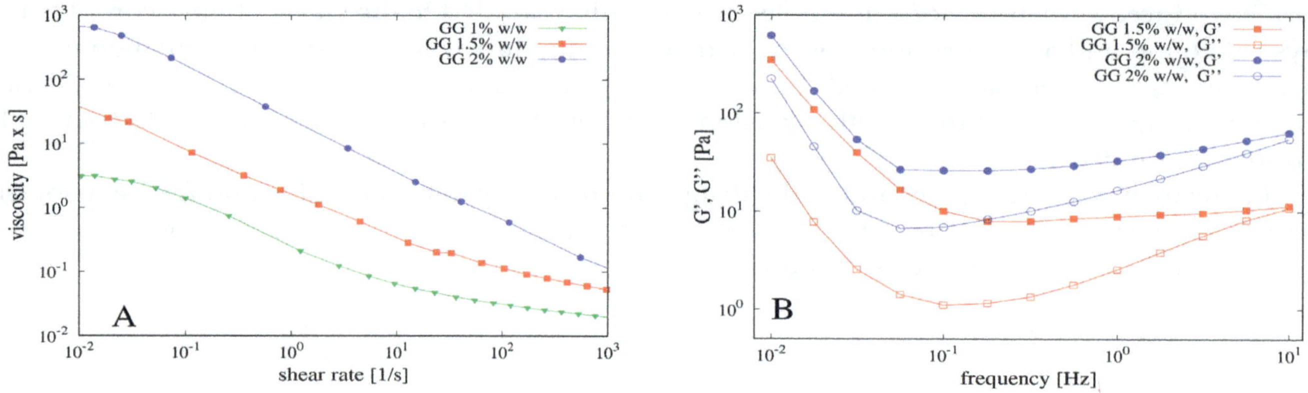

Figure 4. (**A**) Flow curves of gellan gum (GG) at different concentrations 1%, 1.5% and 2% *w/w*; (**B**) corresponding mechanical spectra.

Mechanical spectra were also recorded in the region of linear viscoelasticity and reported in Figure 4B. The polymeric solution at 1.0% *w/w* of GG showed a G′ smaller than G″, behaving as an entanglement network (data not shown). By increasing the GG concentration, the polymeric solution evolves towards a weak gel behavior, with G′ bigger than G″ and slightly dependent on the frequency. During the cooling, GG undergoes a series of structural changes in aqueous solution from random coiled chains to double helices, which then aggregate together thus forming a three-dimensional network. This behavior is well known as the gelation mechanism of gellan gum alone or in the presence of cations has been extensively investigated by different techniques, such as rheological, DSC and light scattering measurements and reviewed in [31].

Preliminary experiments were carried out in order to verify if the three solutions could flow through a syringe needle. GG solutions were loaded into the syringe at 40 °C. This temperature value was chosen in order to avoid any possible thermal damage when drugs are loaded inside the systems. GG concentrations greater than 1.5% *w/w* resulted in a highly viscous solution that caused clogging of the syringe needle, so that only the solutions at 1.0% and 1.5% *w/w* GG were used to prepare the beads.

The morphology of the forming beads by ionotropic gelation strongly depends on the amount of gellan gum in the initial mixture [32–34]. The lower the polymer content, the more deformed and irregular the beads, due to the matrix-forming function of gellan. Moreover, if the GG concentration is too low, the beads lost their spherical shape during the drying process, as already observed in [34]. In fact, both polymer and cross-linker concentrations have major effects on morphology as well as on other properties of the resulting beads, as reviewed in [10], because both concentrations affect the kinetic of the crosslinking process.

Our preliminary tests showed that the polymer concentration represents the main factor controlling the morphology of the beads. For GG concentrations lower than 1.5% *w/w*, the solution was unable to produce stable spherical beads, most likely because the low viscosity of the solution does not allow to keep the spherical shape of the drops when in contact with the cross-linking solution. For this reason, concentrations of GG below 1% *w/w* were not further investigated and the GG concentration of 1.5% *w/w* was chosen (see Section 4.2).

The effect of clay on the rheological properties of GG was also investigated. To this end, 1.0% *w/w* of laponite was added to the GG solution at 1.5% *w/w*. Flow curves and mechanical spectra performed on the polymeric solution containing the clay are shown in Figure 5A,B.

The presence of laponite induces a small decrease of viscosity of the polymeric solution as well as of the G′ value, most likely because the clay interacts with the gellan chains, thus partially destroying the double helix structure and causing the formation of a weaker gel. Indeed, the mechanical spectrum of the GG solution shows a weak gel behavior with the modulus G′ higher than G″ in the entire range of frequencies analyzed. On the contrary, the GG solution with laponite shows an intersection point of the G′ and the G″ curves at frequency of about 1 Hz, thus behaving as a solution (with G″ > G′) for higher values of the applied frequency.

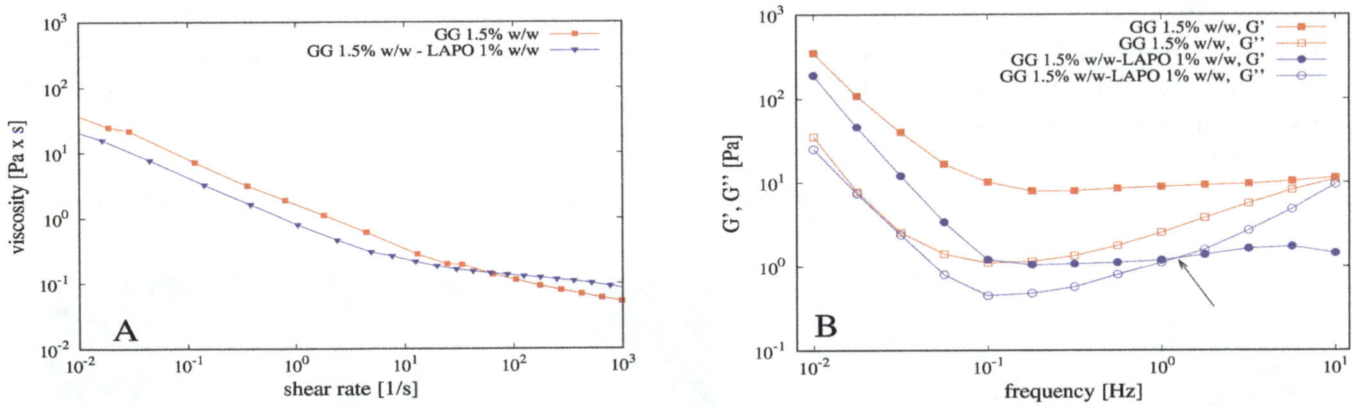

Figure 5. (**A**) Flow curves of GG solution with and without laponite and (**B**) mechanical spectra of the same solutions. Arrow indicates the inversion point G″ ≈ G′ at a frequency of about 1 Hz for the mechanical spectra of the GG solution including laponite.

4.2. Beads Preparation

Based on the rheological properties of its solutions, different GG beads were prepared dropping GG solution at 1% *w*/*w* and 1.5% *w*/*w* into $CaCl_2$ solutions at different concentrations in order to evaluate the effect of the cross-linking agent on the properties of the resulting beads.

The crosslinking process involves calcium ions and carboxylic groups of D-glucuronic acid of GG. More specifically, every calcium ion can electrostatically interact with two carboxylic groups; therefore, it interacts with two D-glucuronic acids of two different repetitive units of the polymer.

The crosslinking concentration always exceeded the concentration of the polymer as molar ratios GG:Ca^{2+} of 1:5, 1:7.5, 1:10 and 1:15 mol:mol were investigated. Regular and spherical beads were obtained with GG concentration 1.5% *w*/*w* for 1:5 and 1:10 GG:Ca^{2+} molar ratios, corresponding to $CaCl_2$ concentrations of 0.3% *w*/*w* and 0.6% *w*/*w*, respectively. Concentrations of $CaCl_2$ < 0.3% *w*/*w* have not produced stable and spherical beads. GG solution 1.0% *w*/*w* gave irregular beads even for higher GG:Ca^{2+} molar ratios 1:7 and 1:15. Based on these results, concentrations of GG below 1% *w*/*w* were not further investigated and the GG concentration of 1.5% *w*/*w* with $CaCl_2$ concentrations of 0.3% *w*/*w* and 0.6% *w*/*w* were adopted because these concentrations did not cause clogging of the syringe needle and produced regular and spherical beads. Further formulations were prepared by adding laponite to GG solution before beads formation. In this case, the beads were formed using the GG solution 1.5% *w*/*w* with laponite 1% *w*/*w* and with the lower concentration 0.3% *w*/*w* of $CaCl_2$, which was chosen by considering that the clay is able to act as cross-linker itself, thus contributing to the polymeric network formation.

The beads were recovered by filtration and characterized immediately after preparation in their fresh form and after the freeze-drying process. Specifically, they were observed at the optical microscope and their diameters measured and reported in Table 1.

Table 1. Diameter values of different bead formulations before and after freeze-drying.

Beads Formulation	Beads Diameter (mm ± SD)	Freeze-Dried Beads Diameter (mm ± SD)
GG/Ca 0.3%	2.41 ± 0.06	1.63 ± 0.03
GG/Ca 0.6%	2.44 ± 0.07	1.56 ± 0.09
GG/LAPO/Ca 0.3%	2.79 ± 0.11	2.06 ± 0.08

Different formulations lead to beads with different dimensions: the cross-linker concentration does not influence significantly the particle diameter, whereas the presence of laponite leads to an increase of the particle diameter. For all formulations, the bead population appear homogeneous and with spherical shape (see Figure 6A) characterized by an aspect ratio of about 1.02. The beads containing laponite (Figure 6D) have a smoother and regular surface with respect to the other ones (Figure 6B,C which differ for the $CaCl_2$, concentration), most likely because the clay, acting as filler, increases the particle surface compactness.

Particle density after freeze-drying ρ_b is extremely low and comparable for all formulations. Specifically, $\rho_b = 0.109 \pm 0.02$ g/cm^3 for GG/Ca 0.3% and $\rho_b = 0.0926 \pm 0.02$ g/cm^3 for GG/LAPO/Ca 0.3%.

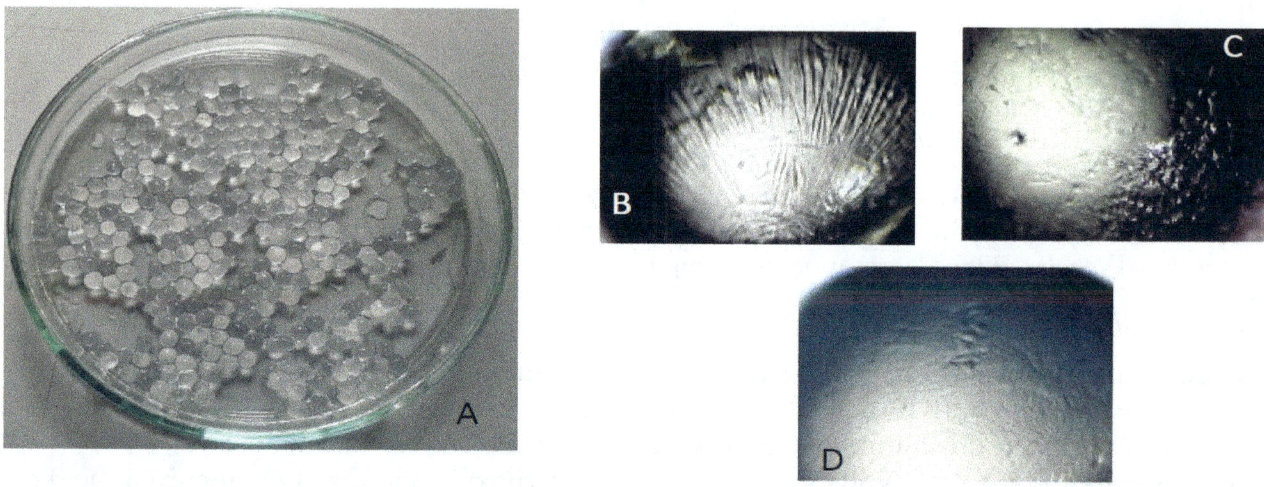

Figure 6. (**A**) Pictures of beads of GG/LAPO/Ca 0.3%; pictures of beads at the optical microscope; (**B**) GG/Ca 0.3%; (**C**) GG/Ca 0.6%; (**D**) GG/LAPO/Ca 0.3%.

4.3. Swelling Experiments

A crucial property of the polymeric beads is the ability to swell in aqueous environments. The results of swelling experiments are reported in Table 2 in terms of the swelling degree at equilibrium S_{eq} (after 24 h).

Table 2. Swelling degree at equilibrium S_{eq} (measured after 24 h) and effective solvent diffusion coefficient D_s^{sg} of different bead formulations in Simulated Gastric Fluid (SGF; HCl 0.1 M) and Simulated Intestinal Fluid (SIF; phosphate buffer 0.044 M, pH 7.4).

Beads Formulation	S_{eq} in SGF	S_{eq} in SIF	D_s^{sg} in SGF [m^2/s]	D_s^{sg} in SIF [m^2/s]
GG/Ca 0.3%	9.08 ± 0.3	45.80 ± 0.9	$(8.8 \pm 0.3) \times 10^{-10}$	$(1.5 \pm 0.1) \times 10^{-9}$
GG/Ca 0.6%	8.97 ± 0.2	25.44 ± 0.6	-	-
GG/LAPO/Ca 0.3%	9.14 ± 0.3	20.60 ± 0.3	$(6.5 \pm 0.3) \times 10^{-10}$	$(1.1 \pm 0.1) \times 10^{-9}$

In general, the swelling degree decreases in both swelling media as the amount of cross-linker is increased. The significant differences observed in swelling degree values in SGF and SIF are related to the nature of GG. The carboxylic groups of GG exist in a protonated form in HCl. This allows the network chains to stay closer to each other, resulting in a smaller swelling degree in acid medium. The beads in SIF exhibit a larger swelling degree as the carboxylic groups are deprotonated, resulting in a repulsion effect between network chains.

The presence of laponite causes a remarkable decrease of the equilibrium value S_{eq} as already observed in [17] dealing with beads made of pH sensitive laponite/alginate/$CaCl_2$ hybrid hydrogel. In agreement with experimental findings reported in [17], the effect of clay is not only to decrease the equilibrium swelling degree but also to reduce the solvent diffusion coefficient D_s^{sg} in both media, as reported in Table 2. In agreement with swelling degrees at equilibrium, Table 2 also shows that D_s^{sg} is larger for SIF than for SGF for particles with and without clay. The values of D_s^{sg} reported in Table 2 for different beads and different media are obtained from the best-fit of experimental data for the time evolution of the swelling degree *S(t)* with the swelling model developed in Section 3.1.

Figure 7 shows the comparison between experimental data for *S(t)* and the swelling model predictions where:

(1) the parameter β has been set to the value $\beta = 2$ in order to account for the large porosity/small density of beads;

(2) the solvent volume fraction (SGF or SIF) at equilibrium φ_{eq} is directly estimated from the equilibrium swelling degree S_{eq} as

$$\varphi_{eq} = \frac{x_{eq}/\rho_s}{\left(1-x_{eq}\right)/\rho_b + x_{eq}/\rho_s},\quad x_{eq} = 1 - 1/\left(1+S_{eq}\right), \tag{17}$$

where x_{eq} is the solvent weight fraction at equilibrium and ρ_b is the dry particle density;

(3) φ_G has been set to $\varphi_G = 0.1\varphi_{eq}$, given the ease of beads re-hydration after freeze-drying.

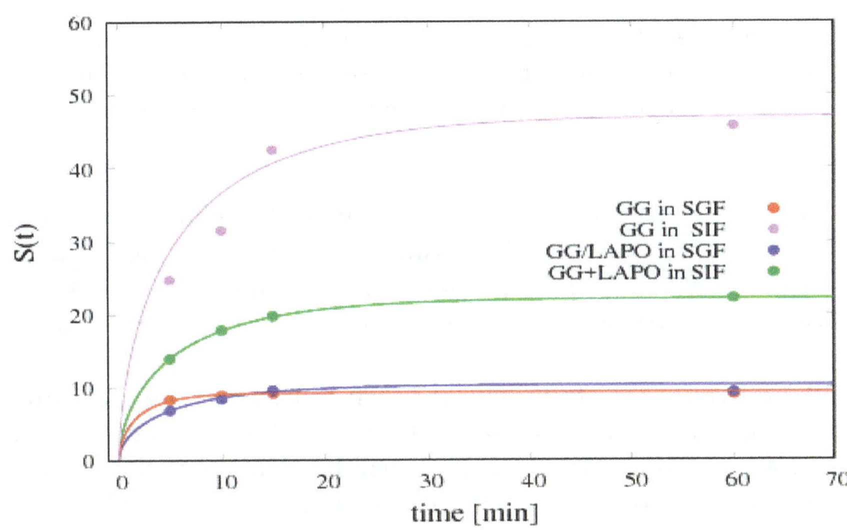

Figure 7. Comparison between the swelling model predictions (continuous lines) and experimental data (points) for the temporal evolution of the swelling degree *S(t)* for two different bead formulations (GG/Ca 0.3% and GG/LAPO/Ca 0.3%) and two different swelling media (SGF and SIF). The best fit values for the solvent diffusion coefficient in the swollen gel D_s^{sg} are reported in Table 2.

Figure 8 shows the time evolution of particle diameter as predicted by the swelling model and the satisfactory agreement with experimental data for particle diameter at equilibrium. It can be observed that dry particles, given the high porosity and the small density, are able to absorb a large amount of solvent, e.g., about 50 times their initial weight for GG/Ca 0.3% formulation in SIF, while the diameter at equilibrium at the most doubles its initial value. The swelling model, being able to account for the high particle porosity, furnishes a reliable forecasting estimate of the equilibrium diameter and of the time-scale for reaching equilibrium conditions, approximately 15–20 min for all the different formulations in the two media.

It is important to point out that, even if the increase in the particle diameter is not so large, it is however extremely important to adopt a release model that takes into account the swelling and the variation of the diameter of the particle over time, as the estimate of the effective drug diffusivity is based mainly on the analysis of release curves at short time scales and is strongly influenced by the variation of the diffusional lengths. Adopting a fixed boundary model leads to an error of the drug diffusion coefficient at least of a factor $(d_{eq}/d_0)^2$ where d_{eq} and d_0 are the equilibrium and initial particle diameter, respectively.

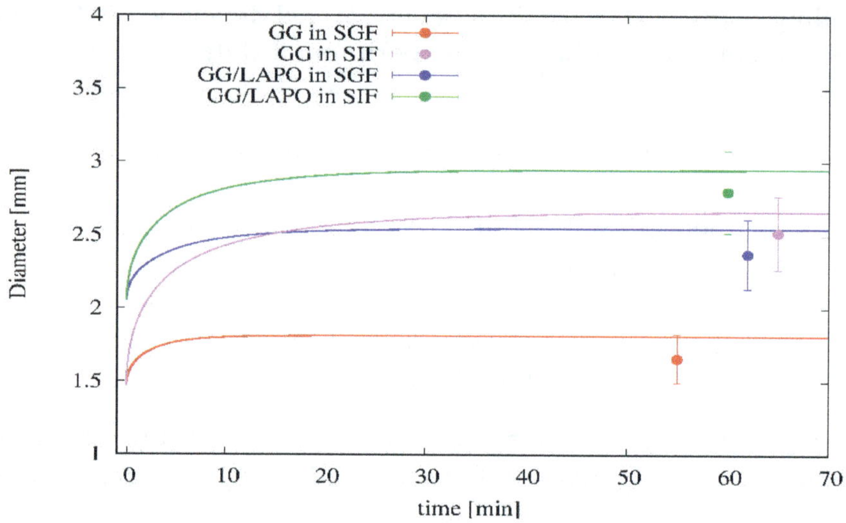

Figure 8. Comparison between the swelling model predictions (continuous lines) and experimental data (points) for the temporal evolution of the particle diameter for two different bead formulations (GG/Ca 0.3% and GG/LAPO/Ca 0.3%) and two different swelling media (SGF and SIF).

4.4. Entrapment Efficiency

Two model drugs of different molecular weights and dimensions were loaded into the beads, namely theophylline (MW 180, van der Waals radius 3.7 Å, aqueous solubility 8.3 mg/mL; pKa 8.6 [35]) and vitamin B12 (MW 1356, van der Waals radius 21 Å, aqueous solubility 10–33 mg/mL, pKa = 3.28 [36]) in order to verify the possible use of freeze-dried beads for the oral administration of drugs.

Table 3 reports the entrapment efficiency of the two drug molecules into two different bead formulations, GG/Ca 0.3% *w/w* and GG/LAPO/Ca 0.3% *w/w*. It is evident that the entrapment efficiency is influenced by both the bead structure and the steric hindrance of the loaded molecule. Indeed, theophylline, smaller than vitamin B12, is less retained by both bead formulations, whereas the presence of laponite increases the entrapment efficiency of both drug molecules. This will reflect in drug-release data analyzed in the next section. The fact that the presence of laponite increases the drug entrapment efficiency has been already observed in [17] for methylene blue loaded laponite/alginate beads.

Table 3. Entrapment efficiency of two model drug molecules, theophylline and vitamin B12.

Beads	Drug Molecule	Entrapment Efficiency (%)
GG/Ca 0.3%	Vitamin B12	53.62
GG/LAPO/Ca 0.3%	Vitamin B12	61.26
GG/Ca 0.3%	Theophylline	20.26
GG/LAPO/Ca 0.3%	Theophylline	36.49

4.5. Release Data Analysis

4.5.1. Theophylline Release

We preliminary analyzed release data of theophylline from beads GG/Ca 0.3% *w/w* without laponite in both media SGF and SIF. Release data are shown in Figure 9A,B in terms of the withdrawal concentration C_{res} $(t_w{}^i)$, from now on referred to as differential release curve, and of the integral release curve M_t/M_∞.

It can be observed that integral release curves exhibit typical Fickian behavior in both media and any type of physical/chemical drug/polymer interaction can be excluded. Continuous lines represent theoretical predictions obtained with the no-drug-polymer interaction model Equations (11)–(13) developed in Section 3.2, numerically solved together with the swelling model Equations (6)–(9) for which the parameter values, specifically D_s^{sg} and β, reported in Section 4.3, were estimated from independent swelling measurements. The only best-fit parameter entering the drug release model is the theophylline diffusivity in the swollen gel D_d^{sg}, whose values are reported in Table 4 for both media.

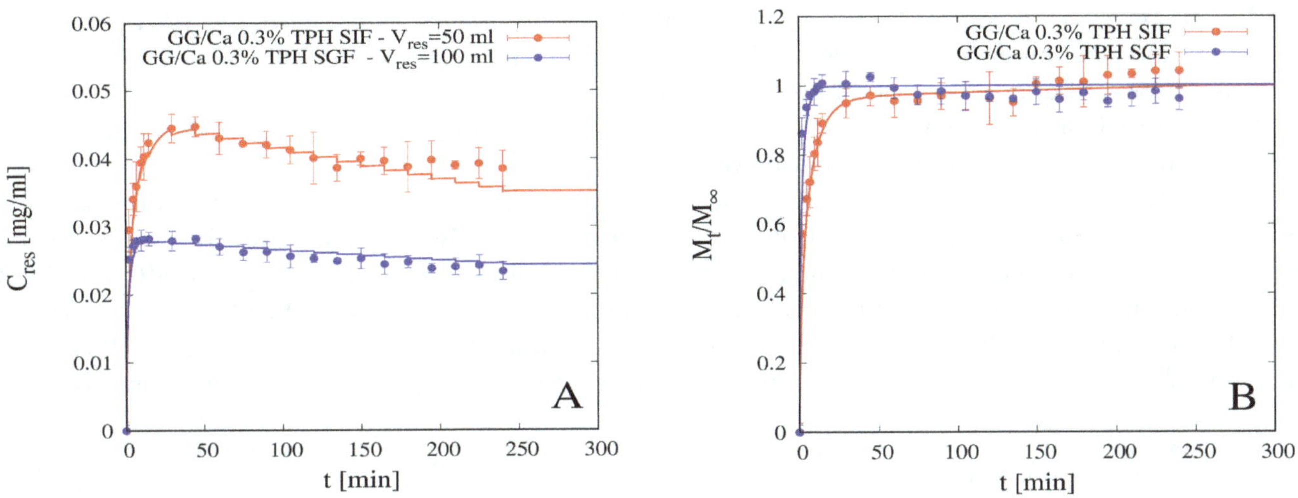

Figure 9. Differential (**A**) and integral release curves (**B**) for theophylline (TPH) from beads GG/Ca 0.3% *w/w* without laponite in SGF and SIF. Continuous lines represent model predictions Equations (11)–(13). Estimated values of the TPH effective diffusivity D_d^{sg} are reported in Table 4.

It is important to point out that, for an accurate estimate of D_d^{sg}, the model best-fit must be performed on differential experimental data of $C_{res}(t_w^i)$, instead of on the integral release curve M_t/M_∞, $C_{res}(t_w^i)$ data being more sensitive to D_d^{sg} both in the initial phase of rapid concentration rise and in the subsequent phase where the effect of withdrawals become significant and not negligible.

The finite volume V_{res} of the reservoir is explicitly taken into account in model formulation, as well as the withdrawals, as can be observed from the sawtooth behavior of the differential release model curve. In fact, smaller values of V_{res}, which do not guarantee the perfect sink condition, are to be preferred as they ensure better mixing and greater uniformity of drug concentration in the reservoir. Imperfect mixing is difficult to model and leads to a withdrawal drug concentration that may depend on the withdrawal point. On the contrary, the non-negligible drug concentration in the perfectly mixed reservoir ($C_{res} > 0$, no sink condition) can be easily modeled by means of a macroscopic balance equation (see Equation (13)). The only requirement is that V_{res} must be greater than a minimum value that guarantees that the maximum value attained by $C_{res}(t)$ during the release experiment is significantly lower than drug solubility in the release medium. This condition is always fulfilled in our release experiments for both drugs and for all V_{res} analyzed.

Table 4. Theophylline diffusivity in the swollen gel D_d^{sg} for two different bead formulations (with and without laponite) and two different media SGF and SIF.

Beads	**D_d^{sg} in SGF [m²/s]**	**D_d^{sg} in SIF [m²/s]**
GG/Ca 0.3%	$(4.26 \pm 0.15) \times 10^{-10}$	$(2.62 \pm 0.2) \times 10^{-10}$
GG/LAPO/Ca 0.3%	$(2.73 \pm 0.3) \times 10^{-11}$	$(1.43 \pm 0.1) \times 10^{-10}$

From integral release data shown in Figure 9B and diffusivity values reported in Table 4 it can be readily observed that theophylline release from beads without clay, despite the larger degree of swelling in SIF than in SGF, is faster in SGF than in SIF. Theophylline effective diffusivity in the bead swollen in SGF is about half the value in aqueous solution $D_{TPH} \approx 8.2 \times 10^{-10}$ m^2/s, while it reduces to a quarter of D_{TPH} in the bead swollen in SIF. This can be explained in terms of the screening effect of the COO^- groups of GG by the ions in SGF solution, thus reducing the possible interaction between theophylline and the charged polymer. A similar phenomenon has been observed by Coviello et al. (1999) [37] for theophylline in sclerox, a polycarboxylated derivative of scleroglucan.

In [37] the authors reported that theophylline diffusion rate in sclerox, without crosslinker, was increased in acid medium with respect to that in SIF, while a diffusion rate lower in acid medium than in SIF was observed in sclerox in the presence of alkane dihalides as crosslinker. We observed the same inversion phenomenon from release data of theophylline in GG beads with and without laponite, acting as a crosslinker as supported by swelling data.

Figure 10A,B shows release data for theophylline from beads GG/LAPO/Ca 0.3% in SGF and SIF and the comparison with model predictions with the corresponding effective diffusion coefficients $D_d{}^{sg}$ reported in Table 4. In the presence of clay, theophylline diffusivity reduces by an order of magnitude with respect to D_{TPH} in both media, but it is significantly smaller in SGF than in SIF. In this case, diffusivity values are in agreement with swelling data, S_{eq} being significantly larger in SIF than in SGF for GG beads including laponite (see Table 2). Therefore, the screening effect of the COO^- groups of GG by the ions in SGF solution, although still present, is balanced and overcome by the reduced mesh size of the network, this last observation being supported by swelling data in Figure 7 and Table 2.

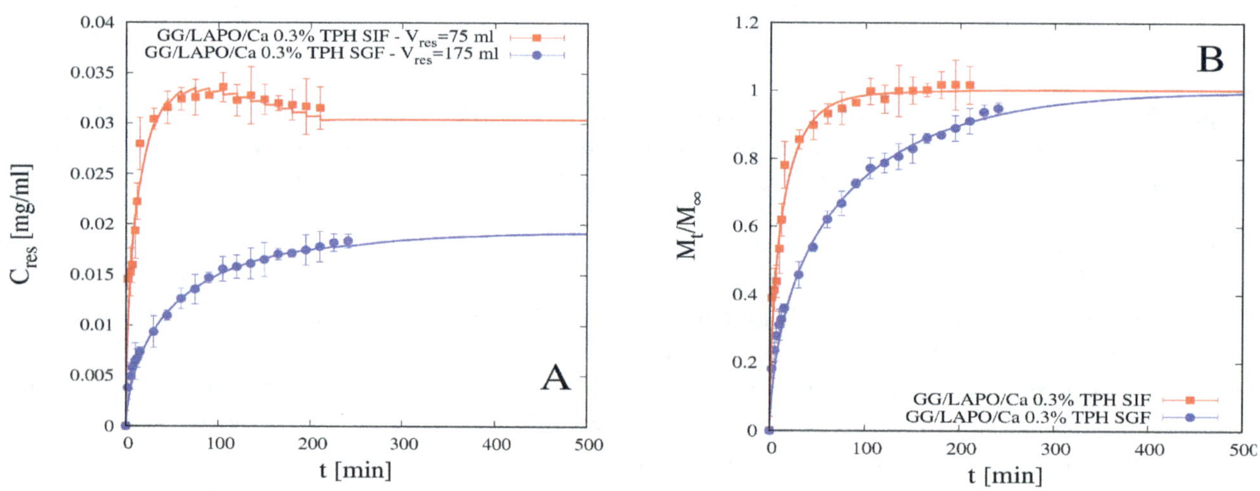

Figure 10. Differential (**A**) and integral release curves (**B**) for theophylline (TPH) from beads GG/LAPO/Ca 0.3% with laponite in SGF and SIF. Continuous lines represent model predictions from Equations (11)–(13). Estimated values of the TPH diffusivity $D_d{}^{sg}$ are reported in Table 4.

This observation is in agreement with experimental findings reported in [17] focusing on drug release (methylene blue) from beads made of pH sensitive laponite/alginate/$CaCl_2$ hybrid hydrogel. These authors observed that the presence of laponite induced a significant slowing down of the release kinetic of hydrophilic drugs especially in acid medium.

Reliability and accuracy of the experimental release curves above presented, as well the predictive ability of the release model proposed, are confirmed by the analysis of gastrointestinal release data, i.e., release data obtained by immersing the beads sequentially first in SGF for 120 min and subsequently in SIF for 120 min, thus simulating the gastrointestinal release in-vitro.

Figure 11A–D shows the differential (A and C) and the integral (B and D) gastrointestinal release curves of theophylline from beads GG/Ca 0.3% (A,B) without laponite and GG/LAPO/Ca 0.3% with laponite (C,D). Continuous lines show the excellent agreement between experimental data and theoretical curves obtained from the release model used in a fully predictive way, by making use of the TPH diffusivity values $D_d{}^{sg}$ previously estimated and reported in Table 4.

It can be observed that TPH release from beads without laponite is so fast in SGF that 95% of the drug is released in acid medium in the first 120 min. On the contrary, the presence of laponite significantly slows down TPH release in SGF, so that about 70% of drug is released in acid medium, and the remaining 30% is slowly released in the intestinal tract. We conclude that bead formulation including laponite represents a release medium capable of supporting the controlled release of a small non-interacting drug as theophylline.

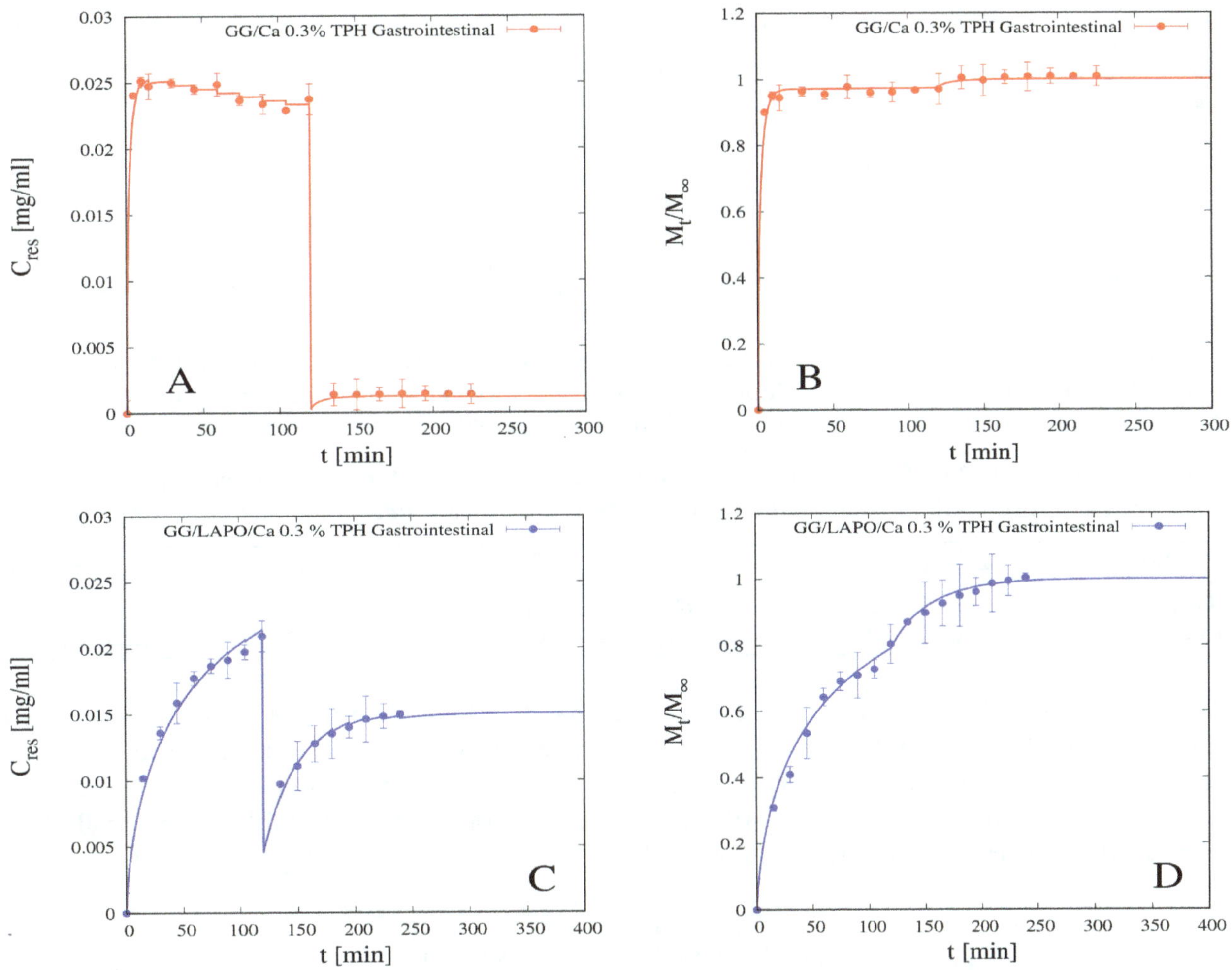

Figure 11. Gastrointestinal differential (**A**,**C**) and integral release curves (**B**,**D**) for theophylline (TPH) from beads GG/Ca 0.3% without laponite (**A**,**B**) and GG/LAPO/Ca 0.3% with laponite (**C**,**D**), $p < 0.001$. Continuous lines represent model predictions from Equations (11)–(13) with TPH diffusivity $D_d{}^{sg}$ reported in Table 4.

4.5.2. Vitamin B12 Release

We preliminary analyzed release data of vitamin B12 from beads GG/Ca 0.3% without laponite in both media SGF and SIF. Differential and integral release data are shown in Figure 12A,B respectively. Additionally, for vitamin B12, as for theophylline, integral release curves from bead formulation without laponite exhibit typical Fickian behavior in both media. Continuous lines represent theoretical predictions obtained with the no-drug-polymer interaction model in Equations (11)–(13) developed in Section 3.2. B12 diffusivity values $D_d{}^{sg}$ in SGF and SIF are reported in Table 5.

It can be observed that B12 diffusivities in both media are: (1) smaller than the corresponding ones for theophylline, as expected given the larger dimension of vitamin B12 and the bigger steric hindrance; (2) comparable in SIF and SGF, despite the larger differences between swelling degrees, as the screening effect in acid medium compensates the reduced mesh size of the network. Moreover, vitamin B12 diffusivity in SIF is in quantitative agreement with diffusivity value $D_{B12} \approx 2.1 \times 10^{-10}$ m^2/s reported in [38] for vitamin B12 in scleroglucan/borax hydrogel swollen in distilled water (pH 5.4).

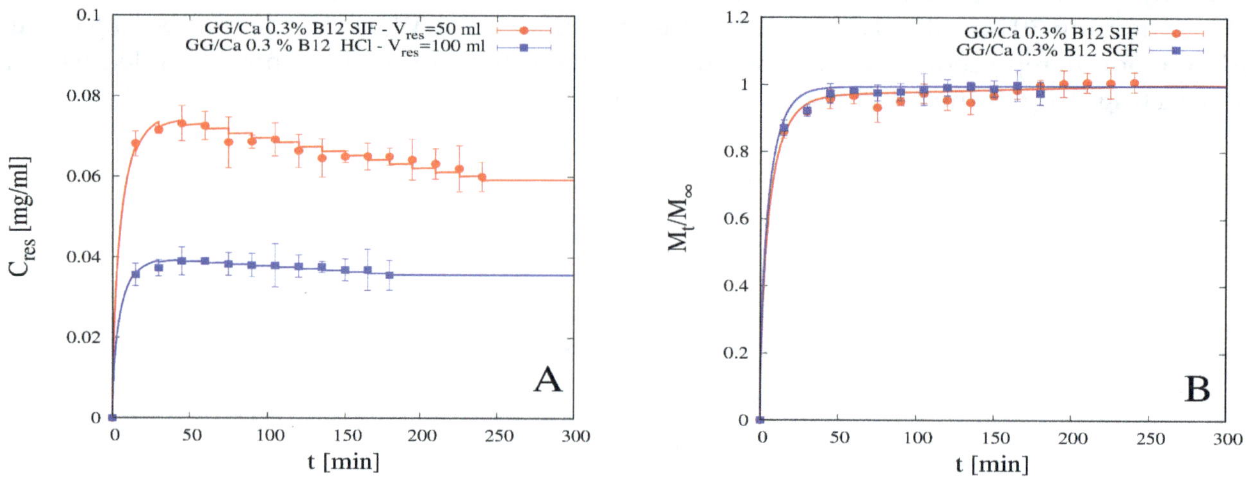

Figure 12. Differential (**A**) and integral release curves (**B**) for vitamin B12 from beads GG/Ca 0.3% without laponite in SGF and SIF. Continuous lines represent model predictions from Equations (11)–(13). Estimated values of the B12 diffusivity D_d^{sg} are reported in Table 5.

Table 5. Vitamin B12 diffusivity in the swollen gel D_d^{sg} and transfer rate coefficient k_{bg}^{sg} for two different bead formulations (with and without laponite) and two different media SGF and SIF.

Beads	D_d^{sg} in SGF [m^2/s]	D_d^{sg} in SIF [m^2/s]	k_{bg}^{sg} in SGF [1/s]	k_{bg}^{sg} in SIF [1/s]
GG/Ca 0.3%	$(1.53 \pm 0.15) \times 10^{-10}$	$(1.85 \pm 0.15) \times 10^{-10}$	-	-
GG/LAPO/Ca 0.3%	$(2.87 \pm 0.1) \times 10^{-11}$	$(5.33 \pm 0.1) \times 10^{-11}$	2.35×10^{-4}	4.12×10^{-3}

Like for theophylline, vitamin B12 release from beads without clay in SGF is fast enough so that the gastrointestinal release data shown in Figure 13 present an almost complete drug release in the gastric tract (98% of drug released after 120 min in SGF) and almost no drug is left to be released in the intestinal tract. Therefore, the bead formulation without laponite is not suitable for controlled release of a medium/large non-interacting drug molecule.

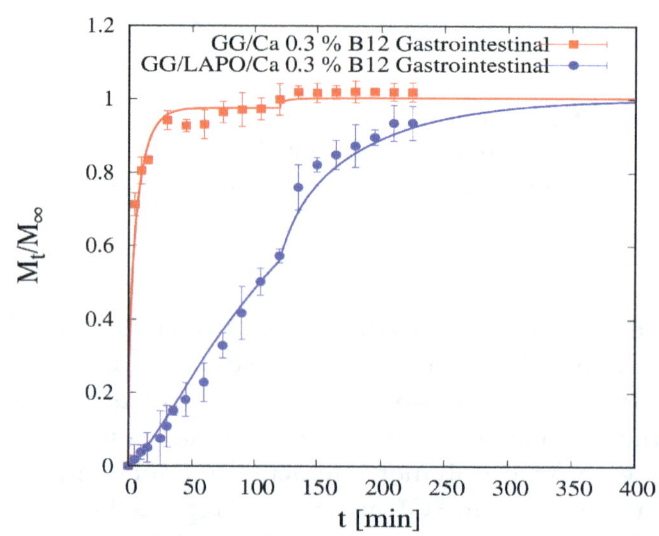

Figure 13. Gastrointestinal integral release curve for vitamin B12 from beads GG/Ca 0.3% with and without laponite ($p < 0.001$). Continuous lines represent model predictions for the Fickian release model from Equations (11)–(13) and for the two-phase release model from Equations (13)–(16) with model parameters reported in Table 5.

A completely different scenario opens up when laponite is included in bead formulation and vitamin B12 release data are analyzed. Figure 14 shows integral release data of vitamin B12 from beads GG/LAPO/Ca 0.3% including laponite in SIF and SGF. It can be readily observed that drug release in SGF exhibits non-Fickian behavior $M_t/M_\infty \approx t^n$ with an exponent $n = 1.2$ much bigger than $\frac{1}{2}$.

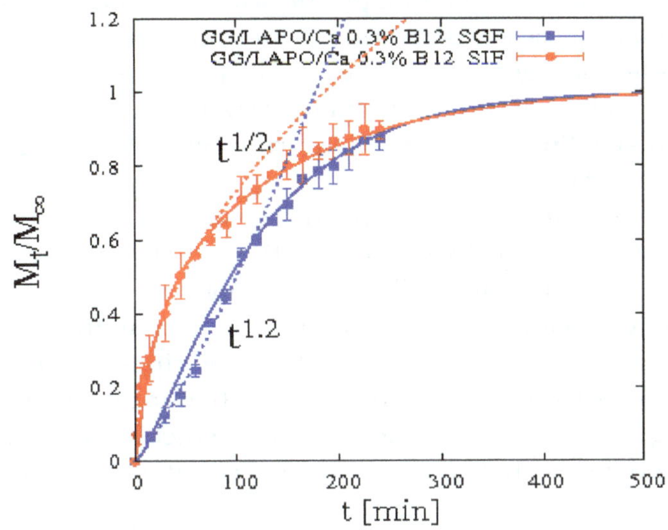

Figure 14. Integral release curve for vitamin B12 from beads GG/LAPO/Ca 0.3% with laponite in SGF and SIF. Dotted curves highlight the Fickian and non-Fickian behaviors in SIF and in SGF, respectively. Continuous lines represent model predictions from Equations (13)–(16).

This is a clear symptom that an interaction occurs between vitamin B12 and the polymer/clay complex. This interaction is strongly weakened by the enlarged mesh size of the network induced by matrix swelling in SIF while it is stronger and sustained by the reduced swelling in SGF.

For this reason, we adopted the two-phase model developed in Section 3.3 describing drug/clay-polymer interaction in terms of a linear transfer rate from a bounded phase, in which drug molecules are initially entrapped, to a gel phase in which drug molecules are free to diffuse and exit the swelling bead. Figure 14 shows good agreement between integral release data and the two-phase model predictions Equations (13)–(16). Best-fit values of vitamin B12 diffusivity ${D_d}^{sg}$ and transfer rate constant ${k_{bg}}^{sg}$ in SIF and SGF are reported in Table 5.

The transfer rate coefficient ${k_{bg}}^{sg}$ for vitamin B12 in SGF is one order of magnitude smaller than that in SIF. The diffusivity $\mathrm{D_d}^{sg}$ is smaller in SGF than in SIF.

By analyzing these findings in terms of the Thiele modulus Φ^2 (introduced in Section 3.3), we observe that Φ^2 for vitamin B12 in GG/LAPO/Ca 0.3% attains the following values: $\Phi^2 \approx 80$ in SIF and $\Phi^2 \approx 9$ in SGF. Therefore, Φ^2 in SGF is one order of magnitude smaller than Φ^2 in SIF. This quantitatively explains why drug-polymer/clay complex interaction leads to a strong non-Fickian behavior in SGF, characterized by a slower release at short time scale because the diffusion time-scale is comparable to the transfer time scale, while a Fickian behavior is observed for vitamin B12 in SIF because diffusion is definitely the rate controlling step.

Diffusivity values ${D_d}^{sg}$ for vitamin B12 are actually much lower in the beads with laponite in both media, and this, together with drug interaction with the polymer/clay complex, reflects in the gastrointestinal release curve shown in Figure 13 together with the corresponding vitamin B12 release curve from beads without laponite. The continuous blue curve represents the two-phase model prediction, from Equations (13)–(16), of the gastrointestinal release without any adjustable parameters.

In the presence of laponite, only 60% of the loaded vitamin B12 is released in the gastric tract (first 120 min), and also the remaining 40% is slowly released in the intestinal tract, as the complete release requires about 280 min in SIF medium. Therefore, the bead formulation including laponite is suitable for sustained release of a medium/large interacting drug molecule.

5. Conclusions

Gellan gum, a natural polysaccharide, was employed together with calcium chloride, selected as cross-linker, in order to prepare beads using the ionotropic gelation method. Laponite, a synthetic clay, was also included in the formulations. Stable and spherical beads (aspect ratio ≈ 1.02) were obtained from GG solutions (GG 0.15 % *w/w*) and GG/laponite solutions (GG 0.15% *w/w*, laponite 0.1% *w/w*) with $CaCl_2$ 0.3% *w/w*. Gellan gum beads including laponite have shown a smoother and regular surface and a larger diameter, namely $d_0 \approx 2.8$ mm and $d_0 \approx 2.1$ mm before and after freeze-drying, respectively. The ability to swell in different media mimicking biological fluids, namely SGF and SIF, was investigated. The bead swelling degree at equilibrium was lower in SGF than in SIF and further reduced in the presence of laponite.

Two model drugs, theophylline and vitamin B12, having different molecular weight and steric hindrance, were loaded into different bead formulations. The presence of laponite in the bead formulation increased the drug entrapment efficiency for both model drugs. Sustained release of both model drugs was obtained from beads including laponite, as a small fraction of the incorporated drugs was released in the gastric medium. This suggests that laponite may be an effective additive in the development of GG beads for sustained release of drugs. Better results in terms of sustained release were obtained for vitamin B12 as it exhibited a significant interaction with the clay/polymer composites in SGF. In the absence of laponite, both drugs were almost completely released in the first two hours of residence in SGF.

The swelling model with "diffuse interface" and the corresponding drug release models developed for polymer/clay beads no-interacting and interacting drugs have proved to be able to correctly describe all the phenomena experimentally observed and to furnish reliable drug diffusivity values in agreement with literature data for the same drugs in similar physical hydrogels.

Author Contributions: Conceptualization, A.A., L.D.M. and M.A.C.; Data curation, L.D.M.; Formal analysis, A.A.; Funding acquisition, A.A., P.P., I.T. and M.A.C.; Investigation, A.A., P.P., S.P., L.D.M., J.T., S.C., I.T. and M.A.C.; Methodology, P.P., S.P., L.D.M. and M.A.C.; Project administration, A.A., I.T. and M.A.C.; Resources, A.A., P.P., I.T. and M.A.C.; Software, A.A.; Supervision, A.A., P.P., S.P., I.T. and M.A.C.; Validation, A.A. and M.A.C.; Visualization, I.T. and M.A.C.; Writing—original draft, A.A. and M.A.C.; Writing—review & editing, A.A., I.T. and M.A.C.

References

1. Debotton, N.; Dahan, A. Applications of Polymers as Pharmaceutical Excipients in Solid Oral Dosage Forms. *Med. Res. Rev.* **2017**, *37*, 52–97. [CrossRef] [PubMed]
2. Borges, A.F.; Silva, C.; Coelho, J.F.J.; Simoes, S. Oral films: Current status and future perspectives: I-Galenical development and quality attributes. *J. Control. Release* **2015**, *206*, 1–19. [CrossRef]
3. Qui, Y.; Park, K. Environment sensitive hydrogels for drug delivery. *Adv. Drug Deliv. Rev.* **2012**, *64*, 49–60.
4. Giannuzzo, M.; Feeney, M.; Paolicelli, P.; Casadei, M.A. pH-sensitive hydrogels of dextran. *J. Drug Deliv. Sci. Technol.* **2006**, *16*, 49–54. [CrossRef]
5. Singh, B.N.; Kim, K.H. Floating drug delivery systems: An approach to oral controlled drug delivery via gastric retention. *J. Control. Release* **2000**, *63*, 235–259. [CrossRef]
6. Bardonnet, P.L.; Faivre, V.; Pugh, W.J.; Piffaretti, J.C.; Falson, F. Gastro-retentive dosage forms: Overview and special case of Helicobacter pylori. *J. Control. Release* **2006**, *111*, 1–18. [CrossRef] [PubMed]
7. Bera, H.; Boddupalli, S.; Nandikonda, S.; Kumar, S.; Nayak, A.K. Alginate gel-coated oil-entrapped alginate-tamarind gum-magnesium stearate buoyant beads of risperidone. *Int. J. Biol. Macromol.* **2015**, *78*, 102–111. [CrossRef] [PubMed]
8. Baumgartner, S.; Kristil, J.; Vrecer, F.; Vodopivec, P.; Zorko, B. Optimization of floating matrix tablets and evalutation of their gastric residence time. *Int. J. Pharm.* **2000**, *195*, 125–135. [CrossRef]
9. Osmałek, T.; Froelich, A.; Tasarek, S. Application of gellan gum in pharmacy and medicine. *Int. J. Pharm.* **2014**, *466*, 328–340.
10. Patil, P.; Chavanke, D.; Wagh, M. A review on ionotropic gelation method: Novel approach for controlled gastroretentive gelispheres. *Int. J. Pharm. Pharm. Sci.* **2012**, *4*, 27–32.

11. Lopez-Cebral, R.; Paolicelli, P.; Romero-Caamaño, V.; Sejio, B.; Casadei, M.A.; Sanchez, A. Spermidine cross-linked hydrogels as novel potential platforms for pharmaceutical applications. *J. Pharm. Sci.* **2013**, *102*, 2632–2643. [CrossRef] [PubMed]
12. Patela, A.M.; Mohamed, H.H.; Schryer-Pragaa, J.V.; Chadwicka, K. The effect of ionotropic gelation residence time on alginate cross-linking and properties. *Carbohydr. Polym.* **2017**, *155*, 362–371. [CrossRef]
13. Cerciello, A.; Del Gaudio, P.; Granatac, V.; Sala, M.; Aquino, R.P.; Russo, P. Synergistic effect of divalent cations in improving technological properties of cross-linked alginate beads. *Int. J. Biol. Macromol.* **2017**, *101*, 100–106. [CrossRef] [PubMed]
14. Benfattoum, K.; Haddadine, N.; Bouslah, N.; Benaboura, A.; Maincent, P.; Barillé, R.; Sapin-Minet, A.; El-Shall, M.S. Formulation characterization and in vitro evaluation of acacia gum–calcium alginate beads for oral drug delivery systems. *Polym. Adv. Technol.* **2018**, *29*, 884–895. [CrossRef]
15. Gupta, K.C.; Ravi, K.M.N.V. Drug release behavior of beads and microgranules of chitosan. *Biomaterials* **2000**, *21*, 1115–1119. [CrossRef]
16. Meirelles, L.M.A.; Raffin, F.N. Clay and Polymer-Based Composites Applied to Drug Release: A Scientific and Technological Prospection. *J. Pharm. Pharm. Sci.* **2017**, *20*, 115–134. [CrossRef]
17. Li, Y.; Maciel, D.; Tom, H.; Rodrigues, J.; Ma, H.; Shi, X. pH sensitive Laponite/alginate hybrid hydrogels: Swelling behaviour and release mechanism. *Soft Matter* **2011**, *7*, 6231–6238. [CrossRef]
18. Wu, C.J.; Gaharwar, A.K.; Schexnailder, P.J.; Schmidt, G. Development of Biomedical Polymer-Silicate Nanocomposites: A Materials Science Perspective. *Materials* **2010**, *3*, 2986–3005. [CrossRef]
19. Haraguchi, K.; Takehisa, T. Nanocomposite Hydrogels: A Unique Organic–Inorganic Network Structure with Extraordinary Mechanical, Optical, and Swelling/De-swelling Properties. *Adv. Mater.* **2002**, *14*, 1120–1124. [CrossRef]
20. Raut, S.Y.; Gahane, A.; Joshi, M.B.; Kalthur, G.; Mutalik, S. Nanocomposite clay-polymer microbeads for oral controlled drug delivery: Development and, in vitro and in vivo evaluations. *J. Drug Deliv. Sci. Technol.* **2019**, *51*, 234–243. [CrossRef]
21. Yang, H.; Hua, S.; Wang, W.; Wang, A. Composite hydrogel beads based on chitosan and laponite: Preparation, swelling, and drug release behavior. *Iran. Polym. J.* **2011**, *20*, 479–490.
22. Li, P.; Siddaramaiah; Kim, N.H.; Yoo, G.H.; Lee, J.H. Poly(acrylamide/laponite) nanocomposite hydrogels: Swelling and cationic dye adsorption properties. *J. Appl. Polym. Sci.* **2009**, *111*, 1786–1798. [CrossRef]
23. Pacelli, S.; Paolicelli, P.; Moretti, G.; Petralito, S.; Di Giacomo, S.; Vitalone, A.; Casadei, M.A. Gellan gum methacrylate and laponite as an innovative nanocomposite hydrogel for biomedical applications. *Eur. Polym. J.* **2016**, *77*, 114–126. [CrossRef]
24. Haraguchi, K. Synthesis and properties of soft nanocomposite materials with novel organic/inorganic network structures. *Polym. J.* **2011**, *43*, 223–241. [CrossRef]
25. Da Silva Fernandes, R.; de Moura, M.R.; Glenn, G.M.; Aouada, F.A. Thermal, microstructural, and spectroscopic analysis of Ca2+ alginate/clay nanocomposite hydrogel beads. *J. Mol. Liq.* **2018**, *265*, 327–336. [CrossRef]
26. Papanu, J.S.; Soane, D.S.; Bell, A.T.; Hess, D.M. Transport Models for swelling and dissolution of thin polymer films. *J. Appl. Polym. Sci.* **1989**, *38*, 859–885. [CrossRef]
27. Adrover, A.; Nobili, M. Release kinetics from oral thin films: Theory and experiments. *Chem. Eng. Res. Des.* **2015**, *98*, 188–211. [CrossRef]
28. Adrover, A.; Varani, G.; Paolicelli, P.; Petralito, S.; Di Muzio, L.; Casadei, M.A.; Tho, I. Experimental and Modeling Study of Drug Release from HPMC-Based Erodible Oral Thin Films. *Pharmaceutics* **2018**, *10*, 222. [CrossRef] [PubMed]
29. Singh, M.; Lumpkin, J.A.; Rosenblatt, J. Mathematical modeling of drug release from hydrogel matrices via a diffusion coupled with desorption mechanism. *J. Control. Release* **1994**, *32*, 17–25. [CrossRef]
30. Paolicelli, P.; Varani, G.; Pacelli, S.; Ogliani, E.; Nardoni, M.; Petralito, S.; Adrover, A.; Casadei, M.A. Design and characterization of a biocompatible physical hydrogel based on scleroglucan for topical drug delivery. *Carbohydr. Polym.* **2017**, *174*, 960–969. [CrossRef] [PubMed]
31. Morris, E.R.; Nishinari, K.; Rinaudo, M. Gelation of gellan—A review. *Food Hydrocoll.* **2012**, *28*, 373–411. [CrossRef]

32. Osmałek, T.; Milanowski, B.; Froelich, A.; Szybowicz, M.; Białowąs, W.; Kapela, M.; Gadziński, P.; Ancukiewicz, K. Design and characteristics of gellan gum beads for modified release of meloxicam. *Drug. Dev. Ind. Pharm.* **2017**, *43*, 1314–1329. [CrossRef] [PubMed]
33. Narkar, M.; Sher, P.; Pawar, A. Stomach-specific controlled release gellan beads of acid-soluble drug prepared by ionotropic gelation method. *AAPS PharmSciTech* **2010**, *11*, 267–277. [CrossRef] [PubMed]
34. Babu, R.J.; Sathigari, S.; Kumar, M.T.; Pandit, J.K. Formulation of controlled release gellan gum macro beads of amoxicillin. *Curr. Drug Deliv.* **2010**, *7*, 36–43. [CrossRef]
35. Cohen, J.L. Theophylline. *Anal. Profiles Drug Subst.* **1975**, *4*, 466–493.
36. Kirschbaum, J. Cyanocobalamin. *Anal. Profiles Drug Subst.* **1981**, *10*, 183–288.
37. Coviello, T.; Grassi, M.; Rambone, G.; Santucci, E.; Carafa, M.; Murtas, E.; Riccieri, F.M.; Alhaique, F. Novel hydrogel system from scleroglucan: Synthesis and characterization. *J. Control. Release* **1999**, *60*, 367–378. [CrossRef]
38. Coviello, T.; Grassi, M.; Palleschi, A.; Bocchinfuso, G.; Coluzzi, G.; Banishoeib, F.; Alhaique, F. A new scleroglucan/borax hydrogel: Swelling and drug release studies. *Int. J. Pharm.* **2005**, *289*, 97–107. [CrossRef] [PubMed]

12

An In Vitro Study of the Influence of *Curcuma longa* Extracts on the Microbiota Modulation Process in Patients with Hypertension

Emanuel Vamanu [1,*], Florentina Gatea [2], Ionela Sârbu [3] and Diana Pelinescu [3]

1 Faculty of Biotechnology, University of Agronomic Science and Veterinary Medicine, 59 Marasti blvd, 1 district, 011464 Bucharest, Romania

2 Centre of Bioanalysis, National Institute for Biological Sciences, 296 Spl. Independentei, 060031 Bucharest, Romania; florentina.gatea@incdsb.ro

3 Department of Genetics, ICUB-Research Institute of the University of Bucharest, 36-46 Bd. M. Kogalniceanu, 5th District, 050107 Bucharest, Romania; ionela.sarbu@bio.unibuc.ro (I.S.); diana.pelinescu@bio.unibuc.ro (D.P.)

* Correspondence: email@emanuelvamanu.ro

Abstract: The multiple causes of cardiovascular diseases signify a major incidence and developmental risk of this pathology. One of the processes accountable for this pathologic development is the instauration of dysbiosis and its connection with an inflammatory process. Low antioxidant colonic protection encourages the progression of inflammation, with cardiovascular dysfunctions being a secondary consequence of the dysbiosis. Curcumin is one of the bioactive compounds displaying promising results for the reduction of an inflammatory process. The present study aims at demonstrating the capacity of three extracts drawn from *Curcuma* (*C.*) *longa* through an in vitro simulation process, for microbiota modulation in patients with hypertension. The acidic pH in the extraction process determined a high curcumin content in the extracts. The major phenolic compound identified was curcumin III, 622 ± 6.88 μg/mL for the ethanol/water/acetic acid extract. Low EC50 values were associated (0.2 μg/mL for DPPH scavenging activity) with the presence of curcumin isomers. A metabolic pattern became evident because the relationship between the short-chain fatty acids acted as a clinical biomarker. The curcumin present stimulated the formation of butyric and propionic acids. Microbiota activity control included a high degree of curcumin degradation and biotransformation in the other phenolic compounds. This developmental process was supported by the progression in the enterobacteria with a corresponding escalation in the pH level. The metabolomic pattern demonstrated a performance similar to the administration of dietary fibre, with the positive effects being dose-dependent.

Keywords: anti-inflammatory; butyric acid; curcumin; modulation; in vivo

1. Introduction

Cardiovascular disease management is long-lasting, and involves several medications because in most cases it is allied to other pathologies [1]. However, in its treatment, the vegetable supplements (herbs, mushrooms, spices, etc.) act as a non-toxic alternative [2]. The development of chronic disease often starts with the occurrence of an inflammatory process that indirectly results in physiological dysfunctions [3]. Oxidative stress, among all the processes, is the chief culprit that determines the development of cardiovascular pathologies. In this context, the role of cerebral oxidative stress in the manifestation of hypertension has been demonstrated [4]. The interest shown towards and reasons for the selection of *Curcuma longa* in this study arises from certain health benefits, which result from its anti-inflammatory and antioxidant properties [5]. Besides, the curcumin isomers possess many biological activities, not clearly studied as yet, involving the interactions with human microbiota [6].

Further, the influence exerted by the microbiota on host homeostasis is the critical point of the brain-gut axis [7]. Thus, the interest in the complex action of the microbiota has escalated, with particular emphasis on the explicit characterisation of the fingerprint of the microbiota of patients with cardiovascular diseases. Further correlation of this aspect was done with the metabolomic profile. Specific biomarker molecules have been identified that are directly involved in the development of heart disease [8]. Due to the significant progress made in molecular biology, it is now possible to recognise the preventive risk factors, such as colon microbiota, that play a role in the development of cardiovascular diseases.

Interaction of microbiota with bioactive compounds (especially phenolics) from medicinal plants extracts is due to the large quantity that reaches the colon, but only a small part is absorbed in ascending segments of the human digestive tract [9]. There are few in vivo studies that directly show the effect of the microbiota pattern on the bioavailability of the polyphenolic fraction. By in vitro/in vivo correlation, it has been demonstrated that the biological effect is a selective one, characteristic of each subclass of phenolic compounds. This is the result of a series of biotransformations, which changes the expected effect [10]. Curcumin is an example in this regard because it is a well-tolerated compound, although there is little evidence in vivo. Meta-analyses of clinical uses have shown that administration has a positive effect in patients with irritable bowel syndrome, and microbiota modulation has been based on correlation with antioxidant and anti-inflammatory activities [11–13].

Thus, the dysbiosis begins with an inflammatory process promoted by the low antioxidant potential at the microbiota level [14]. Dysbiosis may be caused by any of the following, viz., genetic heritage, food consumption or the occurrence and progress of cardiovascular diseases [15]. However, the favorable strains, at the level of Bacteroides sp., govern the strong response during oxidative stress [16]. The study is based on the following findings: (i) Cardiovascular dysfunctions (in those patients with hypertension and dyslipidemia) are correlated and frequently determined by the microbiota dysbiosis, (ii) the decrease in the favorable strains may be connected to the development of cardiovascular risk, (iii) the metabolomic profile is vital to cardiovascular management, and (iv) the microbiota profile signifies a biomarker that can determine early intervention and thus reduce the risk of mortality [17]. The present study aimed at controlling the in vitro effect of the consumption of *C. longa* extracts on the microbiota of a target group, which included hypertensive patients. The research presents a metabolomic profile of the microbiota fingerprint modification, correlated with the in vitro and in vivo characterization of the extracts.

2. Materials and Methods

2.1. Chemicals

Ethanol, methanol, acetic acid, glycerol, 2,2-diphenyl-1-picrylhydrazyl, Folin–Ciocalteu reagent, ascorbic acid, ferrozine disodium salt, ferrous chloride, ethylenediaminetetraacetic acid (EDTA), glucose, peptone, yeast extract, sodium chloride, hydrogen peroxide, sodium hydroxide, sodium tetraborate, methylene chloride, ferulic acid, vanillin, sodium dodecyl sulphate, hydrochloric acid, phosphoric acid, calcium carbonate, agarose, TBE buffer, and cetrimonium bromide were purchased from Sigma-Aldrich GmbH (Sternheim, Germany). Maltodextrin was purchased from Agnex, Bialystok, Poland (17% dextrose index). Peptone water and MRS broth media were purchased from Oxoid Ltd. (Hampshire, U.K.). All reagents were of analytical grade.

2.2. Extraction Process

Dried *C. longa* powder (Kotanyi Condimente SRL, Bucharest, Romania), was used to obtain the three extracts. The extraction was performed in Duran bottles (24 h, at room temperature under stirring) at a concentration of 1% turmeric with the following three solvent mixtures (*v*/*v*):

(a) Ethanol/water = 50/50, (b) ethanol/water/acetic acid = 50/49.5/0.5, and (c) ethanol/acetic acid = 99.5/0.5 [18]. Subsequently, after the extraction process, the mixture was filtered under vacuum using Whatman filter paper no. 1 [19]. The extract was then mixed with 7% maltodextrin until total homogenisation was complete and freeze-drying achieved [17]. Moreover, before conducting the experiments, the dried extracts were dissolved, in 50% (*v*/*v*) ethanol, in a series of dilutions ranging from 0.01 to 0.1%. The freeze-drying process was performed in aseptic condition in order to eliminate the possible interactions with the in vitro research.

2.3. In Vitro Simulation Process

All the in vitro tests were performed in a single-stage culture system GIS1 simulator (http://gissystems.ro/gis-technology/). The in vitro colonic simulation system involved the use of three Duran borosilicate glass bottles (500 mL capacity) having a removable screw cap [20]. The principle of the GIS1 system operations has been described in a previous study [21], and was, utilised as a continuous fermentation process [20].

First, the hypertensive patients' microbiome was reconstituted after 7.0 days mean interval and this process followed the protocol described earlier [22]. Volunteers between 40 years and 70 years of age were drawn from both sexes. Care was taken to ensure that these individuals had not received any treatment with antibiotics or other interfering drugs over the past 6.0 months, as these agents might alter the microbiome fingerprint. The samples (feces) were handled in accordance with the UASVM Bucharest ethical guidelines (ColHumB Registration number: 1418/23.11.2017; www.colhumb.com) and individually analyzed. Feces samples were collected twice from each volunteer and treated separately without any pooling ($N = 3$). Informed consent was obtained from each participant for the sample, storage after the collection. Samples were collected in 20% glycerol and stored at −15 °C until use [18,19]. Following the removal of large particles, the microbiota was reconstituted in peptone water [23]. Microbiota obtained (in the same conditions) from healthy persons was used as a control. The second control was obtained from the same hypertensive patients' untreated with *C. longa* extracts (hpu control).

First, the sampling, at the level of each colonic segment of the simulation process was accomplished, in the case of each product addition. Further, to examine the effect of the atomised extracts on the evolution of microbial communities, three identical series of treatments were performed by adding one dose (capsule) every 6.0 h in the in vitro simulator. Moreover, for the effective delivery of the products in the colon, enteric-coated capsules were used (size 0; BSC, Wenzhou, China) instead of direct addition of the extract. The capsules were directly added in the simulated environment under sterile conditions [17]. When the simulation was completed, each sample was centrifuged, (4000× *g*, 15 min, Hettich Universal 320, Hettich GmbH & Co., Kirchlengern, Germany) and the sediment (microbial fingerprint) was placed in glycerol 20% for qPCR analysis [20]. Control tests were run with ethanol, and capsules with maltodextrin only in order to establish whether solvent traces or lack extracts affect microbiota response.

2.4. Antioxidant Activity Quantification

2.4.1. In Vitro Analysis

To determine the antiradical potential, the DPPH (2,2-diphenyl-1-picrylhydrazyl) radicals were utilised according to the spectrophotometric protocol, for which the readings of the optical density of the reaction mixtures at 517 nm Helios γ (Thermo Fisher Scientific, Waltham, MA, USA) were also required. The antiradical potential was expressed in terms of the effective concentration (EC50), which was the extract concentration (µg/mL) required to inhibit the DPPH activity by 50% after at least 30 min of incubation [24]. Ascorbic acid was used as positive control.

Subsequently, the reduction power was determined spectrophotometrically at 700 nm wavelength (Helios γ, Thermo Fisher Scientific, Waltham, MA, USA), with the results being expressed as the value of the extract concentration (μg/mL) necessary to obtain an optical density of 0.5, at the specified wavelength [25]. Ascorbic acid was used as a positive control.

Further, the chelating activity was determined by using ferrozine (5 mmol/L) as the reagent. The absorbance was spectrophotometrically measured at 562 nm (Helios γ, Thermo Fisher Scientific, Waltham, MA, USA). The chelating activity was expressed as the effective concentration (EC50), which represented the concentration of the extract (μg/mL) required to obtain a 50% value [26]. EDTA was used as a positive control.

The choice of methods to evaluate the antioxidant activity was performed according to the reaction mechanism and the existing reference data [27–29].

2.4.2. In Vivo Antioxidant Potential

To determine the antioxidant potential in vivo, a modified protocol of dos Santos Andrade et al., 2011 [30] was employed. *Saccharomyces* (*S.*) *boulardii*, a probiotic yeast obtained from the University of Lille, Lille, France, was used as the in vivo model. The biomass was obtained using the YPG medium (2% glucose, 2% peptone, and 1% yeast extract) and further cultivated in the lab shaker incubator at 30 ° C, for 48 hh, at 150 rpm. The yeast cells were separated through centrifugation at 4500× *g* for 5 min and washed twice with NaCl 0.9% (sterile). Finally, the yeast cells were diluted with the same solution, whose optical density (OD) was 1.0 at 600 nm [31]. Further, to obtain the critical concentration, which is defined as the cross between the viability and mortality lines, the following mixture was used: 0.1 mL sample, 0.1 mL yeast cells in a sterile saline solution, and 0.2 mL H_2O_2 (different concentrations–0.001%, 0.005%, 0.01%, 0.2%, 0.3%). The mixture was made on a honeycomb plate and incubated at 30 °C for 1 h by using Bioscreen C MBR (Oy Growth Curves Ab Ltd., Helsinki, Finland). The cells were diluted by serial dilutions, then plated on a solid YPG and finally incubated for 48–72 h at 30 °C in an incubator (Memmert Model 100-800, Memmert GmbH & Co., Schwabach, Germany). The results were expressed as a percentage of the viability and mortality, through the use of a control sample without extract as a protection against oxidative stress [32].

2.5. Metabolomic Profile.

2.5.1. Quantification of the Curcuminoids

The experiments were performed with an Agilent capillary electrophoresis (CE) instrument equipped with a diode array detector (DAD) and CE standard bare fused silica capillary (Agilent Technologies, Germany) with a 50 μm internal diameter and 72 cm effective length. Prior to use, the capillary was washed successively with basic solutions: 10 min with 1 N NaOH, 10 min with 0.1 N NaOH, followed by ultrapure water for 10 min, and running buffer for 20 min. The capillary was flushed between runs with 0.1 M NaOH for 1 min, H_2O for 1 min, and background electrolyte (BGE) for 2 min. Moreover, after three consecutive runs, the BGE was refreshed. Data acquisition and processing were performed with ChemStation software. Sample injection was performed using the hydrodynamic mode (35 mbar/12 s), while the capillary was maintained at a constant temperature of 300 C.

The method selected to quantify the curcuminoids is based on Yuan and Weng (2005) with some variations [33]. The separation of the curcuminoid compounds was obtained using 15 mM tetraborate buffer, pH = 10.64 (adjusted with 1 M NaOH) as the background electrolyte. The BGE was filtered through 0.2 μm membranes (Millipore, Bedford, MA, USA) and degassed before use. Using 30 kV voltage and direct UV-Vis absorption, detection was performed from 200 nm to 450 nm, with the samples being quantified at 262 nm.

Sample Preparation

First, 2 mL of each initial extract (ethanol/water; ethanol/water/acetic acid; ethanol/acetic acid) was vortexed with 15 mL of methylene chloride for 5 min and subsequently centrifuged for 10 min at 6000× *g* at 4 °C. The organic layer was separated and evaporated to dryness in a nitrogen atmosphere.

The residue was dissolved in 250 μL methanol and analyzed by capillary electrophoresis. Similarly, 5 mL of each sample resulting from colon simulation was processed and the residue which was taken in 100 μL of methanol was subsequently analysed by CE.

2.5.2. Ferulic Acid and Vanillin Quantification by CE

The ferulic acid and vanillin in the samples obtained after colon simulation were analyzed using a previously published method [34]. The analysis was done with an Agilent CE instrument equipped with a diode array detector (DAD) and CE standard bare fused silica capillary (Agilent Technologies, Waldbronn, Germany) having an internal diameter of 50 μm and an effective length of 72 cm. As a migration electrolyte (BGE), 45 mM tetraborate buffer was used with 0.9 mM sodium dodecyl sulphate (SDS), adjusted to a pH of 9.35 with 1 M HCl. The method required the use of 30 kV voltage, constant temperature of 300 °C, and direct UV absorption at 280 nm.

Sample preparation: First, 15 mL of each sample was purified through solid phase extraction with a C18 cartridge (Bond Elut Plexa, Agilent, Waldbronn, Germany). The cartridge was preconditioned with methanol (10 mL) and washed with water (5 mL), after which the sample was applied. After the sample passed through, the cartridge was washed with 5 mL water and finally with 5 mL methanol (solvent for the extraction of the polyphenols). The methanolic effluent thus collected was concentrated to 1 mL, filtered through 0.2 μm membranes (Millipore, Bedford, MA, USA) and degassed before injection. Standard addition was further employed, to evaluate the extraction efficiency.

2.5.3. Organic Acids Analysis by CE

The organic acid analysis was done based on the earlier published method [35]. A standard bare fused silica capillary (Agilent Technologies, Waldbronn, Germany) with an internal diameter of 50 μm and an effective length of 72 cm was used. The migration electrolyte (BGE) was 0.5 M H_3PO_4, 0.5 mM of CTAB (pH adjusted with NaOH at 6.24), and 15% vol. of methanol as an organic modifier. In this method 25 kV voltage was applied at a constant temperature of 25 °C, and direct UV absorption at 200 nm. The samples obtained after colon simulation were filtered through 0.2 μm membranes (Millipore, Bedford, MA, USA) and degassed prior to injection.

2.6. The qPCR Profile of the Microbiota

After the samples passed through the GIS1 colon simulator, quantification of the microbial community was done. Further, the principal bacterial groups from the human gut were analyzed using the quantitative polymerase chain reaction (qPCR) technique. Specific primers for phylum Firmicutes, the Bacteroides-Prevotella-Porphyromonas group, Enterobacteriaceae family, Lactobacillus-Lactococcus-Pediococcus group, and genus Bifidobacterium have been already revealed in earlier studies. A bacterial universal primer pair was used to determine the bacterial load from each sample [21].

The DNA was extracted from 1 mL of the sample using the PureLink™ Microbiome DNA Purification Kit (Invitrogen, Waltham, MA, USA), while the DNA concentration and purity were measured with the NanoVue Plus spectrophotometer (GE, Boston, MA, USA).

The qPCR analysis was conducted on a 7900 real-time PCR equipment (Applied Biosystems, Foster City, CA, USA) using the Power SYBR Green PCR Master Mix (Applied Biosystems, Waltham, MA, USA) and 40 ng of the DNA template was introduced in each reaction. Based on the results obtained after the amplification reaction optimisation, the primer concentration was between 0.2–0.5 μM [20].

The reference strains: *Escherichia (E.) coli* ATCC 10536, *Lactobacillus (L.) plantarum* ATCC 8014, *Bifidobacterium (B.) breve* ATCC 15700, *B. fragilis* DSM 2151, and *Enterococcus (E.) faecalis* ATCC 51299 were used for the standard curve. All the samples were run in triplicate [21].

2.7. Phylogenetic Diversity of the LAB Strains

Dilutions from each sample were cultured on the MRS + $CaCO_3$ plates for 48 h at 37 °C. Five colonies were randomly selected from the plate and cultivated in 1 mL MRS broth for 24 h at 37 °C.

The cultures were centrifuged for 5 min at 10,000× *g*, followed by a one-time wash with sterile distilled water (SDW) with subsequent resuspension in 400 μL SDW, and frozen for 1 h at −70 °C. The PCR Master Mix (Promega, Madison, WI, USA), 0.2 μM of the primers (5′-CTG CTG CGT CTG CTG-3′), and 1 μL of the lysate culture were introduced in a 25 μL PCR reaction. The PCR amplifications were done in Mastercycler Nexus (Eppendorf, Hamburg, Germany). The amplification programme involved initial DNA denaturation for 7 min at 95 °C, 30 cycles of DNA denaturation for 1 min at 94 °C, annealing for 1 min at 53 °C, an extension for 8 min at 65 °C, and a final incubation for 16 min at 65 °C.

The PCR products were separated in 1.7% agarose gel electrophoresis with 1X TBE buffer. Migration was performed at 65 V for 2 h.

The genetic profiles were analyzed with PyElph 1.4 using the WPGMA clustering method. *L. plantarum* ATCC 8014, *E. faecalis* ATCC 51299, *Lc. lactis subsp. lactis* DSM 20729, and *L. acidophilus* ATCC 314 were used as the reference strains [21].

2.8. Statistical Analysis

Evaluations of all the parameters investigated were performed in triplicate, with the results expressed as the mean ± standard deviation (SD) values of three observations. The mean and SD values were calculated using the IBM SPSS Statistics 23 software package (IBM Corporation, Armonk, NY, USA). To do the calculations, the significance level was set at: Significant = $p \leq 0.05$; very significant = $p \leq 0.01$; and highly significant = $p \leq 0.001$ using the normal distribution of the variables. The differences were analyzed by ANOVA followed by a Tukey post hoc analysis. The IBM SPSS Statistics software package (IBM Corporation, Armonk, NY, USA) was used to analyze and correlate the experimental data [18].

2.9. Sample Availability

Samples of the three extracts are available from the corresponding author (in certain conditions).

3. Results

3.1. The In Vitro and In Vivo Antioxidant Activity

Figure 1 depicts the in vitro antioxidant activity of all the three extracts. These determinations revealed that the capacity of the extracts to respond via biological activities is directly dependent upon the presence of the principal compound. The results also demonstrated the lowest EC50 value for the ethanol/water/acetic acid extract. Further, from the Figure it is evident that the antiradical activity was the lowest with an EC50 of a maximum of 1 μg/mL when ethanol/water was used as the solvent. By contrast, this value was around 50% higher than when an acidic extracting medium was used (Figure 1).

The EC50 values of chelating capacity were lower by more than 50% compared to the control, behavior recorded for all three extracts. Ethanol/water/acetic acid extract had an EC50 value of 0.20 μg/mL, $p < 0.01$. The results demonstrated that the lack of water did not determine the presence of compounds that can increase chelating capacity in vitro. For the reduction power, the values were relatively equal, with a minimum of 0.4 μg/mL ($p < 0.05$) for the ethanol/water/acetic acid extract. This value, 20% lower than the rest of the extracts, was obtained in the absence of water as a solvent.

Figure 2 represents the in vivo activity. The critical point (red arrow in Figure 2) was marked as indicated by the use of the graphics model. The acid extraction, however, determined a similar level of peroxide concentration at which the strain tested was able to survive. In fact, it was observed to be approximately 30% lower than the first solvent and is explicably based on the concentration of the extracted components. Thus, the acetic acid determined the presence of compounds which solubilize only in this medium and which have raised the degree of resistance to oxidative stress.

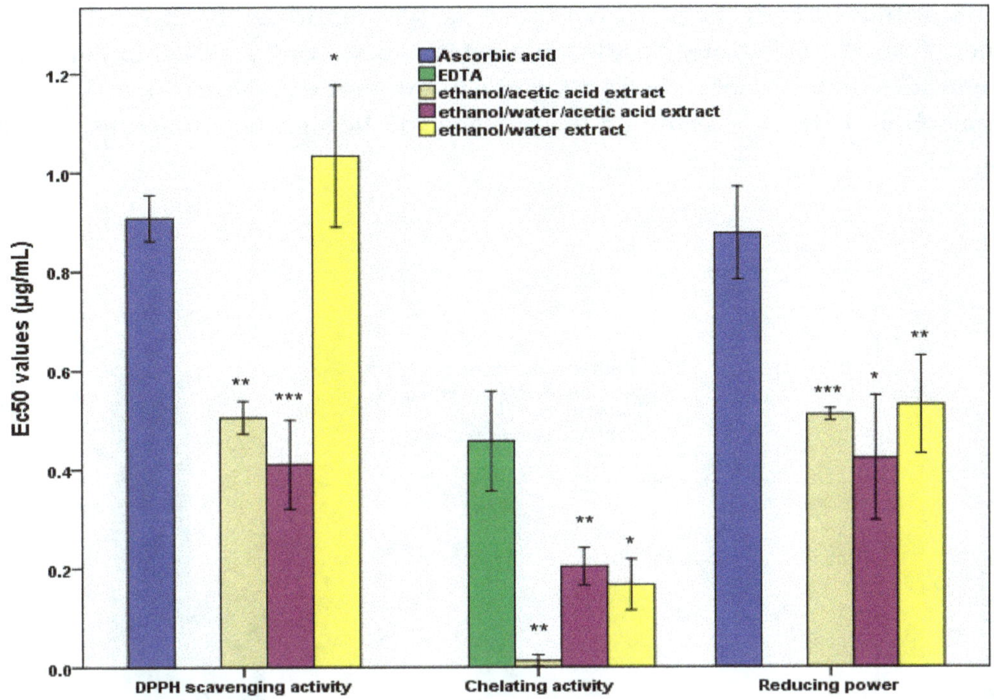

Figure 1. The figure represents the effective concentration (EC50) values for in vitro antioxidant activity as a measure of the impact of curcuma extract after the simulations in the GIS1 system. Different letters mean significant statistical differences (($* = p \leq 0.05$; $** = p \leq 0.01$; $*** = p \leq 0.001$), $n = 3$).

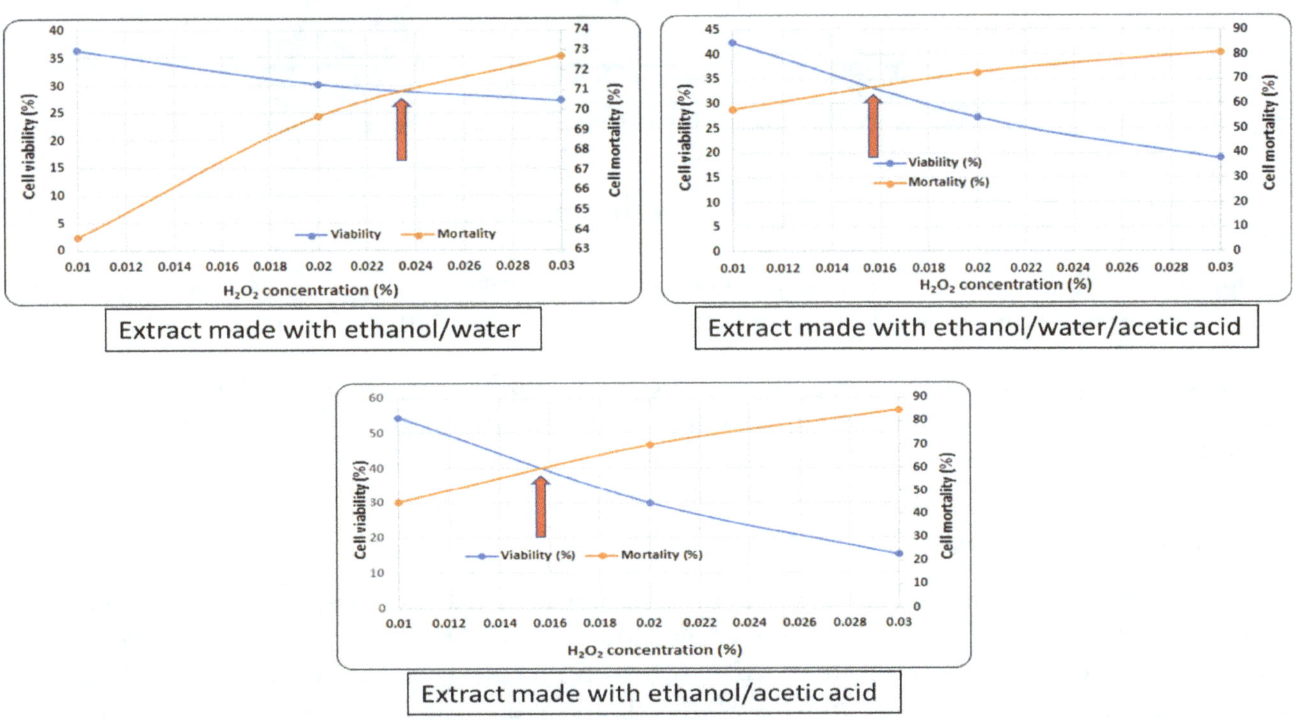

Figure 2. The cell viability as a parameter of the in vivo antioxidant activity in the presence of *C. longa* extracts.

3.2. Determination of the Quantities of Curcumin, Ferulic acid, and Vanillin

Predominantly, curcumin III was found to be the major constituent in the acetic acid-based extractions. For the three-solvent extract, the level was 622.5 µg/mL, around 35% more than the presence of only ethanol and acid. Although curcumin is water insoluble, the presence of water determined the solubilisation of the other compounds, which indirectly assisted in the release of the curcumin isomers from the substrate. Besides, the extracts also contained other compounds, although they were in quantities that did not directly affect the in vitro study (Figure 3). According to the earlier data, the hydroalcoholic extract determined the presence of the significant oleoresins, which explained the EC50 values [36].

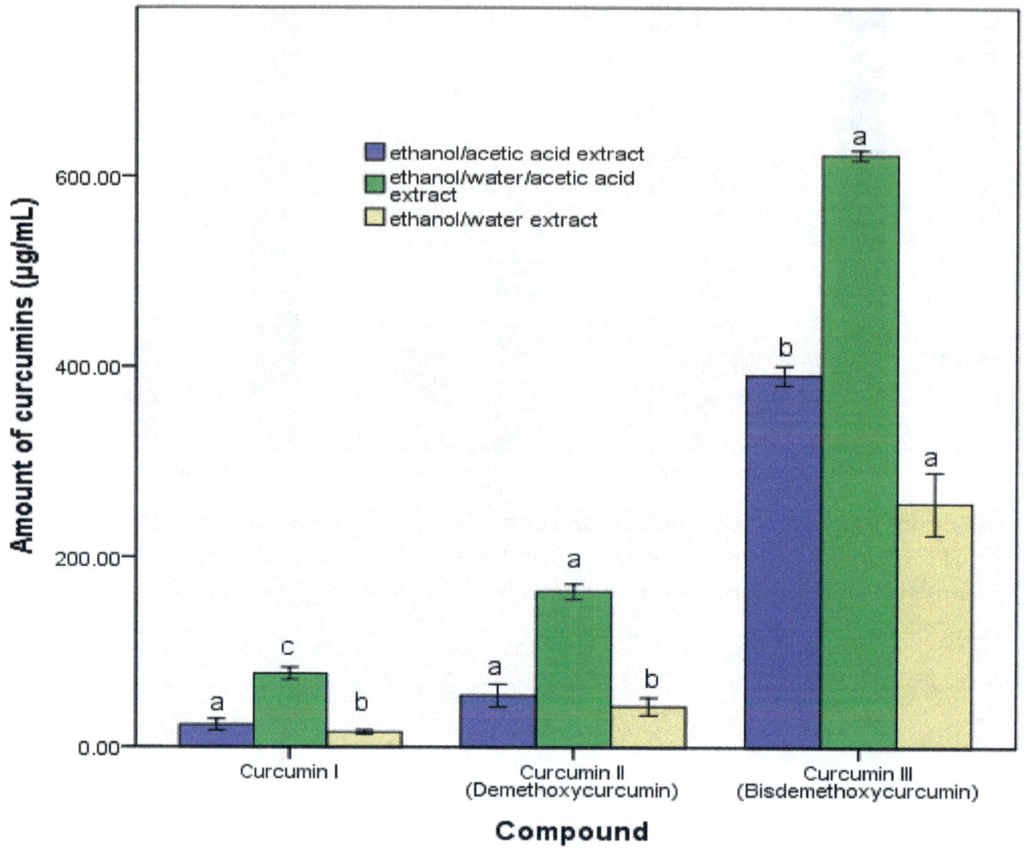

Figure 3. The total amount of curcumins in the three extracts. Within each group of samples, different letters mean significant statistical differences ((a = $p \leq 0.05$; b = $p \leq 0.01$; c = $p \leq 0.001$), $n = 3$).

Curcumin degradation products (ferulic acid or/and vanillin) [37] were not identified in any of the samples, which in turn led to the assumption that curcumin and its derivatives had been metabolised by the microbiota.

3.3. Microbiota Fingerprint Response

Some food ingredients directly impact human health by their capacity to modify the gut composition. In the present study, we analysed the impact of the curcuma extract on the main microorganism groups from the human gut. According to the spectrophotometric analysis, all the DNA extracts had a concentration of over 150 ng/µL and were uncontaminated by proteins or RNA, thus being suitable for qPCR (data not shown).

As shown in Figure 4, the curcumin extract strongly influences the Enterobacteriaceae group although it affects the Bacteroides-Prevotella-Porphyromonas group to a lesser degree, where the number of the cells remains constant in all the samples. In the ethanol/water extract, the number of Enterobacteriaceace is 10 times lower than it is in the remaining samples.

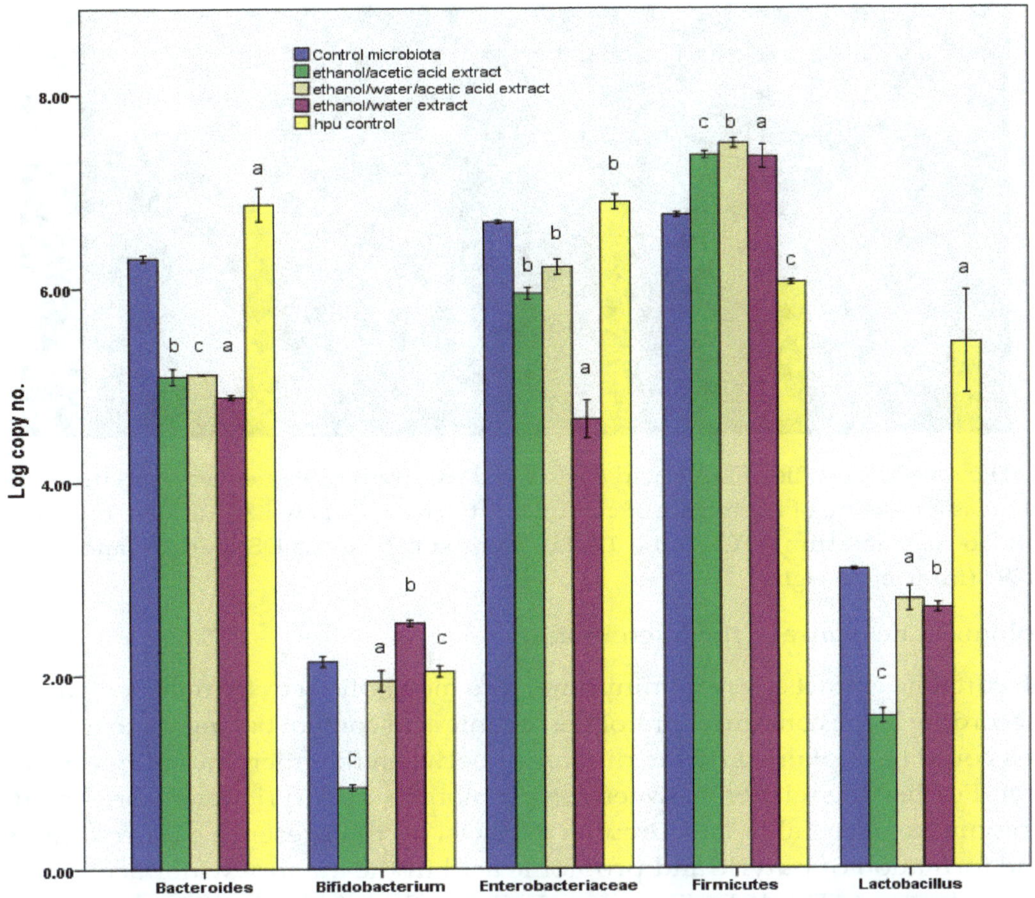

Figure 4. Log of number of copies obtained after in vitro tests through GIS1 as a measure of the impact of curcuma extracts on the number of the main groups of microorganisms from human gut. Different letters mean significant statistical differences ((control microbiota vs. treated samples/hpu; a = $p \leq 0.05$; b = $p \leq 0.01$; c = $p \leq 0.001$), $n = 3$).

At gram-positive bacteria for phylum Firmicutes, which is also the dominant group from the microbiota, the number of cells is higher than control (10^7 genomes/mL), but it is constant among the samples, instead the dynamics within this phylum is different. Therefore, the number of microorganisms in the Lactobacillus-Lactococcus-Pediococcus group is approximately 10 times higher in the ethanol/water extract and ethanol/water/acetic acid extract samples than in the ethanol/acetic acid extract. The number of bifidobacteria is also higher in the first two samples analyzed in the ethanol/water extract and ethanol/water/acetic acid extract.

3.3.1. Phylogenetic Diversity of the LAB Strains

LAB (lactic acid bacteria) strains represent an important microbe group from the human gut, which, several times, has been found in association with host health. As this group includes both beneficial and pathogenic strains, we have analyzed the phylogenetic relations of the strains from each sample by rep-PCR (Figure 5).

Different colonies from the MRS plates were selected and analyzed based on their phylogenetic profile using the PyElph 1.4 program. The phylogenetic analysis revealed the presence of one dominant clone in the ethanol/water extract and ethanol/water/acetic acid extract, which is closer to the phylogenetic on *L. acidophilus* ATCC 314. In the ethanol/acetic acid extract, two different clones were identified, which are part of the same cluster, with one being identified in the other two samples.

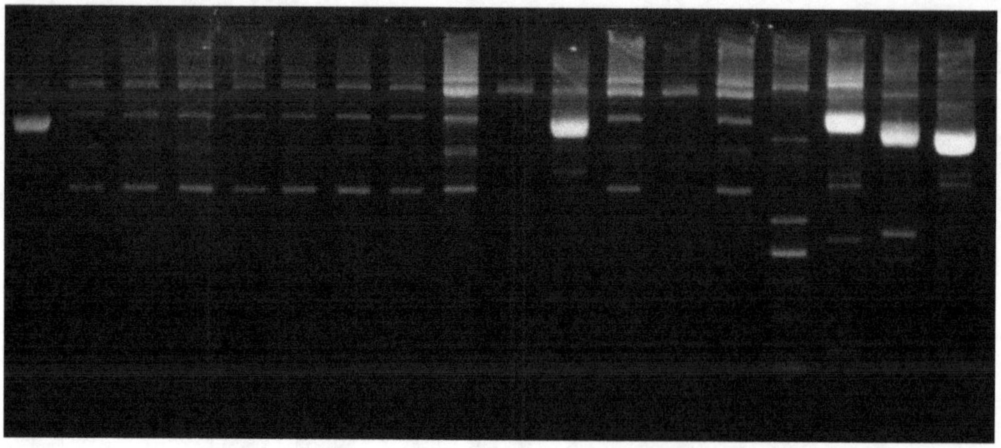

Figure 5. The rep-PCR profile of lactic acid bacteria (LAB) strains obtained after in vitro tests through GIS1 system as a measure of the impact of curcuma extracts. 1–14 new LAB strains, 15- L. acidophilus ATCC 314; 16- L. plantarum ATCC 8014, 17- Lc. lactis subsp. lactis DSM 20729, and 18- E. faecalis ATCC 51299 (from left to right).

3.3.2. Metabolomics: Response of the Microbiota

After the curcuma extracts were administered, the metabolic activity revealed variations between the samples according to the concentrations of the organic acid content belonging to the same microbiota. The variations could be explained by the difference between the microbiota fingerprints and by the curcumin level. Further, the relation between the propionic and butyric acid represented a microbiota modulation biomarker (see Table 1). Curcuma extracts, by the presence of curcumin (see Figure 3), stimulated the formation of butyric and propionic acid in the ethanol/water/acetic acid extract and ethanol/acetic acid extract. This behaviour was similar to the administration of dietary fibre.

Table 1. Organic acids levels (μg/mL) obtained after in vitro tests through the GIS1 system as a measure of the impact of curcuma extracts (administered as capsules) associated with the microbiota metabolic response.

Organic Acids (μg/mL)	Control Microbiota	Hpu Control	Treated Microbiota from Patients with Hypertension		
			Ethanol/Water Extract	Ethanol/Water/Acetic Acid Extract	Ethanol/Acetic Acid Extract
Formic acid	34.21 ± 5.35	nd	284.8 ± 21.07 [a]	362.12 ± 15.00 [a]	301.01 ± 9.00 [b]
Oxalic acid	nd	nd	7.68 ± 0.43 [b]	5.75 ± 0.40 [a]	9.38 ± 0.51 [a]
Succinic acid	nd	nd	62.04 ± 2.21 [b]	39.54 ± 7.05 [c]	31.4 ± 0.45 [c]
Malic acid	nd	nd	nd	nd	20.48 ± 3.19
Tartaric acid	nd	nd	nd	nd	nd
Acetic acid	435.13 ± 6.23	340.50 ± 4.70 [c]	505.16 ± 48.54 [a]	918.97 ± 22.98 [a]	1147.59 ± 73.88 [a]
Citric acid	nd	nd	nd	nd	nd
Propionic acid	145.46 ± 3.45	180.50 ± 0.01 [b]	nd	33.53 ± 3.77 [b]	62.53 ± 3.69 [c]
Lactic acid	330 ± 5.10	390.00 ± 5.60 [c]	534.89 ± 32.60 [c]	415.49 ± 11.32 [a]	449.17 ± 12.53 [d]
Butyric acid	146.65 ± 4.37	37.80 ± 0.76 [c]	117.33 ± 4.68 [b]	322.76 ± 11.59 [a]	247.11 ± 29.84 [a]
Benzoic acid	1.71 ± 0.10	nd	5.72 ± 0.56 [c]	6.44 ± 0.30 [b]	11.48 ± 1.06 [a]
Phenyllacticacid	17.6 ± 0.36	0.55 ± 0.01 [c]	3.48 ± 0.34 [c]	4.27 ± 0.08 [c]	2.84 ± 0.14 [c]
OH Phenyllactic acid	44.58 ± 0.76	40.00 ± 1.80	2.28 ± 0.10 [b]	10.88 ± 0.54 [c]	2.25 ± 0.22 [b]

[a] = $p \leq 0.05$; [b] = $p \leq 0.01$; [c] = $p \leq 0.001$, for control microbiota vs. treated samples/hpu, $n = 3$; nd—not detected.

Also, lack of propionic acid was registered when ethanol/water extract was administered. This diminished pattern of short-chain fatty acids (SCFAs) was also characterized by the smallest amounts of butyric and acetic acids, compared with control microbiota. The high level of lactic acid was correlated with the metabolic activity that increased in the presence of curcuma extracts. In addition, in vitro SCFAs production by the two inocula (Table 1) demonstrated a low microbiota metabolic response compared to treated microbiota.

4. Discussion

The study tested the hypothesis that hypertensive patients have dysbiosis at the microbiota level, based on the progression of an inflammatory process associated with oxidative stress activity. Results have proved that the *C. longa* extracts were associated with a reduction in the oxidative stress effects, modification of the microbiota pattern, and improvement in the level of biomarkers (like butyric acid formation). Further, the in vitro antioxidant effects were not directly correlated with in vivo activity, although the data were relevant for the observation that low EC50 values were linked to the presence of the curcumin isomers.

On comparing the response of the *S. boulardii* cells, the role of specific compounds (especially curcumin) in combating oxidative stress became clear. The critical point indicated the potential of the ethanol/water/acetic acid extract to support the physiological mechanisms of the inhibition of the free radicals [32]. Such analysis may be an easy method of evaluating the effectiveness of a nutraceutical in modulating the response of the human microbiota and intervening in the improvement of inflammatory processes. The coevolution of the microbial pattern with the host's health was supported by the data displayed in Figure 6. The phylogenetic relationships after the administration of the extract were an indicator of the role of the bioactive compounds in the expression of the metabolomic biomarkers (see Table 1). Stimulating bacterial diversity was a factor that promoted the reaction to the inflammatory process. Thus, it can be deduced that the action of oxidative stress induced differences in the microbial pattern [20] through a direct link to the presence of the major bioactive compounds (see Figure 3). Thus, such an extraction pattern expressed a distinct in vitro/in vivo behaviour based on the difference in solvent and the bioavailability of the principal bioactive compound (curcumin). The in vivo response, compared to the in vitro, revealed a pattern that is in direct correlation with the pH of the solvent used.

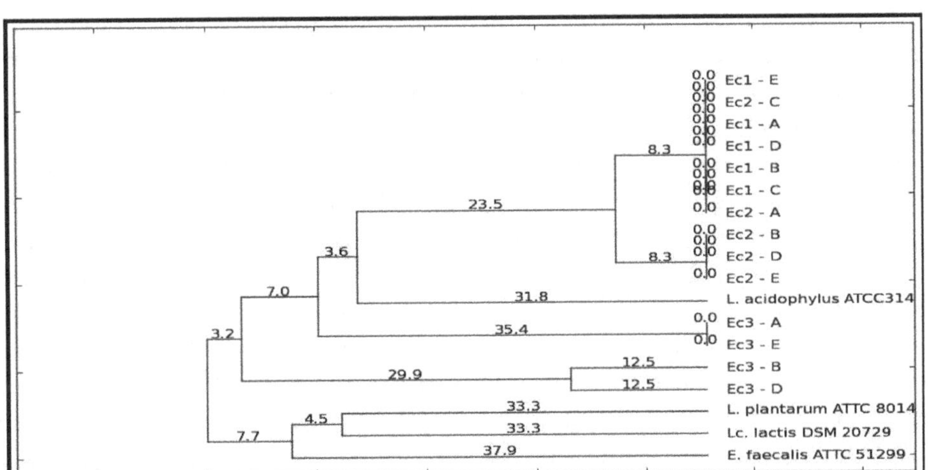

Figure 6. Dendrogram of LAB strains using WPGMA clustering method obtained after in vitro tests through GIS1 system as a measure of the impact of curcuma extracts. EC1 = ethanol/water extract; Ec2 = ethanol/water/acetic acid extract; Ec3 = ethanol/acetic acid extract.

The in vivo response of the *S. boulardii* eukaryotic cell represents the preclinical assessment of the enzymatic mechanisms of hydrogen peroxide reduction as an indicator of the development of degenerative pathologies [38]. The reduction in the accumulation of the oxidised proteins as an effect of the stress caused by hydrogen peroxide decomposition confirms the protection given by the curcumin against the development of degenerative pathologies [39]. These data were synchronised with a low EC50 value for the inhibition of lipid peroxidation (see Figure 1). They also revealed a decrease in oxidative damage, confirmed by the value of the critical point in vivo (see Figure 2), particularly for the use of ethanol/water/acetic acid as the solvent.

However, post in vitro simulation, the curcumins identified were absent. This finding could be explained in several ways because trace amounts were found in the other two compounds in which it became transformed. The first cause concerns biotransformation determined by the fermentative activity of the microbiota [11]. It has been noted as well that the low alkaline pH is indicative of high solubilisation and a high bioconversion rate in the other compounds [11] or utilisation as a carbon source [40]. In this context, the earlier research revealed that the curcumin could act as a carbon source for Enterobacteriaceae. In parallel, besides the extracts, a sample containing ethanol alone was run; it was evident that it had exerted no effect on the microbiota pattern. The same effect was observed after the blank sample (capsule + maltodextrin without curcuma extract; Figure 4). This behaviour can thus be interpreted as a response to the curcumin metabolism, which translates into the action of the compounds produced through its degradation. Thus, the pH value, in response to the curcumin action, can be used as a biomarker, which is recognised as a parameter by both the present investigation and prior studies [41]. These results confirmed a previous study (https://aor.ca/blog/curcumin-under-fire-the-root-of-the-problem), which proves the instability of this compound. Based on the highly degrading behaviour it was possible to explain the contradictions observed in this study. Besides, the results could partially explain the pharmacological target of curcumin based on the interaction with the microbiota fingerprint through the metabolomic pattern [6].

Thus, the administration of the extracts was similar to a polypharmacological effect. The in vitro administration was mediated by the degradation products of curcumin, demonstrating a multifactorial action [42]. The fermentative action of the microbiota showed that its low stability induced a multiple, microbiological, and metabolomic response, which was in accordance with the previous studies [43]. Reduced quantities of vanillin and ferulic acid have not been identified as significant degradation compounds. They could also represent biomarkers of the pharmacological action of the *C. longa* extracts [44]. The results of this study highlighted the bioavailability of the curcumin [43]. Pharmacological action was performed by the metabolomic indicators and not directly through increased bioavailability. Thus, this study confirms the impact of the modulating action of the curcumin on the perturbed microbiota. The metabolomic pattern and increase in the microbial diversity (LAB strains) were a pharmacodynamic response of the *C. longa* extracts, which was a good indicator of the physiological and biochemical effects.

The aim of the article was achieved as it demonstrated a correlation between the metabolic products and microbial pattern modulation in the simulated colon (see Table 1). The increase in the quantity of curcumin III from one extract to another was not correlated with the acidity of the solvent (ethanol/acetic acid) [45,46], but can be explained by the reduced acetate/propionate ratio. Moreover, it was found to be around 20%, which corresponds to a progressive decrease in the serum cholesterol [26]. The reduction in cardiovascular risk is a confirmation of the high rate of biotransformation of the phenolic component and favourable microbial proliferation. Thus, the modulation of the microbial pattern can correct the progression of the inflammatory processes of the host, thus reducing the sensitivity to oxidative stress. The reduction in the oxidative stress disorder naturally improves the cardiovascular risk, in particular, maintaining hypertension within optimal limits [30].

The modulation of the metabolomic pattern, by improving the ratio of the SCFAs, showed that the ethanol/water/acetic acid extract has potential therapeutic use against cardiovascular progression. By raising the quantity of curcumin, prebiotic activities were induced, by a modulation of the intestinal microbiota and specific metabolic pathways, contributing towards host health improvement. This effect is similar to that of green tea polyphenols [31]. Clinical data also showed that an increase in the butyrate level, caused by the use of functional products, exerted a positive effect. The presence of curcumin in the in vitro environment (see Figure 3) was correlated to the rise in the butyrate content, particularly in the acid extractions (see Table 1). The level of butyrate plays an important role in responding to different inflammatory processes. Changing the SCFAs profile by stimulating the synthesis of butyrate correlated with curcumin administration [47]. This aspect represented a novelty of the study, demonstrating the altered microbiota response to the presence of curcumin. Even if the direct influence on the microbial pattern was balanced among the three extracts, the quantity of curcumin and the quantitative distribution between the isomers influenced the outcomes of the study. Thus, the differences between the isomers have also been translated by a modulation of the metabolic response of the microbiota. This is a significant factor in preclinical studies because the presence of various forms of the biomarkers plays a crucial role in reconstituting the pattern of the microbiota in hypertensive patients [33].

Also, an increase in the number of organic acids in the simulated environment was a health status indicator in accordance with a previous study [37]. This behaviour was correlated with the curcumin level and represented an indicator of an anti-inflammatory response [48].

5. Conclusions

Our study proved that the inhibitory concentrations towards more strains were reached by the administration of curcuma extracts. The in vitro experiments proved that the poor bioavailability does not mean that the curcumin was not metabolized by the gut bacteria. The effects of the *C. longa* extracts were correlated with the antioxidant potential and fingerprint microbiota modulation. The results showed a decrease in the microbiota dysbiosis for the ethanol/water/acetic acid extraction. The large curcumin quantity was correlated to a decrease in the unfavorable strain. The property of the curcuma extracts in reducing the oxidative stress is dependent upon their ability to enhance the antioxidant potential at the colon level. Valorisation of the favorable strains will result in a lowered inflammatory process, which is dose-dependent.

Author Contributions: E.V. designed the experiments, analyzed the data and wrote the paper; F.G. performed the CZE analysis; I.S. and D.P. contributed with qPCR analysis of the samples after in vitro simulations. The authors discussed and made comments on the results.

References

1. Iciar, M.T.; Sevillano-Collantes, C.; Segura-Galindo, A.; del Cañizo-Gómez, F.J. Type 2 diabetes and cardiovascular disease: Have all risk factors the same strength? *World J. Diabetes* **2014**, *5*, 444–470. [CrossRef]
2. Dias, D.A.; Urban, S.; Roessner, U. A historical overview of natural products in drug discovery. *Metabolites* **2012**, *2*, 303–336. [CrossRef]
3. Straub, R.H.; Schradin, C. Chronic inflammatory systemic diseases: An evolutionary trade-off between acutely beneficial but chronically harmful programs. *Evol. Med. Public Health* **2016**, *1*, 37–51. [CrossRef] [PubMed]
4. Kishi, T.; Hirooka, Y. Oxidative stress in the brain causes hypertension via sympathoexcitation. *Front. Physiol.* **2012**, *17*, 335. [CrossRef]
5. Hewlings, S.J.; Kalman, D.S. Curcumin: A Review of Its' Effects on Human Health. *Foods* **2017**, *6*, 92. [CrossRef]
6. Peterson, C.T.; Vaughn, A.R.; Sharma, V.; Chopra, D.; Mills, P.J.; Peterson, S.N.; Sivamani, R.K. Effects of turmeric and curcumin dietary supplementation on human gut microbiota: A double-blind, randomized, placebo-controlled pilot study. *J. Evid. Based Integr. Med.* **2018**, *23*. [CrossRef] [PubMed]
7. Clark, A.; Mach, N. Exercise-induced stress behavior, gut-microbiota-brain axis and diet: A systematic review for athletes. *J. Int. Soc. Sports Nutr.* **2016**, *13*, 43. [CrossRef] [PubMed]
8. Ahmadmehrabi, S.; Tang, W.H.W. Gut microbiome and its role in cardiovascular diseases. *Curr. Opin. Cardiol.* **2017**, *32*, 761–766. [CrossRef] [PubMed]
9. Selma, M.V.; Espin, J.C.; Tomas-Barberan, F.A. Interaction between phenolics and gut microbiota: Role in human health. *J. Agric. Food Chem.* **2009**, *57*, 6485–6501. [CrossRef]

10. Ozdal, T.; Sela, D.A.; Xiao, J.; Boyacioglu, D.; Chen, F.; Capanoglu, E. The reciprocal interactions between polyphenols and gut microbiota and effects on bioaccessibility. *Nutrients* **2016**, *8*, 78. [CrossRef]
11. Ng, Q.X.; Soh, A.Y.S.; Loke, W.; Venkatanarayanan, N. Do a meta-analysis of the clinical use of curcumin for irritable bowel syndrome (IBS). *J. Clin. Med.* **2018**, *7*, 298. [CrossRef] [PubMed]
12. Boulangé, C.L.; Neves, A.L.; Chilloux, J.; Nicholson, J.K.; Dumas, M.E. Impact of the gut microbiota on inflammation, obesity, and metabolic disease. *Genome Med.* **2016**, *8*, 42. [CrossRef] [PubMed]
13. Zhi, Y.K.; Sunil, K.L. The human gut microbiome—A potential controller a wellness and disease. *Front. Microbiol.* **2018**, *9*, 1835. [CrossRef]
14. Henson, M.A.; Phalak, P. Microbiota dysbiosis in inflammatory bowel diseases: In silico investigation of the oxygen hypothesis. *BMC Syst. Biol.* **2017**, *11*, 145. [CrossRef] [PubMed]
15. Mangge, H.; Becker, K.; Fuchs, D.; Gostner, J.M. Antioxidants, inflammation and cardiovascular disease. *World J. Cardiol.* **2014**, *6*, 462–477. [CrossRef]
16. Wexler, A.G.; Goodman, A.L. An insider's perspective: Bacteroides as a window into the microbiome. *Nat. Microbiol.* **2017**, *2*, 17026. [CrossRef] [PubMed]
17. Xiao, S.; Zhao, L. Gut microbiota-based translational biomarkers to prevent metabolic syndrome via nutritional modulation. *FEMS Microbiol. Ecol.* **2013**, *87*, 303–314. [CrossRef]
18. Boeing, J.S.; Barizão, É.O.; e Silva, B.C.; Montanher, P.F.; de Cinque Almeida, V.; Visentainer, J.V. Evaluation of solvent effect on the extraction of phenolic compounds and antioxidant capacities from the berries: Application of principal component analysis. *Chem. Cent. J.* **2014**, *8*, 48. [CrossRef]
19. Tanvir, E.M.; Hossen, M.S.; Hossain, M.F.; Afroz, R.; Gan, S.H.; Khalil, M.I.; Karim, N. Antioxidant properties of popular turmeric (*Curcuma longa*) varieties from Bangladesh. *J. Food Qual.* **2017**, *2017*, 8471785. [CrossRef]
20. Vamanu, E.; Gatea, F.; Sârbu, I. In vitro ecological response of the human gut microbiome to bioactive extracts from edible wild mushrooms. *Molecules* **2018**, *23*, 2128. [CrossRef]
21. Vamanu, E.; Ene, M.; Biță, B.; Ionescu, C.; Crăciun, L.; Sârbu, I. In vitro human microbiota response to exposure to silver nanoparticles biosynthesized with mushroom extract. *Nutrients* **2018**, *10*, 607. [CrossRef] [PubMed]
22. Vamanu, E.; Pelinescu, D.; Sarbu, I. Comparative fingerprinting of the human microbiota in diabetes and cardiovascular disease. *J. Med. Food* **2016**, *19*, 1188–1195. [CrossRef] [PubMed]
23. Vamanu, E.; Pelinescu, D. Effects of mushroom consumption on the microbiota of different target groups–Impact of polyphenolic composition and mitigation on the microbiome fingerprint. *LWT-Food Sci. Technol.* **2017**, *85*, 262–268. [CrossRef]
24. Olugbami, J.O.; Gbadegesin, M.A.; Odunola, O.A. In vitro free radical scavenging and antioxidant properties of ethanol extract of *Terminalia glaucescens*. *Pharmacogn. Res.* **2015**, *7*, 49–56. [CrossRef]
25. Alam, M.N.; Bristi, N.J.; Rafiquzzaman, M. Review on in vivo and in vitro methods evaluation of antioxidant activity. *Saudi Pharm. J.* **2012**, *21*, 143–152. [CrossRef] [PubMed]
26. Vamanu, E.; Nita, S. Antioxidant capacity and the correlation with major phenolic compounds, anthocyanin, and tocopherol content in various extracts from the wild edible *Boletus edulis* mushroom. *BioMed Res. Int.* **2013**, *2013*, 313905. [CrossRef] [PubMed]
27. Das, K.C.; Das, C.K. Curcumin (diferuloylmethane), a singlet oxygen ($^1O_2$) quencher. *Biochem. Biophys. Res. Commun.* **2002**, *295*, 62–66. [CrossRef]
28. Alter, J.; Hossain, M.A.; Takara, K.; Islam, M.Z.; Hou, D.X. Antioxidant activity of different species and varieties of turmeric (*Curcuma* spp): Isolation of active compounds. *Comp. Biochem. Physiol. Part C Toxicol. Pharmacol.* **2019**, *215*, 9–17. [CrossRef]
29. Ashraf, K.; Sultan, S. A comprehensive review on *Curcuma longa* Linn.: Phytochemical, pharmacological, and molecular study. *Int. J. Green Pharm.* **2017**, *11*, S671.
30. Dos Santos Andrade, T.J.A.; Araújo, B.Q.; das Graças Lopes Citó, A.M.; da Silva, J.; Saffi, J.; Richter, M.F.; de Barros Falcão Ferraz, A. Antioxidant properties and chemical composition of technical cashew nut shell liquid (tCNSL). *Food Chem.* **2011**, *126*, 1044–1048. [CrossRef]
31. Brandão, R.L.; Rosa, J.C.C.; Nicoli, J.R.; Almeida, M.V.S.; do Carmo, A.P.; Queiros, H.T.; Castro, I.M. Investigating acid stress response in different *Saccharomyces* strains. *J. Mycol.* **2014**, *2014*, 178274. [CrossRef]

32. Kos, B.; Suskovic, J.; Goreta, J.; Matocic, S. Effect of protectors on the viability of *Lactobacillus acidophilus* M92 in simulated gastrointestinal conditions. *Food Technol. Biotechnol.* **2000**, *38*, 121–127.
33. Yuan, K.; Weng, Q.; Zhang, H.; Xiong, J.; Xu, G. Application of capillary zone electrophoresis in the separation and determination of the curcuminoids in urine. *J. Pharm. Biomed. Anal.* **2005**, *38*, 133–138. [CrossRef]
34. Matei, A.O.; Gatea, F.; Teodor, E.D.; Radu, G.L. Polyphenols analysis from different medicinal plants extracts using capillary zone electrophoresis (CZE). *Rev. Chim.* **2016**, *67*, 1051–1105.
35. Gatea, F.; Teodor, E.D.; Paun, G.; Matei, A.O.; Radu, G.L. Capillary electrophoresis method validation for organic acids assessment in probiotics. *Food Anal. Meth.* **2015**, *8*, 1335–1340. [CrossRef]
36. Ombra, M.N.; d'Acierno, A.; Nazzaro, F.; Riccardi, R.; Spigno, P.; Zaccardelli, M.; Pane, C.; Maione, M.; Fratianni, F. Phenolic composition and antioxidant and antiproliferative activities of the extracts of twelve common bean (*Phaseolus vulgaris* L.) endemic ecotypes of southern Italy before and after cooking. *Oxid. Med. Cell. Longev.* **2016**, *2016*, 1398298. [CrossRef]
37. Shen, L.; Ji, H.F. The pharmacology of curcumin: Is it the degradation products? *Trends Mol. Med.* **2012**, *18*, 138–144. [CrossRef]
38. Pothoulakis, C. Review article: Anti-inflammatory mechanisms of action of *Saccharomyces boulardii*. *Aliment. Pharmacol. Ther.* **2008**, *30*, 826–833. [CrossRef]
39. Poljsak, B. Strategies for reducing or preventing the generation of oxidative stress. *Oxid. Med. Cell. Longev.* **2011**, *2011*, 194586. [CrossRef]
40. Edwards, C.A.; Havlik, J.; Cong, W.; Mullen, W.; Preston, T.; Morrison, D.J.; Combet, E. Polyphenols and health: Interactions between fibre, plant polyphenols and the gut microbiota. *Nutr. Bull.* **2017**, *42*, 356–360. [CrossRef]
41. Meddeb, W.; Rezig, L.; Zarrouk, A.; Nury, T.; Vejux, A.; Prost, M.; Bretillon, L.; Mejri, M.; Lizard, G. Cytoprotective activities of milk thistle seed oil used in traditional Tunisian medicine on 7-ketocholesterol and 24S-hydroxycholesterol-induced toxicity on 158N murine oligodendrocytes. *Antioxidants* **2018**, *7*, 95. [CrossRef]
42. Stiru, O.; Dorobanțu, L.F.; Pasare, A.; Bubenek, Ș.; Filipescu, D.; Moldovan, H.; Iliescu, V.A. Acute type A aortic dissection. A single center experience. *Rom. J. Cardiol.* **2014**, *24*, 251–259.
43. Shen, L.; Liu, L.; Ji, H.F. Regulative effects of curcumin spice administration on gut microbiota and its pharmacological implications. *Food Nutr. Res.* **2017**, *61*, 1361780. [CrossRef]
44. Nelson, K.M.; Dahlin, J.L.; Bisson, J.; Graham, J.; Pauli, G.F.; Walters, M.A. The essential medicinal chemistry of curcumin. *J. Med. Chem.* **2017**, *60*, 1620–1637. [CrossRef] [PubMed]
45. Kumavat, S.D.; Chaudhari, Y.S.; Borole, P.; Mishra, P.; Shenghani, K.; Duvvuri, P. Degradation studies of curcumin. *Int. J. Pharm. Rev. Res.* **2013**, *3*, 50–55.
46. Schneider, C.; Gordon, O.N.; Edwards, R.L.; Luis, P.B. Degradation of curcumin: From mechanism to biological implications. *J. Agric. Food Chem.* **2015**, *9*, 7606–7614. [CrossRef]
47. Ohira, H.; Tsutsui, W.; Fujioka, Y. Are Short Chain Fatty Acids in Gut Microbiota Defensive Players for Inflammation and Atherosclerosis? *J. Atheroscler. Thromb.* **2017**, *24*, 660–672. [CrossRef]
48. Salehi, B.; Stojanović-Radić, Z.; Matejić, J.; Sharifi-Rad, M.; Anil Kumar, N.V.; Martins, N.; Sharifi-Rad, J. The therapeutic potential of Curcumin: A review of clinical trials. *Eur. J. Med. Chem.* **2018**. [CrossRef] [PubMed]

Permissions

All chapters in this book were first published by MDPI; hereby published with permission under the Creative Commons Attribution License or equivalent. Every chapter published in this book has been scrutinized by our experts. Their significance has been extensively debated. The topics covered herein carry significant findings which will fuel the growth of the discipline. They may even be implemented as practical applications or may be referred to as a beginning point for another development.

The contributors of this book come from diverse backgrounds, making this book a truly international effort. This book will bring forth new frontiers with its revolutionizing research information and detailed analysis of the nascent developments around the world.

We would like to thank all the contributing authors for lending their expertise to make the book truly unique. They have played a crucial role in the development of this book. Without their invaluable contributions this book wouldn't have been possible. They have made vital efforts to compile up to date information on the varied aspects of this subject to make this book a valuable addition to the collection of many professionals and students.

This book was conceptualized with the vision of imparting up-to-date information and advanced data in this field. To ensure the same, a matchless editorial board was set up. Every individual on the board went through rigorous rounds of assessment to prove their worth. After which they invested a large part of their time researching and compiling the most relevant data for our readers.

The editorial board has been involved in producing this book since its inception. They have spent rigorous hours researching and exploring the diverse topics which have resulted in the successful publishing of this book. They have passed on their knowledge of decades through this book. To expedite this challenging task, the publisher supported the team at every step. A small team of assistant editors was also appointed to further simplify the editing procedure and attain best results for the readers.

Apart from the editorial board, the designing team has also invested a significant amount of their time in understanding the subject and creating the most relevant covers. They scrutinized every image to scout for the most suitable representation of the subject and create an appropriate cover for the book.

The publishing team has been an ardent support to the editorial, designing and production team. Their endless efforts to recruit the best for this project, has resulted in the accomplishment of this book. They are a veteran in the field of academics and their pool of knowledge is as vast as their experience in printing. Their expertise and guidance has proved useful at every step. Their uncompromising quality standards have made this book an exceptional effort. Their encouragement from time to time has been an inspiration for everyone.

The publisher and the editorial board hope that this book will prove to be a valuable piece of knowledge for researchers, students, practitioners and scholars across the globe.

List of Contributors

Milica Markovic, Moran Zur, Inna Ragatsky and Arik Dahan
Department of Clinical Pharmacology, School of Pharmacy, Faculty of Health Sciences, Ben-Gurion University of the Negev, Beer-Sheva 8410501, Israel

Sandra Cvijić
Department of Pharmaceutical Technology and Cosmetology, Faculty of Pharmacy, University of Belgrade, Vojvode Stepe 450, 11221 Belgrade, Serbia

Reem Abou Assi and Ibrahim M. Abdulbaqi
The Discipline of Pharmaceutical Technology, School of Pharmaceutical Sciences, Universiti Sains Malaysia, Penang 11800, Malaysia
The Discipline of Pharmaceutical Technology, College of Pharmacy, Al-Kitab University, Altun kupri, Kirkuk 36001, Iraq

Toh Seok Ming, Chan Siok Yee, Habibah A. Wahab and Yusrida Darwis
The Discipline of Pharmaceutical Technology, School of Pharmaceutical Sciences, Universiti Sains Malaysia, Penang 11800, Malaysia

Shaik Mohammed Asif
The Discipline of Pharmaceutical Technology, School of Pharmaceutical Sciences, Universiti Sains Malaysia, Penang 11800, Malaysia
Pharma Research, Wockhardt Research Center, Aurangabad 431002, India

Sarah Sulaiman and Luca Marciani
Nottingham Digestive Diseases Centre and National Institute for Health Research (NIHR) Nottingham Biomedical Research Centre, Nottingham University Hospitals NHS Trust and University of Nottingham, Nottingham NG7 2UH, UK

David Dahlgren and Hans Lennernäs
Department of Pharmacy, Uppsala University, Uppsala, Sweden

Marcelo Dutra Duque
Department of Pharmacy, Faculty of Pharmaceutical Sciences, Universidade de São Paulo—USP, Av. Prof. Lineu Prestes, 580, São Paulo—SP 05508-000, Brazil
Department of Pharmaceutical Sciences, Institute of Environmental, Chemical and Pharmaceutical Sciences, Universidade Federal de São Paulo—UNIFESP, Rua São Nicolau, 210, Centro, Diadema—SP 09913-030, Brazil

Daniela Amaral Silva
Department of Pharmacy, Faculty of Pharmaceutical Sciences, Universidade de São Paulo—USP, Av. Prof. Lineu Prestes, 580, São Paulo—SP 05508-000, Brazil
Faculty of Pharmacy & Pharmaceutical Sciences, Katz Group-Rexall Centre for Pharmacy & Health Research, University of Alberta, 11361 - 87 Avenue, Edmonton, AB T6G 2E1, Canada

Michele Georges Issa, Valentina Porta and Humberto Gomes Ferraz
Department of Pharmacy, Faculty of Pharmaceutical Sciences, Universidade de São Paulo—USP, Av. Prof. Lineu Prestes, 580, São Paulo—SP 05508-000, Brazil

Raimar Löbenberg
Faculty of Pharmacy & Pharmaceutical Sciences, Katz Group-Rexall Centre for Pharmacy & Health Research, University of Alberta, 11361 - 87 Avenue, Edmonton, AB T6G 2E1, Canada

Lu Xiao
Department of Basic Medicine, Zunyi Medical University, Zhuhai Campus, Zhuhai 519041, China

Ying Liu
Pharmacy Department, Wuhan Medical Treatment Center, Wuhan 430023, China

Tao Yi
School of Health Sciences, Macao Polytechnic Institute, Macau 999078, China

Yvonne E. Arnold and Yogeshvar N. Kalia
School of Pharmaceutical Sciences, University of Geneva & University of Lausanne, CMU-1 rue Michel Servet, 1211 Geneva 4, Switzerland

Stéphane Bernard
Debiopharm International SA, Chemin Messidor 5-7, 1006 Lausanne, Switzerland

Julien Thorens
Debiopharm International SA, Chemin Messidor 5-7, 1006 Lausanne, Switzerland
Pharmacie des ins, 3 rue de Frontenex, 74000 Annecy, France

Gislaine Kuminek, Gregory E. Amidon, Nair Rodriguez-Hornedo and Gordon L. Amidon
Department of Pharmaceutical Sciences, College of Pharmacy, University of Michigan, Ann Arbor, MI 48109, USA

Marival Bermejo
Department of Pharmaceutical Sciences, College of Pharmacy, University of Michigan, Ann Arbor, MI 48109, USA
Department Engineering Pharmacy Section, Miguel Hernandez University, San Juan de Alicante, 03550 Alicante, Spain

Jozef Al-Gousous
Department of Pharmaceutical Sciences, College of Pharmacy, University of Michigan, Ann Arbor, MI 48109, USA
Department of Biopharmaceutics and Pharmaceutical Technology, Johannes Gutenberg Universität Mainz, D-55099 Mainz, Germany

Alejandro Ruiz-Picazo and Isabel González-Alvarez
Department Engineering Pharmacy Section, Miguel Hernandez University, San Juan de Alicante, 03550 Alicante, Spain

Yasuhiro Tsume
Department of Pharmaceutical Sciences, College of Pharmacy, University of Michigan, Ann Arbor, MI 48109, USA
Merck and Co., Inc., 126 E Lincoln Ave, Rahway, NJ 07065, USA

Alfredo Garcia-Arieta
Service on Pharmacokinetics and Generic Medicines, Division of Pharmacology and Clinical Evaluation, Department of Human Use Medicines, Spanish Agency for Medicines and Health Care Products, 28022 Madrid, Spain

Bart Hens
Department of Pharmaceutical Sciences, College of Pharmacy, University of Michigan, Ann Arbor, MI 48109, USA
Department of Pharmaceutical and Pharmacological Sciences, KU Leuven, Herestraat 49, 3000 Leuven, Belgium

Deanna Mudie
Department of Pharmaceutical Sciences, College of Pharmacy, University of Michigan, Ann Arbor, MI 48109, USA
Drug Product Development and Innovation, Lonza Pharma and Biotech, Bend, OR 97703, USA

Marie Wahlgren, Magdalena Axenstrand, Åsa Håkansson and Ali Marefati
Department of Food technology engineering and nutrition, Lund University, 221 00 Lund, Sweden

Betty Lomstein Pedersen
Ferring International PharmaScience Center (IPC), Kay Fiskers Plads 11, 2300 Copenhagen, Denmark

Constantin Mircioiu
Department of Applied Mathematics and Biostatistics, Faculty of Pharmacy, "Carol Davila" University of Medicine and Pharmacy, 020956 Bucharest, Romania

Valentina Anuta
Department of Physical and Colloidal Chemistry, Faculty of Pharmacy, "Carol Davila" University of Medicine and Pharmacy, 020956 Bucharest, Romania

Ion Mircioiu
Department of Biopharmacy and Pharmacokinetics, Titu Maiorescu University, 004051 Bucharest, Romania

Adrian Nicolescu
Department of Medicine, Queen's University, Kingston, ON K7L 3N6, Canada

Nikoletta Fotaki
Department of Pharmacy and Pharmacology, University of Bath, Claverton Down, Bath BA2 7AY, UK

Alessandra Adrover
Dipartimento di Ingegneria Chimica, Materiali e Ambiente, Sapienza Universitá di Roma, Via Eudossiana 18, 00184 Rome, Italy

Patrizia Paolicelli, Stefania Petralito, Laura Di Muzio, Jordan Trilli, Stefania Cesa and Maria Antonietta Casadei
Dipartimento di Chimica e Tecnologie del Farmaco, Sapienza Universitá di Roma, Piazzale Aldo Moro 5, 00185 Rome, Italy

Ingunn Tho
Department of Pharmacy, University of Oslo, 0316 Oslo, Norway

Emanuel Vamanu
Faculty of Biotechnology, University of Agronomic Science and Veterinary Medicine, 59 Marasti blvd, 1 district, 011464 Bucharest, Romania

Florentina Gatea
Centre of Bioanalysis, National Institute for Biological Sciences, 296 Spl. Independentei, 060031 Bucharest, Romania

Ionela Sârbu and Diana Pelinescu
Department of Genetics, ICUB-Research Institute of the University of Bucharest, 36-46 Bd. M. Kogalniceanu, 5th District, 050107 Bucharest, Romania

Index

M

O

P

R

S

T

U

V

W

www.ingramcontent.com/pod-product-compliance
Lightning Source LLC
LaVergne TN
LVHW060552210926
848485LV00005B/1304
9781639276745